RESEARCH AND REVOLUTION IN THE FIELD OF MEDICINE

CAUSE OF THE DISEASE

DR.K.DEIVAMANI MANI

DR.DEIVAMANI

ISBN:9798694765466

Cover design by: Art Painter
Library of Congress Control Number: 2018675309
Printed in the United States of America

Dedicated to,

- *Dhanwantri [AYURVEDHA - INDIA]*
- *Hippocrates [FATHER OF MEDICINE – GREEK]*
- *Avicenna [HAKIM IBN SINA] [UNANI MEDICINE-GREEK]*
- *Agasthiyar [FATHER SIDHA MEDICINE -TAMILNADU-INDIA]*
- *Hahnemann [FATHER OF HOMEOPATHY MEDICINE-GERMAN]*
- *Sebastian Kneipp [NATUROPATHY-GERMAN].*
- *Acu puncture , acu pressure treatment [CHINA]*
- *Saragar , Susurudhar [FATHER OF SURGERY - INDIA]*
Saint , Therasa

I adore our great Masters, they created Individual medical system for the suffering Human being and I dedicate this work for them , Dedicate this book to all doctors in the world, dedicate this work to those who dedicate their life for medical service like nurses and All Health care workers including Pharmacist and co workers involved in cleaning and maintaining the hygiene & all those who involving in disease preventing aspect directly and indirectly.

DR. Hahnemann and all Allopathy Doctors almost reaching to one point to discover what causes disease but I am coming at final and I am completing the work and taking your effort and work and dedication all in my name. What I learned, what I searched, what I discovered all taken from earlier incomplete research works of homeopathy and allopathy.

A special thanks to politicians and government , Public for promoting health sector.

"DISEASE FREE WORLD IS MISSION"
"MISSION 2050 ERADICATION OF ALL THE DISEASE"

CONTENTS

PREFACE

Why I Have To Read Research I Am Not A Student Or Researcher Or Doctor ?

Research is boring and heavy subject matter, most of the people in the same research field does not willing to read that, but here the research is most fundamental and day to day problems is discussed and most of the human body and their disease discussed and not much huge collection of research papper submission but i have written like normal medical text. Research included in the regular medical book formet so dont hesitate just by reading the word research.

The book has been written in two mode like a doctor, reseasercher explaining and discussing the disease and treatment and in another mode is like a leader or your higher official scolding and warning and guiding what the doctors suppose to do in present and future to save the patient life and to offer a good health.

This book is written in the aim of reaching the discovery to every common man and women in the world. So, I expect your co operation & help in spread this work. If this work is sleeping in the corner of the book shop then we connot achive Disease free world. Need participation of everybody to achive the Aim.

Most of the time you may think I am keep using the same terminology and repeating the same treatment history but I am just using that to explain some other facts. Like inflammation in the ENT and same inflammation in the GIT and again inflammation in the nerves system. Why this explanation this is totally new concept but we have to explain in each system otherwise it may be missed and again the reading person may think that their disease is not discussed here .

The introduction will discuss what is the major issues in the medical field and the whole text will explain here and there about the issues and solvation in the whole text. The research part is merged with regular medicinal subjects.

Not Just A Cause ,Here The Cause Everything :

Actually, speaking research is all about only to the cause so, when we read about one disease cause is just a one line,so cause may not take major attension, but here the cause is not just a cause, cause is everything. Example typhoid is caused by salmonella, so after reading the cause we have to read about source of salmonella and clinical future and then what is the treatment. But my research about the cause is something different when you read about cause of mayocardial infarct the cause is distracted inflammation then you will come to know prevention and treatment everything is some thing simple and different since here the cause is not something from outside not something internal factors, the problem is at the level of repairing center or curing center , it means the core issue is, disease to the doctor who is given cure, the doctor inside our body is collapsed. So, it is not just a cause the cause is everything here. So, we are not going to read about infection (like salmonella) we are going to read about internal doctor. Why I am using the term it is simple because when we understand some basic facts then all the majority of disease follows same thing, since I use same explanation for most of the disease but for the doctors and public it easy to remember. The reason behind repetation is, It is not 1000 different cause and 1000 different treatment and not 1000 different pathology all the disease just one cause for almost all the non communicable disease (cancer, tumor, arthiritis, diabetes,hypertension,kidney failure ,,,, etc) one pathology and one prevention method. So, the medical field going to be extremely easiest subject here after. Maybe you will be ready for practice within 3 years more then sufficient.

There are lots of new curies and interesting facts are there in the books especially for homeopaths and allopathy and all other doctors the major head ache and confusion to the doctors are solved. A homeoapaths having many interesting facts even in homeopathy subjects and allopathy is having many interesting facts in allopathy system in this book. But public reading this fact you may not get surprice since you are not having any confusion already and you are not passed out and practicing without knowing anything about the disease so it may not surprice you but for the doctor it is greatest surprice. Public have a great surprice in terms of permanent relief from disease ever for them and their family members is a great surprice.

I have not written book to read, I have given easiest solvation to major discomfort,pain and suffering of the human in the world. So, utilize this and enjoy this life without struggle and suffering.

Thanks

DR.K.Deivamani,BHMS.

Chennai,INDIA.

INTRODUCTION

Hai, Welcome,I have discovered cause for diseases, almost for all the diseases. I hope I have completed the research work of many doctors in the world. The discovery is highest beneficial to the humans, we can do treatment plan and prevention of the disease all is possible only if we know the cause of the disease. Many government and private sector spending huge amount to discover cause for one single disease but I have been discovered cause for almost all the disease, it's a happy news for the people in the world. Discovering cause alone may not going to give great benefit to the public, until reform the health sector. Why ? how ?

Many Doctors, a variety of medical treatments like Allopathy & AYUSH (Homeopathy, Ayurveda, Siddha, Unani, Natural medicines and acu puncture) various types of medicines, lots of hospitals and more then sufficient nurses, all we have more or less to the extent necessary. But why there is huge number of incurable cases and why they demanded to take life long medicines ?. there is no cure for the disease so that we can stop the treatment after some-time. Most of the vital organs fall in chronic disease and most of the elders are suffering with Diabetes and Hyper-tension, a greater number of coronary artery (Heart attack) disease and so many deaths due to cardiac diseases and can-cers. Many kidneys failure cases. Huge number of liver failure cases. Death related with infections and lung diseases are in-creasing in children's, sharp raise in allergic and asthmatic cases, cancer incidence is increasing day by day.

The reason behind the failure of the Health sector. (Health sector is failing? Yes, but that is also not revealed by the Doctors globally) .so what is the reason and How to solve it ?

1.   ALLOPATHY Doctors beliving disease are incurable.AYUSH doctors says diseases are curable but support from the government and public is not as expected.So, INTEGRATED MEDI-CINE aproach may over come this issue. Unfortu-nately, patient believing those who says there is no cure. Allopathy doctors retain all the incurable cases with them so number disease in the world is increasing.

Almost 95% of the total diseases are unknown

etiology ,it means doctors may not know the cause of the disease . That's why allopathy doctors say there is no cure. CAUSE OF MANY DISEASE IS NOT DISCOVERED is the core reason why so many incurable dieases.

The allopathic Doctors giving importance to medicinal management (manage the disease till the end of life) and or surgery. They never happy in giving cure OR even attempting the cure. The management is giving so many complications and many new diseases , since they manage the disease till death of patient life.

So, allow the patient to cure first and at the same time educate the patient to seek the allopathy doctors when only in emergency situation since here the management is necessary. Many diseases are curable, most of the disease is preventable. Management need at the maximum 1 week to 1 month not more then that is required. If the case is been kept under management for more then this period unnessarily has to be consider as offence and need punishment.

2.   Prevention is better than cure. The Doctors follows this in infectious disease (disease caused by bacteria, virus) but not in other disease. When we know the cause, then only we can prevent the disease. I have discovered cause of all the disease, CONFUSED INFLAMMATION IS THE CAUSE FOR DISEASES (discussed within the book in detail).

So, prevention is now so easy. Avoid making confused inflammation which is source all non communicable disease [1] .

3.   Unnecessary prescriptions are

globally increasing, India is the top leading country in consuming excessive allopathic drugs. So many drug complications and medicine induced disorders in INDIA. allopathic doctors encouraging patient to take medicines to all the disease including all self-limiting disease and incurable disease. Allopathy doctors prescribing any one medicine just to retain them, even though they are not having any medicine for that condition. Allopathy doctors has to ask yourself why all your medicine act only 6 hours and 24 hours. Why life long medicine almost for all chronic disease ? this is just for sales of medicine nothing more then that.

Send the cases to AYUSH to cure don't encarage life long medicines.

4.   Doctors slowly changing their choice of treatment towards least important disorders then vital important diseases. Like cosmetic,fertility treatment, etc, because it has better money and no risk. Do that treatment but my dear treat the disease which you have been created already and then we will together do the cosmetic and other least dis orders. Educate the society to prevent the disease and cure the vital importand disease and then least importand disease.

5.   Increasing Fake specialty doctors in allopathy. Fake specialist ? then how we can call. A specialist means, me & public is understanding, he knows everything about disease and medicines, but allopathy doctors don't know what is the cause for disease ? there is no medicine to cure. THEN HOW THEY ARE SPECIALIST ?. The simple reason behind the specialist is to cheat the public in the name of specialist.

6.   Without our knowledge there is one more issue is happening. All other systems demanded to read allopathic disease and medicine texts (excluding pharmacology) so their main core aim is distracted due to reading allopathic standard text. So, when allopathy says one disease is incurable AYUSH doctors also will say the disease is incurable. The allopathic text written in such way to convince doctors to prescribe allopathic medicine. So, studying allopathic text book produce confusion to AYUSH Doctors, since AYUSH doctors they have their own concept about health and disease. So, there is need of separate text book for basic medical understanding but without altering fundamental concept of AYUSH or else need integrated approach.

7.At present doctors are paid and getting more services from the government by increasing number of the diseases. A hospital will be opened by a government if they found a greater number of diseases , a surgery usnit is opened if they found more surgical cases and more dialysis unit if more kidney failure ,more eye hospital if the particular locality is having more vision problem. Helping and supporting the health sector is very good approach but keep some measurement. Like before opening the hospital what is the number of cases and what is the yearly achievement how many vision losses recovered how many vision losses prevented. How many kidney failures cured and how many kidney failures prevented? Is that over all the cases is falling down or increasing. If the liver failure and kidney failure is not prevented and number of vision loss is increasing suspend the doctors and provide negative marks and if the situation is same status in further years terminate them from medical profession life long. This is the right approach, followed in every field but doctors are paid if they create a greater number of caeses this is reality I am not exaggerating the true facts.

8.Law in favoure of consumer a patient is strongly belives the doctor who is treating him. But doctors are utilizing this option to earn money and giving new diseases and not curing him is the current trend. So, need a law to regulate the doctors if I am the patient what will be my maximum expectation number 1. I have to be cured and come out of this disease then 2. I don't want any disease complications when I am treated 3. I have to be warned before I am getting the disease like if I do this, I will get this disease such a warning I need, so that I don't get illness and I never going to be got many more new diseases when I am going to treated.

The doctors have to be punished or warned if the number diseases incidence is increasing especially if the disease is preventable and the disease spreading due to less awareness about the disease, this has to be considered as a negligence by doctors in the particular locality. Since there is no advertisement and education about the disease that's is the reason the patient is getting the disease. At present the disease spread is utilized to earn money and not preventing the disease. It means indirectly paid for disease spread. Actually, in india we have lots of disease controle progromme. Allopathy doctors are not co operating with them.

Either they are allopathy or homeopathy

they must know the remedy to prevent and remedy to cure and either they have to cure themselves or guide them to proper doctors since patient does not know who is best. So, the doctors utilizing the option to treat without having any medicine to cure that this malpractice is done by allopathy universally is highly condemnable. Need warnining notice and punishment if they just managing the disease without curing the disease.

9. FUTURE Aim of doctors is to remove all the disease from the people and achieving disease free world.

"I AM NOT SIMPLY LISTING THE PROBLEMS , I SOLVE THE PROBLEMS, WHAT I HAVE TO SOLVE. BUT I EXPECT YOU (Rest of the Doctors , all others in health sector and people and government and politicians) TO PARTICIPATE TO SOLVE THE PROBLEMS FROM YOUR PART ".

Cause for Disease

When asking Doctors to cure the disease, without knowing the cause of the disease is something foolish. But in the medical field full of unknown disease. It means doctors may not know how this disease has come , then how they attempting to treat the disease is something strange, but it is true allopathy and all pathy does not know how the disease attacking the humans ?. Medical field is full of dark.

If a doctor knows the cause of the disease, He can say easily that I can prevent and cure the disease, but when someone does not know, how he will say I will cure.

DR.Hahnemann after discovering the homeopathy he started practice but he found there are disease which keep recurring so he started searching on this aspect he discovered many facts ; he wrote this in the text book of CHRONIC DISEASE [1828]. He is discovered fundamental cause for disease. Since he is come to the conclusion without knowing the cause of the disease it is wast to treat the case we connot give complete cure so he did research and found the cause of the disease but allopathy doctors never attempt to find the cause for the disease and they are not even consider Hahnemann concept of chronic disease till date so his discovery is at present limited only to the homeopaths. What he discovered when treating the sexually transmited disease (gonorrhea and syphilis) by allopathy the disease symptoms disappeared but the disease spread from one location to all over the body and produce sickness to the person now and his generation. he added one basic chronic disease called deficiency disorder called psora and he says this psora is the fundamental cause for the disease and this psora is the mother of all the disease since psora makes the foundation then only the sycosis (the proliferation disease – sycosis will develop) the destructive disease sysphilis will develop only after psora is started their manifestation. what is sycosis ? syscosis is one of the chronic disease syndromes , which has the proliferation is the basic core this disease is arising due to suppression of gonorrhea. What is syphilis ? syphilis is collection of syndromes predominantly having destruction which is arising due to suppression or mal treatment of syphilis. Psora eventhough said as a deficiency disorder, Hahnemann says psoric miams formed after suppression/ mal treatment of the skin disease.

Almost I am started doing research by following foot print of doctor Hahnemann since now days there are many more new disease and massive allopathic domination since homeopaths also in confusion to saying what is the cause for the disease of the current medical terminology say example what is the cause for psoriyasis homeopathys will reply it is combination of all 3 miasm . ok then explain what is that how this mias is the cause for the psoriyasis. Mostly there is no much great answere and if at all he says it is happening due to wrong treatment of allopathy it is may not be complete and better explanation of the medical profession.

Hahnemann discoveries and my discoveries are not having any great difference but I have written by current medical terminology plus many additional research works. My research work will help the medical field to cure maximum number of disease and this research is mainly about cause of disease and how to prevent that.

What is the cause for diabetes again psora, syphilis and sycosis? explain how ? no idea. Allopathy doctors not having any idea how the disease arises but homeopaths know to some extend but it is not practically easy to grasp. Most of the eminent homepaths only following Hahnemann miasm for their treatment. Nearly 90 % homeopaths in india and world homeopaths ignores the Hahnemann chronic disease concept when treating the disease so they will not complete their cure.

DR.Hahnemann chronic disease is highly completed and finest research of 18 the century. It is need further elaboration need more reaserch to support Hahnemann chronic disease at present medical concept. It is ignored since homeopaths reading modern pathology of allopathy and general medicine,allopathy theory says something and at the same time studying homeopathy concept of the disease so there is confusion but most of the homeopaths choose the allopathy disease concept since it is easy (but forgetting that allopathy concept is highly incomplete guess work not coming to the conclusion or not doing any research,everywhere they written as unknown etiology any way it is easy to current situation, the labs and patient language everything is allopathic pathology and general medicine style so early homeopaths adapts allopathic style eventhough it is incomplete science. So, this text book is considering many main objects like completing the incomplete works of the allopathy and homeopathy and making better platform for understanding how the disease arising and how to prevent that.

KNOWING THE CAUSE OF THE DISEASE WILL HELP US TO CURE. THE CAUSE OF THE DISEASE IS UNKNOWN THEN THE TREATMENT MAY NOT BE EFFECTIVE CURE THEN NUMBER NEW DISEASE WILL ARAISE WHILE GIVINNG TEATMENT. WHEN WE REGULATE THE TREATMENT, THE FUTURE GENARATION WILL ESCAPE FROM FALL IN DISEASE. PREVENTION IS BETTER THAN CURE, PREVENT ALOPATHY UNSCIENTIFIC TREATMENT SAVE THE PUBLIC.

The cause for all the disease is discovered now, there is no much trouble in curing the disease hereafter. **Confused inflammation is the cause for all the disease this is happen due to prescription of allopathy medicine by stopping inflammation and immunity.**

No Target to the Doctors, No Demand to Cure

" Either you are cured or destroyed, that is not my problem, I am safe and earning well, why I have to worry about you. Who is going to ask question? When I am getting degree, itself I am professional and I am looking by the public as if I am the great, even though I am not doing anything here ". SO, this attitude is the current trend of doctors so that they forgot the medical field is having many failures, we haave to be recover and reform that. SO DEMAND THE DOCTOR OF ALL FIELD.TO CURE THE DISEASE.SAY TO DOCTORS , I DON'T WANT TO TAKE THE MEDICINE LIFE LONG or at least choose the doctor who is saying I will cure.

Homeopathy says and believes the diseases are curable.

People giving high priority to health, we cannot say its simple high priority, it's a fearful high priority. People and the government are paying more money for health, but they are not getting enough service from the health care sectors. They are not cured fully they are not recovered fully. How many more doctors you need ? how much extra money you need to control the disease and give the effective cure and make the sick free world. Or at least reduce the number of chronic diseases is the quastion. It is not related with money they need a clarification what is happening in and around how they can change themselves from disease producer to curing the disease and making perfect health by reading this book.

The diet and regiment will reduce some disease occurrences, cleanness and hygiene in toilet habits prevent some disease, proper drainage, preventing the open defecation will prevent few diseases , , etc. But what about remaining huge number of diseases, they respond only with medicine. It may not go by doing regular exercise, dieting all will give less improvement need a good medicinal aproach to recover and cure fully need to eliminate what treatment approach make many diseases.

All the diseases are curable or recoverable if the condition is not too much worse. There are lots of incurable cases in India and world but this cases never attempted.They made this world to accept the pain and suffering life long trained the public to take medicine life long. So, public forget that disease is curable running behind the doctors for maintaining the disease they started accepting to take medicine life long, IT IS THE GREATEST SUCCESS OF THE ALLOPATHIC PHARMA INDUSTRY. THIS VICTORY ALL DONE BY A GREAT EFFORT OF ALLOPATHIC DOCTORS AND SPECIALIST. SO THAT LIFE LONG THEY WILL HAVE MONEY FROM PHARMA COMPANY,THEY WILL RUN THEIR

LIFE WITHOUT ANY STRUGGLE. but patient ?

In patient & out patient

Out patient (or) In patient incharge doctors, who is winning ?

The aim of building hospitals is to provide in patient [IP] treatment in an emergency situation. This hospital is fulfilled their aims, but then who failed. There is a great failure in the out patient (OPD) sector. The clinic sector is failed. When the out-patient department has given effective treatment, then there is no disease in the in-patient ward. They managing the disease by prescribing so many medicines, never aimed to cure the disease. Why management, when high possibility is there to cure. How long will you manage ? Till the end of life of the patient.Atleast, will you do the management successfully. NO, the management is again failing. Then what doctors doing ?. Creating fear about disease, then they sale the medicine but disease will grow despite the medicine, they will manage that in the hospital then patient will die one day, due to the same disease. Then what kind of treatment given this many day ?

In patient recovery gives great comfort and confident about the allopathic treatment & doctors so the people expect the same will happen in out patient treatment and clinic, but here allopathy fails greatly.

AYUSH group of doctors achiving great success in OP, But the volountery introduction of patient to allopathy hospitals and clinics is happening in an emergency & delivery & all acute disease. This voluntary introduction is missing for AYUSH doctors. So, no great patient visits volountrily. Almost all the child birth is happening inside the allopathic hospitals so every mother delivering and their relatives gives their entry inside the allopathy hospitals, allopathy doctors good service is really attracting the world. So, the people easily convert themselves for allopathy, but their good service in obsetetric ward may not going to help to cure in other disease is true even they have lots of failure in gynecology but how the patient know this ? this facility is missing for AYUSH doctors.

all the AYUSH Doctors they failed in diverting the cases from allopathy to cure the sickness. The reality goes opposite yes allopathy keep all the incurable disease with themselves. They never refer the cases to cure.They hold nearly 95 % incurable cases with them just less then 5 % cases only treated by all other systems . THE AYUSH FAILED TO DIVERT THE CASES FROM THEM.

SO, THERE IS NO CHANCE TO CURE 95 % , SURE THE NUMBER OF DISEASE OF INDIVIDUAL NEVER GOING TO BE LESS, THE BURDEN OF SPENDING MONEY NEVER GOING TO REDUCE FOR BOTH GOVERNMENT AND FOR PUBLIC.

All other science developed, Medical science under developped

This 21st century All the other department giving effective success to the public. All other sector is giving effective good service to the people like tele communications, civil Engineering , automobile, space research every thing and everybody making the people happy and making the hard taks is simple , practically showing that science is grown you no need to suffer any more. It was the time we are walk for travelling long distance but now every individual no need to worry about the transport. We have effective building and infrastructure. all other branch in the world achieved better service record THEY MADE LIFE EAS-IER AND SIMPLER REALLY THE PEOPLE ARE ENJOYING THE

GROWTH OF THE SCIENCE EXCEPT HEALTH SECTOR. But still the medical field recommending life long medicine to the public many deaths.

There is a better medical science like homeopathy but allopathy is dominating and occypying entire medical field. ITS OUR WEAKNESS AND OUR BLINDESS WE ARE NOT ENCAURAGING RIGHT PERSON TO TAKE CARE OF US WE ALWAYS BELIVE THOSE WHO CHEAT US AND MADE US SICK.

No one is raised the question about this issue ? Why the doctors are failed to give effective treatment and cure from sickness ? Why this field only lagging behind the all other sector because no one is knowing this failure. Allopathy masking this failure by showing some surgical results or some emergency management. Even they never bothered about it because the failure gives the money then who will show interest in cure the sickness. when you cure one single diabetes by one-year medicine then he loss 20–30 years money from one patient, because now patient medicine for diabetes nearly 30-40 years. If you keep the condition same he will be paid pharma company also will pay for him and patient fall so many other sickness and recurrent hospitalization everything is money then how he cure and why he has to cure, who is going to ask or command, because we teached to the world that diabetes will come due to genetics and it will come if your parents are diabetes so public prepared themselves it is like our sin or karma so lets suffer with this public and even doctors does not know that disease not a sin or due to genetics its all created.

Our great grand parents, grand parents our parents and our relatives all will have diabetes, bp and die from that illness many cancer deaths and so many organ failures but still we run behind allopathy, because we never have the thought that this is fake treatment, We are cheated by doctors, we believe life long treatment is right one. we all run to medical college for getting MBBS seat we ready to pay.

People are believing that doctor says all are true, and more than that doctors are strongly believing the diseases are not curable he believes in the text book.The text book says diseases are incurable.

Why he is not sending cases to any other AYUSH Doctors ? because he never considers others are doctors and he strongly believes that what he is doing is the absolute right. He considers allopathy is the only doctors, then to whom he will refer the case.so that is reason for second opinion or theird opinion or thousand opinion he will refere again one allopathy alone not to AYUSH doctors.

The public anyway may not go to ask the question to the doctor. here the decision maker is a doctor so he will make what is best for him rather then what is right to the patient.

It's unavoidable some mistakes and complications will happen to the public. yes of course possibility of complications will happen while treating, but we have to ask the sorry to the patients we feel guilty of doing that act nothing is happen to allopath. We have to explain that it was happened due to medicine so we have to refer them to some AYUSH doctors. But its not happen allopathy hold that patient and try to give treatment even a drug induced hepatitis, drug induced kidney failures.

From where they are trained to do such criminal activities, now a days, so many kidney failures patient they hidden this case as it happen due to diabetes or HTN and they are asking to come to dialysis and then they asking for to come and do kidney transplant.ALL THIS FALL UNDER CRIMINALISAM IN THE FIELD OF MEDICINE DOING JUST SIMPLY IN THE DAY TO DAY PRACTICE BY ALLOPATHY.

Since kidney failures indicates failure of medical system but how doctors feeling opening a Dialysis center.

They will announce as if there is great invention where made to save the public. DIALYSIS CENTER IS NOT A BLOCK MARK IT IS A BLOCK PAINT UPON THE DOCTOR FACE. So, have some basic sense that what you are doing. keep dialysis center,along with hospital attachement and give dialysis silently. BUT SEE HOW FAMOUS YOU ARE,YOU ARE HAPPILY OPENING A DIALISIS CENTER WITH BIG ADVIRTISEMENT PEOPLE AND GOVERNMENT ALSO FEEL HAPPY THAT WE HAVE ONE MORE HOSPITAL TO SAVE THE PUBLIC. Why kidney failed ? why you are not recovered the kidney failure . first say why kidney disease ? any answere ?

Just 15 years before there are great rumor where spreaded across tamilnadu that siddha medicine will cause Kidney failure so allopathy diverted all the cases from siddha treatment.Today for what purpose you are opening dialysis center ? are you having safest medicine in the world ?.

What ever may be the reason patient never allowed to go out and never allowed to meet other system of doctors ? is a new normal in the field of Allopathic medicine.

Cheating in the Name of Specialist

Nephrologist, Urologist, Gastro endrologist, Rheumatologist,,,,,, so many specialists but what is the use of specialist ? what is the purpose of specialist. Is specilist going to cure, if MBBS OR MD does not cure ? No, its not like that he also does not know that but he is specialist this cheap drama is to simply cheat the patient. in what way the specialist differs from other doctors I Don't know. Just to attract the world, attract the people but the reality is nephrologist does not know how the kidney diseases are occurring. Why the people are rushing towards specialist. Because specialist knowing everything about the disease, everything about the treatment and he is more educated he will take care of the patient well.This is the patient thinking but The specialist or the ordinary MBBS are does not know the what is the cause of the disease. They do just medicinal management.Both does not know how to cure the disease fully.

Rheumatologist does not know how the rheumatism has come, how the SLE has come and he does not know how all other connective tissues disorders? then what is the purpose of rheumatologist ?.

Gastroenterologist does not know why the sphincter in the esophagus not closed properly that's the reason for GERD, he does not know many gastrointestinal disorders why happened then what is the purpose of meeting specialist.

The highest innocence from the public is, they bear the fault of the doctors .They know what allopathy doctors doing they bear this since There is no other way ? Here we can clearly make out the AYUSH systems are in a great sleep, the doesn't know what to do now? they don't know how to handle the situation?

MBBS does not know how the diabetes has occurred, MD allopathy not know how the diabetes has occurred. again, a diabetologist may not know how the diabetes has come ? then why specialist ? diabetologist will cure the diabetes? no, no. What is the purpose of specialist ? because it will attract the patient and it helps in divert the patient to the hospitals.

The specialist is not created based on the need of the public but it has been created to convert and divert the cases to hospitals. for every system one specialist and for every disease one specialist.

Why we are discussing this here is in this way they hold all the patient does not allow them to go out and get cured.When the ordinary and the specialist are equal then why the specialist it's cheating the public in the name of the specialist.

It is relating to health sector so that this aspect equally considered in the nation, to provide all the facility to complete the health needs of individual in the country.

I HAVE OBSERVING MANY PROBLEMS IN THE HEALTH SECTOR, ONE OF THE MAIN MOTO OF WRITING THIS BOOK IS TO SOLVE ALL THE ISSUES AND RECTIFY AND RECOVER THE FIELD OF HELTH SECTOR.

Anatomy or Physiology VS
Surgery or Medicine

There are lots of new surgical procedure to attract the patient like laser surgery and laparoscopic surgery. This procedure used to attract the patient and get them extra money by saying this is an advanced technology and simple like that. (Because we can cure and prevent disease no need to wait till surgery) More into a commercial and business-oriented aspects by doctors. It's important to change his business direction to curative aspects. He will allow the disease to mature and show his recent equipment and do business in the name of surgery, he is not showing interest in cure.

He was not joined in the profession for earning money, he was not planning to do surgery. But why he is doing all, because his fundamental principles and his system fundamental concepts taking him slowly a top-listed businessman rather than a professional. Strong and fanatic obsession over anatomy guide him towards surgery and no patience in observing facts and curing.

Allopathy gives the highest importance to anatomy (study of the human body parts and tissues) so that the doctors are convenient in doing surgery then healing and curing. physiology studied just for additional knowledge so that it is not implemented when he practices.

Physiology (study of human functions of the body) explains natural curing power of the human body. Homeopathy gives importance to physiology and strongly believes the natural capability of the human body and the ability to heal themselves. So, homeopathy invite the natural curing power to cure the disease by the medicine. Homeopathy is the only system which is following teaches how body cure themselves and giving cure by inviting the body to cure and recover themselves. So, homeopathy is a best naturopathy. Here the nature it means human body natural curing power it does not mean by using some natural herb to cure the person. There is rule and human body has inbuild automatic capacity of curing themselves. Homeopathy uses that tecniq to cure.

Instead of prevention of the disease, surgery goes in an opposite direction , when a person diagnosed minimal fibroid or small tumor then the surgeon asked you to wait until the tumor is bigger in size so that easy to remove. Allowing to mature so then harvest. Here there is no cure, no prevention only surgery.we all teached to take ultra sound and they give disease we go straight away to gynecologist to do surgery,this is the way we are trained.No thinking about why more are less all the women is getting the fibroid , no question towards the gynecologist since I am your patient for longer time why don't you prevent my disease ? why don't you save my uterus ? why I have to loss my uterus . Then what is the purpose of specialist.

Anatomy and surgery are the top importance reason for failed cure rate, and one of the top most reason for highest treatment cost. One of the importance to medical studence diverting themselves move towards surgery then general physician aiming to cure.

Reduce the syllabus of the anatomy and eucate to cure the patient rather then doing surgery. Both for Allopathy and AYUSH.

vital force

By the time when we discuss either anatomy, physiology DR. Hahnemann gives third aspect of the human life that's **vital force.** [VITAL FORCE GOES OPPOSITE DIRECTION TO ANATOMY].

He gives the introduction to the vital force in the 9th aphorism of the organon.In the healthy condition of the man the spiritual vital force [autocracy], the dynamism that animates the material body [organism] rules with unbounded sway and retains all parts organism in admirable, harmonious, vital operation, as regards both sensation and functions, so that our indwelling, reason gifted mind can freely employ this living, healthy instrument for the higher purpose of our existence.

Medical insurance

Insurance department support need for OPD cure.at present the insurance department spending money only for IP ADMISSION but the money needs to cure the disease so that number in admission will be less in future.

Need financial support to cure the opd patients from insurance department to reduce the number incurable disease in the world.

AT PRSENT INSURANCE DEPARTMENT MONEY UTILISED FULLY BY BY ALLOPATHY,VERY , VERY LESS AMOUNT BY AYURVEDHA OTHERS ARE NOT INCLUDED IN INSURANCE DEPARTMENT.NEED TO INCLUDE ALL AYUSH SYSTEM DOCTORS TO BE ADDED IN INSURANCE CLAIM ELIGIBLITY.MORE THEN 80 % INSURANCE MONEY IS AT PRESENT UTILISED ONLY FOR SURGERY. (UPON THIS NEARLY 40 % MONEY IS USED FOR UNNESSORY DRUG COMPLICATIONS OF ALLOPATHY MEDICINE,30 % MONEY IS USED FOR FAKE AND DUPLICATE CHEATING WAY OR UNNESSORY

OPERATIONS TO CLAIM THE MONEY, ONLY 30 % MONEY IS USED FOR EMERGENCY PURPOSE AND THOSE WHO REALLY NEED IT).

INDIAN INSURANCE COMPANY PAY OVER ALL JUST LESS THEN 1 LAKSH RUPEES TO INDIAN HOMEOA-PATHS IN A YEAR AS INSURANCE CLAIMS.SINCE 99.99 % INSURANCE COMPANY NOT GIVING INSURANCE CLAIM-ING OPTION TO HOMEOPATHS AND NO CLAIMING OP-TIONS FOR OUT PATIENT TREATMENT.

A insurance officer will close his eyes and sanction the claimed amount for kidney failure cases to allopathy doctors (?). PAID FOR MAKING SICKNESS AND KILLING THE PATIENT. (Eventhough the claim settled for the aspect of humanitariyan (understanding condition of the patient) but who is reciving the money ? those who made kidney failure ? shall I take this is a award for creating the kidney failure ? — this is a small example to understand whats happening in medical field.

NO INSURANCE CLAIM OPTION FOR SIDHA AND NATUROPATHY AND HOMEOPATHY at present.

90 % allopathy private hospitals run by insurance money only. It means there is no government and private hospitals even the private hospitals funded by insurance money.

The condition is woulta for ayush doctors in tamilnadu no government support, no insurance support, no public support.

Integrated Medicine

This approach Will attain a great failure, if Allopathy doctors is not willing to changes his mindset and if they do not willing to break their own fake rules and concepts no use in union. The allopathy believe cure is impossible and they laugh if you say you can cure, then what is the use in uniting systems. He needs lots of education regarding the cure and then only, he can allow to join with integrated system.

When discussing about the integrated medicine, uniting allopathy with AYUSH system. Aim of this union is not to shows the world all are equal or something degree related. Social activist and politician and the public think that simple unity will give success rate in curing the sickness.

We have to keep in mind each system of medicine gives the definition in different way to health and causes of disease and treatment . Keeping all doctor under one roof may help patient just to see them all in one place and easily approachable. But what I am expecting is tracing the similarity of the systems from where they can unite really as qualitative union. That union again has to support the cure. Each system has to come forward to eliminate their negative aspect like if the medicine or cure aspect is giving danger to the patient. Since if allopathy ready to eliminate their approach towards stopping the inflammation then sure the whole world will escape from almost 95 % chronic disease.

At present one patient consulting many ayush group of doctors after fed-up with allopathy but there are few getting success many not getting enough result. Why there are many patients running again to allopathy ? Due to taking allopathy and ayush simultaneously allopathy creates the disease and homeopathy cures so patient may not feel any changes. Need proper guide according to the disease.

The integrated medicine is utilizing all the systems but they must pass the eligibility criteria as the biology and physiology descriptions. when says something but it is beyond our knowledge then it can be considered as future research and then use them for practice after completing the research, when remaining all can be used after evaluation.

Remove unnecessary unacceptable and cruel failed and unscientific method of treatment in each system of medicine. Giving importance to curative medicine in each system that princibles and medicine is acceptable by human medical science and then utilize that. Main Aim of integrated medicine is curing the disease and reduce the disease burden without any side effects or main effects.

At present the Homeopathy is explained well by me and it is easy to comprehend. Eventhough Hahnemann says the same I have made that simpler and easier to understand. Homeopathy has been invented an allopathy doctor and scientist Dr.Hahnemann.MD. merging allopathy and homeopathy with allopathy easy. I found Allopathy pharmacology has to be removed massively to save the public but emergency care is needed one for save the life in an emergency medicine. Out patient has to be managed by homeopathy and In patient handled by homeopathy but when ever there is an intervention emergency need allopathy is indicated. So, this is my introduction to integrated medicine for merging allopathy and homeopathy.

Merging and mingling other system is necessary but id ont know much about other system so need to study other system to include here the integration it doesnot mean everyone has to be included within integrated system merging allopathy and homeopathy is more then sufficient but if both system again failed to give the cure patient, then any system which can able to give a cure is selected to merge.

According to my discovery in future there is no kidney failure or liver failure cases in future so there is no need of any pathy treatment. But this is not going to happen as a one-day event so what about the kidney failure and liver failure patient those who present today how we are going to give treatment for the same kidney and liver failure and other organ failure and severe pathology induced disease. Homeopathy is a best medicine for earlier cases and moderate pathological changes so no much cure possibility in advanced pathological changes allopathy is also struggling in the same. Here we have to consider other system to give the cure possibility. Then they included into integrated approach. The basic aim is prevention (possible nearly 95-99

%) if the disease occurred by default using homeopathy to treat that so 100 % we are ready to prevent and curing so earlier. So future is safe this is possible only if the allopathy doctors willing to ban the unnessory disease producing drugs like paracetamol and anti histamines ,,, etc.

The third approach is curing the disease which is present today (possibility is less then 50-60 %). Try to understand once the disease occurred the possibility of recovery is always too less then expected try to prevent disease and support to prevent. This 50 - 60 % is again possible only if allopathy doctors ready to treat diseases by homeopathy or send the cases to homeopathy or other ayush system.

Fourth possibility is giving the way to recover the patient for advanced pathological cases trying to recover as for as possible (less then 10 %) still I belive the percentage what I am writing is too high then reality it is tough to recover the destructed body tissues by diseases. This possibility is luckily more if the cases cured by other system since my knowledge about other system is too less or zero. If they have really better medicine sure the percent may increase further 2-5 % . what are all the other best system for cure the present chronic diseases Acu pressure, Acu puncture, Ayurvedha, Siddha and Unani, Naturopathy, Raiki, Pranic healing, Touch therapy ,,, etc.

When all the system is failing still, I have other choice to complete the recovery from severe pathologicaly advancing cases. Using technology to assist the body recovery instead of removeing the creatining and urea by dialysis trying to build the destructed neprons by inducing body to regenerate their neprons. Its an example.(hoping one or more percentage of cure)

But in anyway we are strongly moving towards preventing the disease since we discovered a cause for the disease, we have to prevent the disease and we have to elim-

inate the causative agent which creating the disease is the top most priority.

Mission 2050 (complete eradication of all disease)

We are going to eradicate all the disease is the main

aim of writing this book.

The human body has the ability to cure all the disease. But there are huge number of diseases in the humans which is not been cured themselves so need some medicinal help. what are all the disease why it happens.CONFUSED INFLAMMATION AND CONFUSED IMMUNITY is the cause for all the disease. The good PROTECTOR inflammation is turned into destroying Confused inflammation by allopathic medicine. (Reaserch observation, explained clearly in confused inflammation chapter).

How body will change like this instead save us it is destroying us. why this confusion. this confusion is made by inappropriate use of allopathy medicines.

SO, BY BANNING ALOPATHY MEDICINES (pharmacology alone) we can save the public and we can prevent future disease creation this is the real and top most prevention in the world . The present incurable disease can be minimized with help of AYUSH group of doctors.

" THE DISEASE-FREE WORLD IS POSSIBLE " .

MISSION OF CURING ALL THE DISEASE BY 2050.

IF ALLOPATHY IS NOT CONTROLED NOW, BY 2050. HE WILL MAKE A 100 % SICK COMMUNITY.

1. IMMUNITY AND NATURAL CURE (DEFENCE)

Human and any living creatures in the world are having their own protecting, adapting, adjusting power to protect from enemy and to adjusting with external environment.

The immunity is the word popularly used by public and doctors. We have inbuild mechanisam to repaire the damage and kill the germs like virus and bacteria, but we are teached by medical profession to consume medicine for everything so they need to hide the immunity and natural curing power. If you attacked by germs and had an infection then within few days you will be saved by killing the germs, this function is carried out by immunity. When we have injury and wound, we have self repairing center, that will repair and heal the wound. But we feel confortable only after applying some ointment to the wound, we belive that ointment is curing wound. If we are not applying that ointment wound will get septic it will not get heal, in this way we are trained to take medicine.

When we learn about our body immune and protecting system, It is structred and well planned to protect us from germ. The immunity will get activated only after the organisam entered inside the body but we have surrounded crores and croes of germs but the immune system is getting activated ocassionally how it is possible because the body has other level protection like hard thick skin in the soles is prevent micro organisam entry inside the body. suppose If the germ entered inside the body fever comes that fever will prevent the germ multiplication and then finaly immune system get activated to kill the germs. So, we have to undetstand that we have many level protections first to prevent entry itself if that is failed then inflammation, if inflammation is failed then immunity. This arrangement is like a preplan eventhough we have external protection we also had internal protection. As a human we must understand what are all the external factors which is protecting us from germs and what are all the internal factore which is protecting us from germs (going to read in this chapter) we have to preserve this functions that is enough we no need to consume medicine all time since medicines are not doing anything great then natural curing power. Since almost all the allopathic drug having worst side effect which is targeting to destroy this natural protecting and immune power, so we suffer one after another disease life long.

The current medical trend is changed in the past 20-30 years. The health sector is fully occupied by business. In this new trend total human germ killing and self recovering power is hidden and explaining to consume allopathy drug. Kind of making drug addiction. Our body immune system is reversed due to the medicine it means it started attacking our own body cells. Initially the doctors hiding the natural curative power from the patient and now they are slowly forgetting the natural curing power. The doctors in the world is keep praised as if he did great, but the reality is opposite. He is utilizing his good name to sales of medicine and for earning. Not to save the life. The business world is trying to use him he is helping them and earning well.

Why this much huge introduction ? the explanation is simple we have natural curing power. If we use that we no need to suffer like this. Since in the world allopathic doctors not invented any better medicine then natural curing power and he is making sickness by killing natural curing power. Then there is no cure and no prevention at all.

He thinking that he is save the life of the patient , true is no. he belives every disease is incurable ? then why he is here,just to manage the disease and peacefull ending to the patient. There are 2 enemy for allopathy doctors one is allopathy pharmacology and 2 is allopathy surgery unit. If he wakes up and if he is having clear brain and if he is understanding what is happening in and around this 2 enemy will loss the job and people in the world will have better life.

If he allowed to natural cure, he is not prescribing anti inflammatory then there is no asthma. If there is asthma if he is cured asthuma the patient will be cured then who will give the money to you. If asthma patient is live without cure then per day allopathy earning is atleast 50 rupees and periodical hospital admission almost during the life time one asthmatic patient provides nearly 1-2 lakh this money will be lost if you cured him. The surgery unit will be closed if he started curing the disease in the early stage. But allopathy basic study itself focused on anatomy and surgery then how he will cure.

The first fault is surgery removes all the major protective functions like removing tonsil and adenoid and nasal mucosa and so an and then recurrent infection and inflammation and immune system keep working now inflammation and immune system is destroyed due to heavy ant inflammation and steroids this is the second fault and then so many new disease due to this now he is considering all the disease is some thing new eventhough its all about distracted or collapsed inflammation and immunity. The third fault is prescribing medicine for unknown disease and managing with superficial relief this gives the possibility of many other disease. He never and ever considers all the failures, he never thinking that why disease keep recurring and people also never imagine why we have to take life long medicine. But doctors having better life since its giving money if he is not cure.

If he preserves the tonsil the infection is affect only as a local disease then patient recover if the tonsil removed then infection spread from throat to lungs easily and produce pneumonia and patient will go to admitted in the hospital frequently. So many childrens losing their life. If the tonsil is remaining in your throat then what is the use of the surgeon. Surgen has to remove the tonsil since it is making sickness. This is what the learning of the doctors.

Immunity

Immunity in the medical terminology is different then the immunity by patient. Patient understanding anything saves him from disease is immunity so in true sense and patient understanding there are 3 immunity .

1. External protecting leyars like skin and thick palms and soles, entry guard like tonsil and adenoid, nasal mucosa, sneezing, cough, urination , tympanic membrane ,,,etc
2. Inflammation - fever and congetion symptoms
3. Internal entry level guards like regional lymph nodes and macrophage and so many protections are there.

If you have injury in the palms and soles then possibility of germ entry inside the body is more so don't use the hands in unhealthy place or make more hygiene will prevent the disease.

If the inflammation is not working then the virus or bacteria will multiply more then septicimic possibility is more.

If the lymph node is removed or under functions then the germs will be allowed to roam all over the body without any ressitance.

In the whole of this book we are going to see what is the natural curing power how we can improve that. What is the role of many inflammation cells and immune cells all together? How inflammation or immunity is changed what happens after the change everything will be discussed.

This chapter going to explai, we have enough curing power and protection then why we have to depend upon medicine for every sickness.we are going to remember some of the basic protecting mechanisam.

The human has developed defense mechanisms to control and to cope with the constant attack of micro organisms (bacteria,virus,fungus), by inducing inflammation and immune system.

• These are a combination of physical and chemical barriers that prevent all types of foreign agents from penetrating the outer layer of the body. Inflammation When body tissues are injured or damaged, a series of events called the inflammatory response occurs (will discuss in detail in this book) ,If any bacteria or virus is entered inside the body then the body will generate the inflammation process to kill the bacteria,How we will know the inflammation is started ?

Below signs and symptoms indicate the inflammation is started.

- Fever
- Pain
- Redness
- Swelling
- Loss of function

The inflammation is a good first line treatment given by the body on its own , it will kill the bacteria or the virus.But with or without our knowledge we stop this inflammation by prescribing many medicines like anti inflammatory (paracetomol) anti allergics (cetrizen,allegra).

Fever or pain or redness or swelling is not an indication for anti-inflammatory. Termination of inflammation is highly contra indicated.

The inflammation signs and symptoms differed in different parts of body.In the nose it will give the symptoms like

This inflammation symptoms either it could be a viral or bacterial infection . Stopping this symptom with different commercial pharma products like cetrizen, cold act or any anti histamine and anti inflammatory stops this symptom abruptly and helps in spread of virus since the anti-histamine and the anti-inflammatory does not have any power to kill the virus or bacteria.

- Fever
- Head ache
- Running nose
- Sneezing
- Nose block
- Throat irritation / pain
- watering of the eyes

Taking anti bacterial along with anti a histamine and anti-inflammatory is also is not a right way keep quit you are trying to stop the treatment which is going inside. Why we have stopped the treatment, is there any strong valid reason for that.

Yes, you will have the body pain. So, take rest. Because the pain demand helps in continue the inflammation and immunity.

Yes, you will have head ache, take the rest.

Yes, you will have the fever, take rest. Because fever demands the inflammation and immunity to continue so allow it to continue.

Running nose and sneezing will annoy you,bear it,since it is help in clearing the virus and bacteria and prevent the germs entry.

All this symptom will subside within one or two days then it will pass two another stage here also some symptoms persist but that will be mild.

My child is cannot bear this can you say some other alternate ,give your child to take care of your parents don't see your child suffering is the best answered.Meet homeopath and he will take care of you. Why homeopath because he does not have any medicine to stop inflammation. he can give some relief.

An allopathic doctor will say you that there are millions of virus or bacteria when you cough and sneez.but he will recommend anti-histamine and anti-inflammatory. Will these 2 medicines will kill this virus , absolutely no. Then why this medicine ? to give comfort.

But patient believing that he is cured.(read the chapter confused inflammation wheather you are cured or getting the sickness you will understand then.)

Forget about HIV medicine, allopathic doctor is not having medicine to kill the ordinary virus which is causing cold and flu symptoms. But why you have to give the medicine ?, when my body is having power to kill the virus .

Diarrhea and vomiting – don't stop that rehydrate give adequate fluid intake and meet homeopathy doctor if needed.

48

- The Immune System ?

Immune system gives the enough fighting cells for killing the germs entered inside the body.The inflammation and immunity are doing more or less same functions protecting the human from the germs. But imunity is having some more additional functions.

IMMUNITY IS A NATURAL CURING POWER EVERY HUMAN HAVING THIS POWER.Inflammation we can experience like pain and fever ,but immunity we may not know the process which will silently cure us and save us.

All the blood cells will directly kill the virus and bacteria directly or indirectly like neutrophil will engulf the bacteriayas. Esonophil and monocytes knows the germs entry so they are reaching the site of germ entry and then call all blood cells to the bacterial entry site and produce inflammation to that particular site.

Bone marrow : its one of the major sources of blood cell production all the white blood cells like neutrophil, esonophil, must cells, monocytes, including lymphocytes all are produced within the bone marrow so the condribution to killing the germs and gives mega support for carry out immune functions. Red blood cells and platelets all are produced within this bone marrow. All the white blood cells having power to kill and digest the germs so bone marrow is the best natural pharmacy which will produce all enough medicine to kill virus,bacteria and fungus.

- THYMUS FUNCTIONS - This

gland produce T lymphocytes and regulate and train the T lymphocytes ; this cell is playing major role in destroying the germs. T lymphocytes will kill the germs and virus so thymus participates immune function this gland bigger and produce many lymphocytes in the neonates and childrens but in old age this gland will become shrink and atrophied replaced by a fat tissue .

•　　　　　Lymphatic system-Similar to artery veins there one more vascular system is there in the body that is called Lymphatic system. Lymphatic system will collect the plasma from the tissues and carry to the local lymph node then to veins and then finally drain to the heart. By doing this functions the germs and micro dead particles waste particles also taken to the regional or local lymph node and it will be destroyed over there.

•　　　　　So the Lymph node act as a local or regional police or military campus which will take the enemy (germs and dead cells and other toxins cancer cells etc) there is trabecular mesh like net work is there within the lymphnodes over there B lymphocytes and T lymphocytes are there and macrophage also present this cells will kill tha germs and then the healthy plasma drained into the veins. The B lymphocytes are doing best functions suppose if the germ entered in to the lymphnodes then the B lymphocytes will produce immunoglobulin called antibody thise antibody play a major role in killing bacteria and virus by attaching with germs. Nearly 750 lymph nodes are there in the body. These lymph nodes are distributed all over the body where ever it is necessary and more muber of lymphocytes present in the neck then rest of the body.

- New lymphocytes are manufactured in the lymph nodes;
- Antibodies (manufactures in the lymph nodes) assist the body to build up an effective immunity to infectious diseases;

- When the inflammation and infection begin then the number of white blood cell count increases (leucocytosis) many folds to overcome the infections and to clear the infections. So many cells which is coming to kill the virus and bacteria.

Macrophage

See how many levels of protection we have.

Monocytes – it's a blood cell it will kill the germs. This monocyte matures as Macrophages. They are much more powerful phagocytes (swallowing a bacterium and killing) , often capable of phagocytizing as many as 100 bacteria at a time. Macrophage also helps in wound healing.

These macrophages are spreaded all over the body and present almost invariably many organs and tissues give good protection against bacteria and virus. Just we will see some macrophage function in the body here,

If the germs enter into the tissues then that will be killed by the tissue macrophage, if that is enters into the circulation then that will be taken into the lymph nodes the macrophage within the lymph node will kill them.

If the germs are not cleared in the upper respiratory tract and enters inside the lungs, then germs will be killed and cleared from the circulation by *Alveolar macrophage.*

What protection we have to save the liver ?

• 		Macrophages (Kupffer Cells) in

the Liver Sinusoids. Still another favorite route by which bacteria invade the body is through the gastrointestinal tract. Large numbers of bacteria from ingested food constantly pass through the gastrointestinal mucosa into the portal blood. Before this blood enters the general circulation, it passes through the sinusoids of the liver; these sinusoids are lined with tissue macrophages called *Kupffer cells,* these cells form such an effective particulate filtration system that almost none of the bacteria from the gastrointestinal tract succeeds in passing from the portal blood into the general systemic circulation.

Is there any guard in the colon to prevent infection?

•   *Payers patches* is patchy lymph cells in the intestine and the colon this will give the protection from the infection.

•   Diarrhea is a simple natural protective mechanism in that all the germs are washed out and cleared from the body. Stopping this causes severe infections. Giving adequate fluid is enough to over come the dehydration.

•   Appendix is a lymphatic organ gives the protecting the colon from germs. The appendix gets infected due to germ entry but the appendix if it is in good condition it will kill the germs.

•   Macrophages of the Spleen and Bone Marrow. If an invading organism succeeds in entering the general circulation, there are other lines of defense by the tissue macro-phage system, especially by macrophages of the spleen and bone marrow. In both these tis-sues, macrophages have become entrapped by the reticular meshwork of the two organs, and when foreign particles come in contact with these macrophages, they are phagocytized.

- Glial cells : in the central nervous system the macrophage is glial cells they protect the cen-tral nervous system .

- Tissue macrophage is histiocytes, most of the tissuse are having histiocytes.

Other then macrocytes is there anything else ? so many other protection which is carried out by our body cells. We will see some of them.

- Destroying abnormal cells (e.g., cancer cells) , Natural Killer Cells(NK cells) Dis-charge destructive enzymes to destroy pathogens too big for phagocytes (e.g., parasitic worms).The steroids will reduce total immune response will causes increase the risk of cancer.

- Defensive Proteins **Interferon Protein** - If A virus enters a cell - The infected cell produces interferon - The interferon binds with other cells that become infected with a virus , and protects it by stimulating the cell to produce anti-viral proteins that prevent the virus from making copies of itself -The interferon attracts and stimu-lates natural killer cells and macrophages to kill cells infected with the virus

"Walling-Off" Effect of Inflammation. One of the first results of inflammation is to "wall off " the area of injury from the remaining tissues. The tissue spaces and the lymphatics in the inflamed area are blocked by fibrinogen clots so that after a while, fluid barely flows through the spaces. This walling-off process delays the spread of bacteria or toxic products.

Anti inflammatory and anti histamine break this walling off effect and allow the inflammation chemicals spread across the body both by spraying pro inflammatory chemicals and by allowing the germs all over the body.

SKIN AND MUCUS MEMBRANES PROTECTIVE MEASURES

There is a protective mechanism which is also assisting in protecting the human body from the external noxious agents.

Dead cells are shed and replaced , taking microbes with them , Cells filled with keratin making skin impenetrable, waterproof and resistant to disruptive toxins and most invaders of the Skin. Sweat produced by glands in the skin wash away microbes and their acidity slowdown the bacterial growth. Hair in the nose act as a coarse filter.

But mucous membranes are more vulnerable than skin .The inner surfaces of the body are guarded by mucous membranes that line the respiratory, digestive, urinary, and reproductive systems and protect the internal lining.

Mucous Membranes Stomach secretes *hydrochloric acid* which helps in breaking the food particles as well as kill the micro organism. *Vomiting* is the physiological protective functions. when a person took some poison or took infected food or accidental ingestion of something not good for health will be through out by a vomiting process.

So, this vomiting process is reducing the possibility of spreading infection and poison by removing this from the stomach so allow the vomiting at least sometimes then you cannot bear consult homeopath.

Saliva and tears contain an enzyme called lysozyme that kills bacteria by rupturing their cell walls.

Cerumen (ear wax) – produced in the ear canal and protects the canal by trapping dirt and dust particles.

2.GOOD
INFLAMMATION AND
GOOD IMMUNITY

INFLAMMATION, IMMUNITY, INFECTION & WOUND HEALING

I have been observed disturbing the inflammation process is the cause for majority of the diseases so understanding about this inflammation ,immunity and wound healing helps in cure those disease and again we will not disturb these basic body protection process unnecessarily.

Usually during infection , inflammation and immunity both work together to kill germs, all this process will pass step by step, each step assessed and controlled by the chemicals and nerve, so if one step completed that is sensed by the nerve endings then proceed to another stage by automatic then that process is completed then it proceeds to next stage. So, this whole process of killing the enemy and after that repairing the damaged body parts during this process and then regenerating the damaged body cells all this stages, end to end clearly planned and highly monitored self regulated mechanism automatic mechanisam.

Inflammation (fire war) and immunity (silent war or cold war) is the basic fundamentals of body protection against external injuries factors.

We search cause for the diseases from outside but almost all disease coming interruption of inflammation and immunity by wrong treatment alone. Huge collection of noncommunicable diseases arises due to interruption of the inflammation and immunity, improper treatment of infections and wound healing. so, it is mandatory to read this chapters in depth.

Inflammation and immunity are same or different ? wound healing also come in the same line ? can you explain what is infection ?

inflammation and immunity are doing the same function of protecting the body from injuries noxious agents, but inflammation is initiating the protective function with pain, fever and redness [fire symptoms] the immunity is involved in body protection little later then inflammation. Fever, pain and redness may not be the marked symptoms in immunity but it will take care of the rest of war by producing special cells immunoglobulin [killing germs]. Inflammation is almost always ready to work at any time, but immunity need some more time [2-3 days] to take active participation in the germ killing, usually we may not experience much signs and symptoms of immunity.

Once the virus or bacteria enters into the body (infection) then inflammation starts and control the virus and bacteria and the immunity will help in complete the germ killing. **In this way the infections controlled well by inflammation and clear completely by immunity.**

Infection is a word which is expressiong the germs presence within the human body like viral infection or bacterial infection. But the inflammation is a process in which germ multiplication controlled and minimised. Immunity is a specialized body protecting process in which the germs killing is completed along with the help of inflammation.

Since the inflammation is giving annoying external symptoms often get medical attention so that the inflammation is terminated prematurely in many cases. Inflammation is the initiator of the immunity when inflammation is terminated before completion then immunity also will not be initiated or need to fight unusually longer than normal time since the controlling power of inflammation [by producing high temperature and killing the bacteria's] in the earlier steps is may not happen so the germs will multiply before the immunity is taking its actions.

An immunity comprises inflammation and immunity both together. But allopathy consider immunity is related only with immunity and they exclude inflammation.

(we take blood or urine culture and identify the germs and then we will see the sensitivity of the antibiotics then we prescribe antibiotic ,but all this thing happening inside the body already that's what the functions of the antibody then why antibiotic ?).

Step by step process of inflammation and immunity

1.Once the virus of bacteria enters inside the body

then this is sensed by a liberation of antigen from the virus body so that esonophil and must cells reach to the germ entered site.

2.must cell break and liberate histamine and bradykinine and other pro inflammatory chemicals over there.

3.proinflammatory chemicals break the blood vessals and attract the white blood cells and initiate the fever.

4.white blood cells now migrate and reached to the site of germ entry and engulf the bacteria or virus.

5.the germ entry also triggers the immune system to activate and immunity participate in killing the germs.

6.germs killing is completed now the tissue injury is there yes lots of tissues in and around the inflammation and immune sites are there that has to be solved, so the body us first destroy the partially damged tissues and cleares completely damaged body cells along with partial damaged body tissues.

7.regenerate the destructed body parts (wound healing).

8.during the inflammation the body functions are stopped or minimized like appetite is reduced,some functions are increased heart rate is more and metabolic rate is more like wise many functions are carried out along with inflammation all these hypo, hyper and stopped functions stablised us normal during the inflammation process itself and this recovering functions may take longer time even 2-3 days after a inflammation process.

So in this way inflammation and immunity act as good protector for using

wound healing is happening in 2 way. Wound healing is a process in which damaged body tissues repaired and regenareting a new tissue.wound healing is supporting the heamostasis by arresting the bleeding and supporting the immunity by regenerating the break in the skin and mucus membrane.

Wound healing in inflammation : Wound healing or repairing the inflammation site is the final step of inflammation. During this process internal body parts damaged so that all the damaged parts has been removed and reconstructed by new tissues and cells. We know that liver will be rebuilder their cells even if we cut and remove part of liver, in the similar way all the body parts and tissues will be regenerated and reconstructed after the enemy is killed. If the wound is deep and loss is heavy then there is no complete reconstruction. The regeneration and reconstruction have limitation.

Wound healing in the injury : When we get injury then the wound healing is happening by arresting bleeding and crust formation in the wound to prevent further germ entry by injured site then the platelets will come and arrest the bleeding then and fibroblast will come and fill the gap of the wound then repair and regeneration of the epitheliyam and other damaged cells now the wound is closed. During this wound healing there are many white blod cells will come like neutrophil and macrophage to protect the wound.

Wound healing in inflammation is the last process of inflammation, it means during the inflammation the tissues are damaged unfortunately so wound healing is one among the inflammation process.

But wound healing in the injury, the inflammation process also is initiated to prevent the germ entry and to kill the germ entry but here the inflammation is one among the wound healing process.

Part - 2 - GENERAL PATHOLOGY

3.BAD
INFLAMMATION
& IMMUNITY

(synonym : Distracted infalammation,Confused inflammation & immunity)

Inflammation we know, but more then inflammation there is one more inflammation present (confused inflammation) in the body. This is most important observation and its going to change the world medical field. This one discovery is going to change the fundamental of the medical field and perception of the disease and recovery.

Inflammation is a basic protective mechanism. Confused inflammation is formed while we stop the inflammation. if we stop the inflammation or immunity the inflammation distracted from focused functions and wandering ailmlessly. We can clearly say there is nothing newly formed here, the inflammation is distracted from main stream by forcible allopathic medication. It creates lots of diseases to the humans that is, we are reading in the pathology reading in general medical text book and practicing in the clinic. All the disease is produced by this confused inflammation alone. The inflammation with 2 different charecters making good and bad is not understood till date as if all are same. So that allopathy pharmacology decides either good or bad stop all inflammation in total so that allopathy strongly objects immunity and want to destroy immunity and inflammation. so, that in one-part allopathy reads and write as inflammation and immunity is good (in the first year MBBS- in physiology fundamental study) then they will read the same inflammation and immunity is enemy for human (from next year onwards).

It looks right decision to stop inflammation but who will protect us from germs and with this wrong decision there are many diseases to humans. By stopping inflammation, the confused inflammation or bad inflammation is strongly more pronouncly formed with clear chereacter. A observation more or less right there is destructive part of inflammation so they have to correct that but decision to stop inflammation in general collapses everything. This is the cause for world suffering till date.

Types of confused inflammation cells :

The confused inflammation cells and chemicals, confused or distracted immune cells and chemicals, confused or distracted wound healing cells and chemicals and suspended or continuing or mal transformed functions of the inflammation origin all included in the confused inflammation. fever and anti - pyreti

Allowing fever is good but actually speaking, the history is not in favor of my observation because there are lot many deaths due to varies type of fever happened so doctors and the patients are afraid of fevers in general and its associated symptoms. But the patient death or severe morbidity is not due to fever but it happening due to already damaged inflammation and immunity system, so stopping the inflammation will double the chance of mortality and morbidity in future fevers. Be cautiouse, by stopping fever today into dangerous life-threatening fever in future. A TRUE INFLAMMATION WILL NEVER KILL YOU; YOUR DEATH IS DUE TO PRESENCE OF CONFUSED INFLAMMATION.

Death is not happening with fever its due to overgrowth of bacteria or virus due to keep prescribing medicine to stop the fever and other body protecting function like simultaneous prescribing anti allergic , cough syrups, steroid and more. fever means just raise of temperature it can happen in all the systemic inflammation BUT TYPHOID, MALARIA, DENGUE IS THE INFECTIONS THAT WILL ALSO HAS THE FEVER THEY ARE INFECTIONS BUT SINCE THE FEVER IS THE DOMINENT FUTURE THIS INFECTIONS ARE CALLED IN THE NAME OF FEVRE , LIKE TYPHOID FEVER, MALARIAL FEVER, DENGUE FEVER. If the person dead due to dengue then the people and doctor will afraid in general to all fevers. So, they stop fever, prescription for stopping the natural protecting power or curing power (fever is a curing or protecting power) causes confused inflammation sure it will kill you since allopathy is not having medicine to cure, they have medicine for spoil you.

If you allow the fever to continue then there may not be severe infection either typhoid or malaria or dengue throat infection or any infections since the multiplications are controlled well and immune system will get activated but prescribing anti-inflammatory drugs, the inflammatory remnants (varies inflammatory chemicals and inflammatory cells) will not be fully destroyed (it will be cleared from the circulation normally) , the chemicals of inflammation are sprayed over the whole body without properly clearing.

The damaged tissues of the body parts have to be regenerated by the end of inflammation process but that also collapsed now, so patient feeling better from suffering by anti inflammatory but really the treatment is collapsed rather than recovery. Over all the prescription of anti inflammatory, anti allergic , anti pyretic will delay the inflammation process unusually longer and he is initiated unresolvable life long pathological inflammation and immunity due to circulating inflammatory cells, dead tissues, inflammatory, immune complex, dead and damaged tissues. The patient will react abnormally to the bacteria and virus from hereafter.

nflammatory / anti pyretic drugs works ?

Once the noxious agents enter inside the body or if there is any injury then this will release the arachidonic acid this will induce the inflammation by producing prostaglandin.So now the arachidonic acids converted into cyclooxygenase [cox] this in turn help in produce prostaglandin. Prostaglandin produces fever, pain and inflammation signs.

Anti inflammatory drugs are block the formation of prostaglandin from cyclooxygenase – 1 or & Cyclo oxygenase – 2. So , there is no inflammation at all. No pain, no fever, no congestions and all further proceedings are stopped.

Same way the inflammation / immune system collapsed in general .but body will not stop by this action it struggles to give the recovery once injured site send the impulse to brain if this action is blocked , then the injury will resend the cyclooxygenase again this process repeats so there is huge collections of cyclooxygenase in the circulation, in the body. So, this augmented huge collection of cyclooxygenases produces the prostaglandin abundantly it is excess then the requirement so the unwanted inflammation (confused inflammation) is arising in this way.

There are 2 main possibility of complications the stimulation of cyclooxygenase production is not been withdrawn properly by body so cyclooxygenase will produced but it will be allowed to roam in the circulation and converted into prostaglandin and produce fever like symptoms for just a over strain or creating lots of neuralgias and so many inflammation like symptoms after the present inflammation is subsided **(confused inflammation disease).**

Sudden conversion of excess cycloxygenase into prostaglandin immediately after stopping anti-inflammatory so it will induce post inflammatory diseases or keep the febrile stage unusually longer time raise the suspicion. When takes the anti-pyretic he will not have fever when he stops then fever will come this will continue for many days then will go for many investigation and patient easily shifts for great analysis in the name of PUO **pyrexia of unknown origin**. Your unscientific prescription only doing all this then how pyrexia of unknown origin ? so the total collapsed patient at last truly catch some infections from the hospital itself then you will do treatment for that.

How anti histamine works ?

Once the germ entered inside the body the Must cells and basophil release the histamine,bradykinine and more inflammatory chemicals. these histamine act as chemotactic factor, this histamine helps in fighting inflammatory cells to reach the germ presenting location. When histamine released ,it will stimulate the nerve ending and transmit the signal to the brain, now the brain understood the enemy entry so it will initiate the inflammation. Now running nose and sneezing then cough will be there (if it is in the nose) then finally we will recover the patient from infection by successfully killing the virus or bacteria without any medicine.

But due to some annoying symptoms of cold, patient consumes anti histamine this anti histamine prevents the nerve temporarily not to sense the histamine , for few hours.

Then what about the histamine released and reached to nerve ending ? do you think that must cells and eosinophil will stop sending histamine again no it will keep send the histamine , since there is no response . This histamine will slowly spread to the entire skin and entire respiratory tract . This excess histamine will produce histamine disorders (ATOPIC DERMATITIS, ASTHMA, HAY FEVER, ALLERGIES, ETC) - HYPERSENSITIVITY TYPE -1 .

Since excess accumulation of histamine (mast cell or eosinophil) in the circulation when any germ or noxious agents enters now will lead on to severe outburst of symptoms ANAPHYLACTIC syndrome or ANGIO NEUROTIC SYNDROME is another notaries complication of preventing inflammation by allopathic medicines.

On the other end, the inflammation process is prevented by anti histamine so the patient will not experience runny nose, no sneezes ,no itching at all. By this time, the germ will spread all over the body and then it will multiply and produce severe illness.in this way patient taken from simple infection to severe life-threatening septicemia and septic shock.

Hypersensitivity and inflammation

SUBSEQUENT ENTRY OR INDUCTION OF THE IN-

FLAMMATION IS WILL ABNORMALLY OVER REACT DUE TO PRESENCE OF EXCESS INFLAMMATORY CHEMICALS ALREADY , BUT DOCTORS THINKING IT IS HAPPEN DUE TO UNKNOWN REASON THEY NAME IT AS HYPERSENSITIVITY .ACCORDING TO ALOPATHY THERE ARE 4 TYPE OF HYPERSENSITIVITY. hypersensitivity is true but that was created by allopathy medicine. will discuss later.

Auto inflammation

Even though allopathic prescription prevents the inflammation process by medicine. We can see the task of inflammation is complete in many situations because we are always administering after the inflammation has been started, so more or less the task will be completed or not but on the other hand the medicine prescribed for arrest the inflammation causes excess accumulation of inflammatory chemicals, which is easily carried throughout the body by the circulatory system and produce the confused inflammation disorders (auto inflammation disease).

This auto inflammation disease mostly considered as new inflammations by a doctor. But, the observation says that consfused inflammation is not doing any goodness here it looks like destructing so record that but in the name of inflammation.

In many situations the confused inflammation produce disease without much inflammation sign. redness and fever and pain will be the classical sign of inflammation if that classical symtoms fails doctors considers as if it is new disease, here they tottaly not suspecting this is as a part of inflammation. example (all the pains including neuralgia and migrain etc are confused inflammation only since there is no fever and redness, they are not suspecting this is as inflammation) either they consider confused inflammation (bad inflammation) as good inflammation. or they never consider as inflammation at all. So, number of unknown diseases is increasing day by day this is the cause for public suffering and huge collection of incurable caeses in the world.

totally the disease considered as non inflammatory diseases ,like vitamin deficiency etc. they never imagine like it will be a inflammation disease in many cases since extremely negligible amount of inflammation chemicals involved there or complete lack of inflammation chemicals or cells. It is tough to understand such great diverse symptoms due to distracting inflammation and it is so easy to track once we learn what happening to inflammation after distracted from the main stream of inflammation (explained in detail in confused inflammation chemicals/cells characters).

Current and post medications greatly confuse the accuracy of the inflammation. Where to begin ? how to run ? When to end ? What the inflammation need all are either excess or less or some other mismanagement due to inappropriate signals or signals coming from many place due to confused inflammation chemicals and cells, It *may initiate the generalized systemic constitutional symptoms [like fever, malaise, reduced appetite,,, etc.]*,it means even a minor trivial inflammatory process can be easily diverted moderate to severe systemic upset due to presence of circulating inflammation chemicals more than excess. (all this notaria's misbehaving is due to prescription of medicine against the body defense function). Allopathic doctor explains this event is happen due to *cytokine storm*, I am explaining this is due to presence of more confused inflammation in the body including cytokines previous to the current inflammation and ready to work stage.

So, if we allow the inflammation process without interference then there is no non communicable disease at all

to the humans. The auto inflammation disease (non communicable) is produced by preventing inflammation.

How steroid works ?

The steroid does the same function of anti inflammatory .steroids reduces total production of the phospholipase - A itself.

- so there by all the chemical mediators will be arrested from the root like no histamine no, arachidonic acid formation totally no inflammation chance at all.
- it will suppress the lymphocyte production.
- antibody formation will be arrested.
- Reduces the collagen tissues formation helps in wound healing.

Usually the prescription of steroid will happen once the chemical mediators are started working so the person will have fever or pain, itching the person will rush to the hospitals, then they prescribe the anti inflammatory not much improvement so they prescribe the steroids later for strong result. at present the inflammatory mediators will be arrested and further inflammatory mediator formation also blocked. But the present inflammatory mediators will induce the confused inflammation very weakly since the steroid is there but will have hyper action once the steroid tapered and/or when suitable time arrives.

When steroid is used longer time during this period over all the immunity is reduced so there by possibility of infections is more , this condition is called low immune status . During this period is a golden time for germs to multiply and produce many serious infections without any resistance .So steroid is not doing good functioning for humans it may ease the sufferings temporarily in many situations but altogether it is working against the natural healing and protecting power of the humans.

How antibiotic works ?

The human protecting inflammation and immune system sense the antigenic property of coating of the virus or bacteria,then antibody (immune globulin) is produced for kill bacteria or virus.

But the days when discovered penicillin that is era of massive low immunity during that time the germs are killing lots of humans. Many people in the world is under nourished so that no sufficient immunity to face infections. (you will have sufficient immunity only when you have good protein and nutritious diet).

In many patients the infections and immune war is never ending. So, there is an absolute need of some remedy for tackle the infections. The discovery of penicillin did wonderful job even today to save the human life. But since there is no governing authority to make a discipline in the prescription doctors of current generation are using this option like anything. The allopathic doctor will prescribe the antibiotic for almost all infection. *But antibiotic usage for this generation or any time need only when the person is not having sufficient immunity to tackle the situation, since the inflammation and immunity will kill any virus and bacteria naturally.* Prescription antibiotic to all the infection patient is blind prescription. A pharmacist will prescribe antibiotic to all fever and infection case. A qualified doctor prescribe medicine only on the basis of requirement not to increase his personal wealth.

Prescribing antibiotic will destroy the bacteria but it will make the immune cells unemployed so this immune cell and the whole inflammation and immune process now in chaotic to whom or for what they came is not there (bacteria killed by antibiotic). So, the immune cells (immune globulin, Lymphocytes) will starts attack the cells and tissues rather then attacking the germs. But allopathy doctor sees the patient complaint and suspect auto immune disease and ask the patient to check immune cells against the body tissues, so he misjudges the case as if the problem is starting just to this case so he diagnosed as auto immune disease. It means the body tissues destroys on its own. why it is happening ? no idea may be some inborn error or some genetic malformation. (But he will not guess or suspect that he only unemployed the immune cells which is came for destroying bacteria in the past but he considers now this disease he assumes new one) this is also my research I have discovered that the immune cells distracted from killing bacteria is doing many damage to human body tissues and produce lots of disease.

Either the immune cells for the specific bacteria will start attack the tissues and organs which is having trace of antigen chemicals killed by antibiotics so there by it gives the way to destruction of the tissues due to enormous immune cells for scanty bacterial antigens still present in the circulation since the antibiotic will not remove the antigens within body.(there are many auto immune diseases suspected bacterial or viral antigens present in the blood vessals and nerves trigger the antibodies to attack the nerve or blood vessals or tissues, but no idea where the bacteria ? just bacterial antigens (that also a guess work may the immunity against the body tissues is triggered by some germ antigen. The commercial antibacterial we use is having power to kill and destroy not to remove permanently. So this is a strongest evidence that prescribing antibiotics will kill the bacteria but the dead bacteria partially digested gives stimulation to regular antibody production as well as the stucking antigen of the particular bacteria induce the auto immunity.

And / or the immune cells came for kill the specific bacteria will roam in the circulation (confused immunoglobulins / lymphocytes) produce diseases by another weak stimulus from the body or it will join to the new virus or bacterial entry or join to the chronic disease which is running already.

ANTI GERM KILLERS

Antibiotics and antiviral, anti fungus and other medicines are useful in case of immune compromised individual and poor immunity patient. A person having good immunity can able to produce enough immunoglobulin against the bacteria and virus then no need of antibacterial medications.

Bacterial infection is not the indication for antibacterial. we have to say the necessity of the antibacterial if already enough immunoglobulin produced to kill the bacteria. antibiotic interrupt the inflammation and immune process.

Normal & Bad inflammation

From now onwards the physician has to differentiate whether the disease is confused inflammation, immunity or True inflammation. So, a doctor has to observe the patient without prescription of medicine.

Other non medicinal supports encouraged. water sponging / IV fluids, vitamins allowed, suituring of the wound but without any much strong antibiotics. If really the situation is worse then homeopathy medicine can be allowed to prescribe. But the aim of the prescription is supporting the natural healing power.

FEVER, COUGH, SNEEZING, RUNINING NOSE, PAIN, LOSS OF APPETITE, GENARALISED BODY PAIN. PHOTOTPHOBIA, LACHRYMATION, SMARTING PAIN IN THE EYES, JOINT PAIN, VOMITING, SOUR, ERUCTATIONS, FLATULENCE, CONSTIPATION, DIARRHEA, BACKPAIN, GIDDINESS, CONVULSIONS, BURNING OR PAINFULL MICTURATION, LEUCORRHEA, acute bronchitis, acute rhinitis ,,,,, ETC when associated with inflammation. Don't interfere allow to recover themselves. (All this symptom more or less fall under true inflammation and immune system)

Hearing loss, visual loss, gangrene, cellulites of any body parts, septicemia, tumors, asthma, chronic bronchitis, tuberculosis, chronic tonsillitis, chronic adenoiditis, chronic sinusitis, chronic arthritis, chronic gastric complaints .chronic neurological ailments,all abnormal bleeding, chronic gynecological ailments. all the chronic skin disease, all the chronic inflammation ,, etc. *all or confused inflammation or effect of confused inflammation and Confused Immunity. But this is just random judgement. T*he better and strong idea you will get only when you reading the confused inflammation cherecteristics.

all chronic disease must be a confused inflammation disease (except if there is maintaining cause persistanly present) since if it is true inflammation it will the germs and will close the function much earlier and again the list is made simple based on inflammation which is destroys instead of killing germs so you no need to memorize anything here, just understand but that understanding like what is inflammation disease, what is confused inflammation disease ? you can easily judge it after reading subsequent chapters.

4.CHARACTER OF BAD INFLAMMATION

C onfused (bad) inflammatory cells, chemicals also produce inflammation. But this will lack many futures of real inflammations but it will produce partial inflammation or incomplete inflammation. the confused inflammation will try to induce the inflammation with available confused inflammation chemicals and cells. Even though it is a inflammation (anyway confused inflammation] the doctors or the researchers missed to identify this or even missed to relate with inflammation because of the partial or incomplete in nature. IN SOME SITUATION THE CONFUSED INFLAMMATION WILL PRODUCE DISEASE BUT TOTTALLY ABSENCE OF INFLAMMATION SIGNS AND SYMPTOMS. Confused inflammation easily diagnosed with the help of signs and symptoms and many more analysis of confused inflammation presence.

1.IRREGULAR SEQUENCE :

Unlike real inflammation, this confused inflammation may begin their inflammation by any **stage**, like swelling is the first stage (usually it's the second stage) or fibrosis may be the first stage (usually its the 3-rd stage in the real inflammation)

it depends upon how we disturbed the normal inflammation and what cells or chemicals at the time of interruptions are worked in the inflammation site.

Example :

Almost all the diseases will follow this cherecter except infections and fresh true inflammation.

1.All the tumers are confused inflammation alone but they busy in constructing the tumer (wound healing last stage of inflammation).

2.Urticarea wheal formation simulate the stage of 2 of inflammation.

3.Ulcers all the ulcers are inflammation alone but will begin in the final stage.

4.keloid starts directly 4th stage of inflammation.

2.Multible stage (OR) Single stage OR new stages of inflammation :

Many diseases may not progress as the sequences of inflammation like congestion stage and swelling stage and finally healing or resolution stage. Instead of usual stages, Only one stage will appear and growing of the disease in that stage only. May subsides in the same stage, will not mature as normal inflammation.

Example—Erythematic stage is the stage one but

in confused inflammation only the congestion will remain, running many months to years in the same stage it never progresses to swelling and resolution stages.

Psoriyasis predominance of erethmatic stage never progress into swelling stage and having regeneration phase of inflammation so that cells abundantly forming and much scaling is formed.

In keloid, a greater number of only fibrinogens will be deposited again and again. it means stay only one stage, histamine dominant disease [like asthma , urticaria] the disease will give pruritus, spasm of smooth muscles wheel formations but never progoross into other stage.

Many new stages of inflammation :

It also looks similar to inflammation; all inflammation stage also presents but gives more then expected inflammation stage many other stages also observed. This is due to presence of excess chemicals of the inflammation causes unusually longer time presence of excess lucotriens and bradykinin breaks the blood vessals excess causes congestive stage mixed heavy bleeding. If excess histamine is present then the pruritus marked along with inflammation.

Trivial and subtle stages take unusually longer so that may also produce extra stage (congetion, effusion, resolution is the normal.)

Just take an example of acne stage of confused inflammation:

Starting as Red painful boil (congestion), swellon (effusion), filled with water and bigger then usual (cystic) and then infected and become pustules then it is filled with excess fibrous cells so that it remain hard indurated nodule (tumor) , surprisingly heal sometimes without any medicinal support but with deep scar (final resolution or recovery stage).

Itching is a inflammation symptoms (it appear usually before the inflammation begins due to histamine release). When using heavy histamine then histamine collectively accumulated and spread all over the body produce itching when new inflammation appears.

Bleeding is inflammation symptoms but it goes unnoticeable but individual taking heavy anti inflammatory then the bleeding disorders starts.

3.Overlaping of the different stages of the inflammation with each other looking like a new stage or new disease.

When two many stages are clubbed together and making sickness erase the identity of the inflammation future . The observer may think this is something irrelevant to inflammation but we will find inflammation or immune cells during microscopic analysis.

Example – lichen planus – itching (first stage of inflammation) and fibrosis (final stage of inflammation).

THIS 3 CHARECTERS MAKES THE APEARANCE AS IF EVERY DISEASE IS NEW DISEASE EVENTHOUGH THEY ALL ARE HAVING SAME ORIGIN CONFUSED INFLAMMATION ; DOCTORS NEVER SUSPECTED THIS CULD BE THE INFLAMMATION except in few diseases.

4. Useless / purposeless / Aimless

4.useless

Inflammation is protector having AIM,but confused inflammation has no aim and never protect.

it may produce either continues USELESS (effect less) inflammation or deep DESTRUCTIVE inflammation but here also there is no purpose to kill any virus or bacteria or remove any toxic material.THE CONFUSED INFLAMMATION WILL NOT HAVE ANY PURPOSE.

Eventhough they protect us this is based on orders they neither target us to destroy nor to target us to kill us directly (our body signals) they obey the command. but its action is like a Robo. If we give command to kill some one, they will obey to us and kill . if this command is lost, they will respond to environment since attraction is based on their chemical property within, the destruction happen as an incident or accident not purposefully. But anyway, the confused inflammation never protects anymore since it has lost its controle from inflammation and immune system.

5.No need of invitation, nosy :

It will start participate without any order or invitation. But the true inflammation usually starts after the call or order from neuro chemical or inflammatory chemical signals, due to this reason the confused inflammation has no controle it will be there as long as the stimulus is there for years together.

SO, NO NEED TO HIT OUR BRAIN IN THE WALL THAT WHY THIS CELLS IS CAME HERE WITHOUT ANY VIRUS OR BACTERIA WHO CALLED IT.

YOU ARE PRODUCED CONFUSED INFLAMMATION BUT YOU DOES NOT KNOW THIS BUT EXPECTING TRUE

INFLAMMATION CHARECETERS. When you know the confused inflammation, then you will understand that, it will have different charecter and you will start observe the new confused inflammation charecters and you will teach me what is confused inflammation in future. So need just introduction to say there is some thing new is happening that's all.

Confused inflammation will not come for or respond for neuro chemical or brain order but will go and attend all the strong environmental stimulus sun heat,cold exposure,ac room and some irritant like smoking.w

When any person expose to an injury then inflammation will be activated but here this confused inflammation readily available with already having access to act so due to this this confused cells may participate for any inflammation and spoil that and it may initiate fake inflammation without any injury also but without body basic inbuild genetic ethics and rules.

6.No recovery, No self cure.

The normal inflammation also do destruction but after the destruction the recovery is happen. Congetion,swelling and resolution phase is the normal function of the inflammation. but here there is no such recovery. The disease may run many stages may produce many destructions but you connot able to see cure or recovery, so the disease run abnormally long period.

If the blood clote is happen that clot will remain same within the blood vessals so gangrene will develop. If the ulcer is developed ulcer will develop longer period no recovery.

If at all the recovery happens it is particular local cells stimulai not because of the proper inflammation recovery so the recovered part is loss the function just looks like normal recovery.

Exception:

Direct involvement never recovers , indirect involvement recovers.

Most of the confused inflammation disease never having the power to recover and self cure. But recovery happens in many instances because confused inflammation triggered normal inflammation or recovery. If the confused inflammation is dominantly present in the particular locality there is no possibility of recovery, but if this c inflammation moved to other part then recovery happens.

Example :

a. a stroke patient mostly recovers since the confused inflammation present within the blood vessals so that the vessal get damaged and leaked so that infarct or clotes within the brain this clotes will be absorbed and patient recoverd within the brain since the confusd inflammation dominant zone is blood vessal of the brain not the brain tissues.

b. But we connot see recovery in Parkinson and other axon and myelin damages since the disease directly attack the nerve cells and mayalines.

(Partial normal cells and partial damages in the multible sclerosis due to the destruction also not a targeted and complete and finest destruction (no sharp and clean destruction and complete apoptosis since this confused inflammation and immunity is not having such target). We can see complete destruction in many place this is not a finest part like true inflammation this is due to presence of excess destructive chemicals or mass blood circulation block like that). I am trying to say true inflammation has planned destruction and complete destruction but the confused inflammation luckily not having such a power to destruct completely)

c. in kidney damage the confused inflammation present within the nephrons so the destruction is progressive and continuase.confused inflammation directly damage the kindy.

d. confused inflammation directly damages the liver parenchyma so chronic liver disease without recovery.

7.Always chronic.

All the body making inflammation will run short period almost complete as a acute or at the maximum sub acute stages. This is achived because the work is completed so the automatic and feed back mechanisam get the signal that the target is finished the work so the nervous system demand to stop the inflammation so the inflammation and immunity is stopped their function the cure is achived.

But since we distract the all inflammation and immune producing chemicals and blood cells which is involved in the inflammation so this distracted inflammation cells has no controlling power so they are free so if they triggered they produce disease and they not having off switch so they keep produce and keep doing their function in unnessory place. This is the one simple answere why chronic disease. The choronicity and long destruction is absolutely confused inflammation no doubt about it. But there are so many explanations this is because of the inborn error kind of susceptibility. Confused inflammation not having any controle usually this cell invited to kill the bacteria and withdrawn after completing the function. No one is invited no one is going to withdraw this confused inflammation so destruction unusually long. there is no susceptibility no inborn error for producing the chronic disease.

Exception:

Choronic disease also possible in normal inflammation when there is a continues presence of the cause when a person keeps exposing to the unhealthy environment then they produce disease continuasly but even if they get adequate immunity then there is no chronic disease. Inheling cotton wool and dust causes asthma is due to the cause which is producing the ailment present still.

EXCEPTION 2 :

Confused inflammation can give acute disease shorter than real inflammation. ramsayhant syndrome – a common disease we see if the person lye down in the cold days in a open air he see the facial paralysis this is happen within a day . this is purely confused inflammation.

A confused inflammation invited by the extreme cold weather to his uncovred part of the face and ear so he developed disease. Once if he had the paralysis after the phycian advice the patient avoid extrem cold weather so no more possibility of same trigger.

All type 1 hypersensitivity disease produced by confused inflammation alone.

Urticaria is produced by confused inflammation.

A confused inflammation able to produce acute and acutely acute and sub acute and most powerfully chronic disease. We have to differentiate them by their other cherecters simply the inflammation do good or bad to us. Good inflammation is true inflammation ,bad and destructinve inflammation is confused inflammation.

But a true inflammation run in short duration mostly acute illness but patient recover fully.

Without knowing the cherecter of the confused inflammation and true inflammation you connot able to recover the patient, you connot able to plan the treatment. The therapeutic success depand upon depth of knowledge of the confused inflammation and true inflammation cherecters.

Either acute or chornic you have to terminate the confused inflammation and remove that from the body. But at the same time the true inflammation zone absolutely phycisian free zone and pharma free zone you are not supposed to stop the true inflammation. if you stopped that true inflammation by paracetamol then the patient will have life long confused inflammation. all acute infections are true inflammation. allopathic doctors and their pharma is not allowed to interfere here. Acute inflammation can be allowed to handle homeopaths if the patient is having mixed true and confused inflammation.

8. Hypersensitive

ALREADY ALLOPATHIC DOCTOR GIVEN ENOUGH EXPLANATION ABOUT THE HYPERSENSITIVE NATURE OF

THE INFLAMMATION BUT WE HAVE TO ADD ONE SMALL CHANGE IN THAT [IT IS NOT A TRUE INFLAMMATION IT IS CONFUSED INFLAMMATION AND IT IS CREATED BY AL-LOPATHY.it means a confused inflammation alone produce hypersensitive reaction not a normal inflammation.

FATHER OF CONFUSED INFLAMMATION ALLOP-ATHY.since he was created it.

INVENTOR OF CONFUSED INFLAMMATION IS DR. DEIVAMANI.

Why hypersensitive ? what exactly the meaning of hypersensitivity. It is not like a ordinary inflammation, this inflammation causes damage that's why they are using the term hypersensitivity.It means allopathic doctors found something different in the inflammation and immunity so that difference is induce them to give new name to differentiate inflammation from this altered confused inflammation/immunity and again they use the term hyper sensitive because they observe it is inflammation or immunity like but doing damage so they use this term. They more sensitive . so, they will destroy rather then save us.

And they further observed that an inflammation or immunity, if it is come second time it will be triggered by anything rather than only germs causing severe damage. Initially the inflammation save us but the subsequent entry causes destruction rather then save us (?).

and they further thinking, its happen because of fault in immune producing glands or some inborn error like that. So, they never probed this theory fully in right way to complete the research or observation.

Ther is a question why this auto immunity to this person alone ? why not for everyone ?. what is the cause for malfunction of the immune glands why they produce self destructing cells ? so auto immunity is again unknown origin.

But this hypersentive theory support them or convince them to prescribe steroids or other drugs to controle the inflammation. BUT MY THEORY OF CONFUSED INFLAMMATION STRONGLY ACCEPT THIS HYPERSENSITIVITY CHARACTER PRESENCE BUT REVEAL TRUE CAUSE OF HYPERSENSITIVITY. IT MEANS PRESCRIPTION OF THE ABOVE ANTI INFLAMMATORY OR THE STEROID IS THE CAUSE FOR HYPERSENSITIVITY ITSELF SO IT WILL SURE HELP THEM TO CALM OR RELIVE TEMPRORILY BUT PRODUCE VERY STRONG HYPERSENSITIVIY AFTER USE of this drugs.

[not the usual allopathic explantion,this is my explanation and true explanation not the guess work].

Hypersensitivity explanation:

Normal inflammation will be produced only after germ entry and again it has many stages if one stage has been completed then next stage inflammation cells or chemicals invited to participate in the inflammation almost all the cells of inflammation and immunity will join together during this process and complete the inflammation and immune function from 3-7 days.

all the cells and chemicals withdrawn then inflamed site invite new cells to repair and regenerate the damaged cells so this process may take another 3-5 days, so over all a moderate infection take few days to few weeks to complete its function.

But since we stop this inflammation by anti inflammatory drugs . the drug used to stop the inflammation having marked effect to distract the inflammation not stop-

ping the inflammation fully. Anti inflammation and anti histamine distract the inflammation never stop the inflammation so there is a more inflammation producing chemicals
readily available in the circulation.

Type – 1 hypersensitivity :

If the person exposes to the same trigger now then
the person develop inflammation but the inflammation plus
confused inflammation also join to this same process so
heavy reactions then normal.

Type – 2 hypersensitivity :

Immune mediated hypersensitivity. Here the im-
munogloubilns destruct the body tissues. The allopathy has
a confusion here how tha anti body will destruct our own
body cells. This is highly possible.

No 1: the target of the immune cells will be
destroid by prescription of the antibiotics.

No 2 : Once the target is destroyed now the immunoglobulin confused and distracted. But not withdrawn,
allowed to roam within the circulation.

No 3. the antigen of the particular bacteria still
presents in the body stuck upon the blood vessals and blood
cells since the anti bacterials kills and may not completely
remove the antigen from the circulation. so the complement system or other markers attach within the blood cells
and marking as blood cells as a target then the immunoglobulin cells bind with blood cells help them to destruct.

So many cases of auto immune thrombocytopenia , and anamia and other cytopenias are happen.
The bacterial antigen will be present in the body for many

years so the blood cells will keep destroyed by the body immune cells for many years.

It is not genetically induced; it is not body abnormal predisposition. it is absolutely induced by prescription of anti biotic.

But still you will not see this type 2 immune mediated hypersensitivity since most of the time allopathy doctors prescribe anti biotic to the viral infection and confused inflammation disease so you will not see any immunoglobulins and you will not see any antigen without germs.

Type 3 hypersensitivity

Antibody (immunoglobulin) and antigen (germ) complex are the cause for this type 3 hypersensitivity. Either prescription of anti biotics is the prescription other anti inflammatory or distracting the wound healing substances reduce the possibility of the clearing the immune complex. so, there are many distracted immune complexes ,this immune complex along with other confused inflammation cells destroy our own body cells.

No : 1 why they name this is as hypersensitivity ? since the immune complex is not removed more then that it making destruction. So, they name this is as a hypersensitive.

No : 2 the immune complex produce inflammation, activate the humoral and followed by cellular immunity . here allopathy explains this could be some hereditary or inborn susceptibility to external environment to consider the environment as enemy so the inflammation and immunity is activated.

The circulating confused inflammation is already activated macrophage and lymphocytes clumped here along with immune complex and produce the disease nothing more here to call upon the suceptability.

The confused inflammation reacts to the external environment not as a susceptibility but due to excess quantity and proinflammation chemicals readily available in excess quantity dialate (sun exposure) or constrict (cold claimate) due to the environment changes this will help in initiate the inflammation here so the stagnation of the confused inflammation causes heperemia, the lucotrians and histamines (confused proinflammation chemicals) remain in the circulation start destroys the blood vessals causes so this partial inflammation triggers the macrophage and activate humoral immunity and then cellular immunity here the immune complex remain in the circulation will come and join. It is not ncessory the immune complex has to destruct the blood vessals and then vascular damages has happened we allowed enough histamin and leucotriens will readily damages the blood vessals and initiate the humoral and cellular immunity.

Prescription of anti histamines and anti inflammation and antibiotics all need to develop this disease but the disease may not develop it may take many weeks to many years to develop disease.

No : 3 then they explain this disease is not completing in short span of time more then that it run very longer course. this chronic nature could be again some susceptibility to external

The chronic nature is one-word explanation all the confused inflammation and immunity is not having controle effect and that is not going to remove from the circulation so there is ever ending disease. The disease may relapse and remit but not lost.

" When the protective functions are stopped now and

creating disease now but allopathic texts saying that all the diseases are happen due to genetics (coming from genetics from many years before) .So, this misguiding makes the all doctors to accept this disease is incurable only. Believing that the disease is something beyond our control so its impossible to cure ".

Deleyed hypersensitivity
type 4 hypersensitivity

Delayed hypersensitivity is induced by cell mediated (lymphocytes) this is purely achived by confused inflammation roaming all over the body will trigger the cellular immunity.

So all this hypersensitivity is not possible if the confused inflammation and immunity is not available in the body this changes never happen due to any inborn suceptability or not because of the hereditary factors.

we allow the inflammation chemical to all over the body all this chemical having already working order so they start produce inflammation or immune function anywhere they stuck or heat or cold or any body chemicals like that.

Further explanation of hypersensitivity :

Every time when you block the natural inflammatory chemicals and they allowed to wander around circulation and roam aimlessly starts react to the external environment or internal hyperfunctions or narrow or closed circulation or catched within the spincters (esophageal,urethral anal spincters or crushed or getting pressured in the elbow or axilla or neck folders or leaning towards back, sun exposure or cold exposure everything and everything trigger to produce disease because of this wandering aimless hyper sensitive cells and chemicals.

So here you no need to wait for must cells has to come and release histamine or tissues injury and then cyclooxygenase has to come, here this chemical is more abundant so just a a fraction of second is enough to create angioneurotic edema and death .enough to produce any disease in the humans causes tissue destructions.

The subsequent steps like neutrophil visits and lymphocytes visits and macrophage immune globulin [probably ready and enter into circulation 3rd or 4 th day of inflammation] everything has its own time space in entry to the participate in TRUE -inflammation. But here all are ready so that the disease quick in response and it is triggered by unusually different day to day normal food and chemicals so it is named hypersensitive.

A hypersensitive theory of allopathy has its drawback only discussing immune disease and blaming the immune producing organ itself producing the cells to destroy the body parts.

But my theory says the same hypersensitivity from inflammation and immunity. So, the histamine,leucotriense and all other chemicals which used for destroying the germs are having higher cabablity of destroying the body parts also is there. when we arrest the inflammation, then auto inflammatory disease is ready because we stop the functions of inflammation by ointments external drops and sprays all these chemicals wander in circulation, they produce disease. This confused inflammation chemicals start destroy the body parts so that immune system either newly activated (mostly cell mediated) or using existing confused inflammation join here (immune mediated – immune complex mostly , immunoglobulin mediated partially).

If the leucotriens damage the blood vessals in an unusual place then automatically the confused immune cells will come and participate or new immune system (humoral and cellular) get activated, I hope there is no fault in immune system production we are doing major fault in inflammatory system. So, AUTO INFLAMMATION THEN AUTO IMMUNITY.

So the pro inflammation chemicals start responding to the external environment and produce the inflammation disease either vaso dialatation,vaso constriction or stagnation of the minimal portion of the blood or leaking of the proinflammation chemicals through the sweating (atopic dermatitis) pressure or friction of the skin considered as vascular damage all is because abundance presence of the pro inflammation chemicals always act as initiater of the disease. There are numerus triggers are there to induce many disease internal as well as external factors.

DIRECT AUTO INFLAMMATION ALSO HAS THE SAME ROLE. like confused inflammation cells attracted towards demanding site.

3.Either inflammation or immunity or wound healing cells Why they produce disease in un unsuall or unwanted parts ?. they are ordered to work in the inflamed site, we stopped and allowed to roam in the circulation.This cells are similar like all other blood cells present in the circulation but they are appointed to work we are distracted.so this special cells always ready to initiate the inflammation functions so they have special power then other cells to initiate the inflammation readily within the body or outside the body any tissues or cells or place in the entire human body parts most importandly without any order from the brain or nerve they work based on stimulus of external or internal (discussed many times). Here no need of germs.

So, no surprice or confusion how the body is attacking on its own,its all our mistake we prescribe and take the medicine to stop the natural functions.

A chemical is used for destroying germs we are allowing them to destroy our body cells.

Type -1 hypersensitity purely confused inflammation dominant disease produce symptoms instant. Immunoglobulin join if it is there but mostly confused inflammation dominant. Type 1 hypersensitivity is comparatively faster than remaining hypersensitivity since this is mostly caused by readily available confused inflammation. in other cases, confused inflammation has to induce the real inflammation so that it takes long time especially type 4 hypersensitivity.

TYPE – 2. Hypersensitivity is less inflammation but full of confused immune cell mediated.

TYPE – 3 mixture of inflammation and immune complex disease purely confused inflammation dominant very less new inflammation and immunity.

TYPE – 4 triggered by confused inflammation but new immune system activated (cell mediated).

9. PHYSIOLOGICAL AUTO INFLAMMATION AND AUTO IMMUNE DESTRUCTION :

if the body parts or blood cells or bone marrow or broken skin or mucus membranre everything or blood cells all are will be regenareted by the body.if the inflammation completed normally.

Yes, my dear friend, all through the inflammation and immunity body destroyes many body parts and tissues but at the end all the damages are regenerated but you have to allow the inflammation to complete,but you will not allow you will terminate with the medicine and patient will suffer because of that.

a.the physiological self destruction also will be stopped and b. the same chemical used for physiological normal self destruction makes the destruction other then needed destruction so that severely alrming diseases are happening.

Inflammation is normal in activity. The confused inflammation is having hypersensitivity.

10.Progress :

The continues growth of the tumor or spreading of the disease created by confused inflammation decided by wheather the previus inflammation was closed or not. If that is still not closed, it may be many years before we distracted the inflammation is still secreting the inflammation cells to the particular part.

we may assume that wound or eczema is cleared at this site by our medicines but we forgot that we scattered the fibrous tissues all over the body and failed to switch of the complete inflammation process (it's a automatic process we cannot stop that) once the body heals on its own it will terminate the inflammation process. Since we terminated before completion of the work, body never get feedback mechanism. so, after few year patient come to meet us with tumor or keloid which is keep growing, size is increasing and new tumors or spots appearing.

There are in other situation tumors will be single and it will stop growing further this is happen because there is only less number of fibrous tissues are there but the inflammation has been shut down on its own.this is the reason many diseases keep troubling with rapidity of spreads and some disease just surface but may not spread (keep the mild phase)

If the confused inflammation triggered and induced immunity and now the immunity and inflammation periodically induce the disease in the same way. It means here the progorss is decided by disease making power of confused inflammation.

tumor is an example but this is what happen in almost all the disease a disease will spread like anything in some situation due to still supply of chemical or cells due to stimulus not withdrawn,

Diseases may stop troubling the patient in some disease due to just very less available confused inflammation chemicals.

11.Prognosis :

The confused inflammation may produce acute ,sub acute and chronic diseases but the confused inflammatory chemical/cells remain inside the body more or less life long. The disease may be vanishing in one place and origin in other place we consider this is as a new disease. The prognosis is utterly poor. The confused inflammation produces many diseases in different part of the body we give the prognosis each disease separately but we have to give the prognosis for the confused inflammation not the each and every disease produced by the confused inflammation.

- The C inflammation and immunity has to be cleared from the circulation as early as possible, at present homeopathy is the only system which has that power so prognosis is excellent.

97

• The allopathic medicine has created this condition and they never have any medicine to recover the confused inflammation prognosis worst since allopathic medicine will enhance more confused inflammation. prognosis is poor and worst in some cases.

• Effect of confused inflammation cure is depending upon the possibility of revert to normal tissues which was damaged already. If the condition already deteriorated prognosis is poor in homeopathy also.

• Some time very worst psychological changes, worst disease like even cancer will happen immediate after taking allopathic medicine and immediate confused inflammation formation, this changes unpredictable and here the prognosis is poor since the rapidity of deterioration. (especially in pediatrics). It is better to stop unnecessary allopathic prescription then producing the disease and then taking treatment.

12. Severity :

A.Severity is decided by trigger and presenting destructive confused inflammation chemicals and cells.

If the trigger is environment mostly it will invite the confused inflammation to wards skin (hot,cold,rain, air-,,,,,,etc) so the disease is not affecting vital part so it is mild to moderate. Within the skin the confused inflammation is just a histamine patient will get itching nothing more then that but if the person having destructive orders or cells then severe ulceration and necrosis so it turns into severe disease.

Either simple or destructive chemical but if the organ inviting the confused inflammation ultimately decide the severity like a brain invite the simple confused inflammation causes some unconscitious and convulsion but patient getting the panic and the doctors also consider this is severe disease. Within that the confused inflammation is having power to infiltrate or indurate or produce tumor due to destructive more severe confused inflammation then that is decide the severity of the disease.

B. Rapid progression and sudden deterioration and generalized systemic spread of violent inflammations will happen if simultaneous **real and confused inflammation together produce the disease. A true inflammation focusses the inflammation limited to the bacteria or virus but the confused inflammation takes the true inflammation where evere they spreaded already so recurrent systemic inflammation is triggered mostly the systemic inflammation gives the moderate to severe disease.**

Confused inflammation produces a chronic disease in that real inflammation starts as an acute disease with proper inflammatory signs, run short duration and end on its own or with medicine and then confused inflammation starts its course.[COPD is the best example chronic confused inflammation, super added acute real infections].

Not all the virus or bacteria usually produce severe complications and all the symptoms .the mild or moderate or severe diseases decided by only presence of confused inflammation.

A flu may kill the person with a severe complica-

tion in some individual due to presence of confused inflammation .a severe lethal microorganism causes simple mild
course infections recover without any medicines indicates
no confused inflammation in his body.

13. Access to all area, No restriction.

In the severity of the disease I have mentioned like
more superficial affection then it is mild severity if it is deep
and vital orgon affected it is more series to saying this we
no need great knowledge any one can say this. But this is not
true in case when you read a protection of the each deep
orgon. A germ not so easily enter inside the deep vital orgon
and produce the disease. A blood brain barrier in the brain
and almost respiratory tract keep lungs deeper and with
many guards a kindy is kept more deeper and with many barriers but all this is true only to the germs. But for the inflammation cells are not having any restrictions so either true
or confused inflammation can easily reach to the kidney and
lungs and brain and heart and they can produce the disease.
Even though bad inflammation but this inflammation has
all acces to go to all the orgon. A lymph node may not block
this a tonsil may not block this a blood brain barrier will not
block the confused inflammation.

14 . Absence of expected symptoms or signs of inflammation : partial incomplete inflammation.(rarely no inflammation future)

IN SOME DISEASE THERE IS A MARKED ABSENCE
OF SOME IMPORTANT SYMPTOMS OR EXPECTED SYMP-
TOMS OR SIGNS INDICATES CONFUSED INFLAMMATION.

Lack of heat even though severe redness , lack of

pain even though severe inflammation, lack of swelling ,,,, etc. (negative symptoms)

Because its not a true inflammation, so a confused inflammation will lack sufficient chemicals to produce Classical true inflammation signs and symptoms. So, that the presentation will look like new disease rather then suspecting this is as an inflammation.

(Neutrophil or inflammatory chemicals and mediators) or will have any one future . A Psoriasis will have redness but will not have fever or pain.

In many situations the confused inflammation also has all classic symptoms of inflammation in this situation we can differentiate this to normal by no purpose or chronic in nature. (for observing this factor, we have to wait without any medicine prescription)

Example we can add many examples because almost all the disease is confused inflammation and again almost all the disease lack of some signs and symptoms in confused inflammation.

15.AUGMENTATION OF CHRONIC INFLAMMATION :

(increasing strength of confused inflammation) :

good and bad inflammation and prescription of anti inflammatory and steroids will make more confused inflammation disease.

The scattered and confused inflammation is attracted and produce the disease by strong environmental or internal factors or medicines or hormones.

The bad inflammation triggers and invite the good immunity to initiate the disease. This are all some of the way the silent bad inflammation get activated and increase themselves more.

16.No Death :

The true is human body does not have power to destroy the chemicals or blood cells appointed for inflammation, immunity until completing the task. After completing the task, the cells, chemicals will undergo degeneration by reorder issued by brain. but when we disturb the inflammatory cells/chemicals by anti pyretic, anti allergic, steroids strong ointments, medicated soaps, creams ,,,,,,, ext. so the confused inflammation chemical or roam around the body till death (by the time it produces lots of disease to human being directly as chronic disease, indirectly by disturbing further inflammation / infection) the blood cells produce destruction until their life span.

17. The destructor.

The confused inflammation is never act as a protector anymore, it will give only disease. The normal real inflammation is fall under physiology helps many ways to the human, but the confused inflammation will produce pathology **DESTRUCTION**. Because this confused inflammation is aimless , purposeless ,not having power to control and terminate their presence . Many diseases arise because of this confused inflammation interact with body tissues, even simple stagnation of this confused inflammation or chemical in one place of the body will make pathological disease.

18. shift and moves

The confused inflammatory cells or chemicals quickly **shift** from one part to other part initially via the lymphatics and blood vassals but over the period of time the spread is decided by strong triggers like claimate,heat or cold, injury, pressure, chemical exposure, allopathic drugs ... it never vanish just shift from place to place with strong allopathic drugs or strong triggers.

Temporary cessation and reappear in the same place [remission and relapse] related with presence and absence of triggering factor so easily or it may be achieved by heavy medications.

(23,migratory nature)

19.No need of any germs or foreign invader to produce the disease.

Confused inflammation alone will produce disease,bacteria or germs is not necessary for producing disease. confused inflammation alone will produce a disesase. But without understanding this allopathy doctors belive that auto immune theory. Occarding to auto immune theory : the body cells has the intension or plan to attack the body / wrongly consider body cells as the enemy. And so many guess works . Enough explanation given don't want to bore you again.

20. Location of disease occurance. local / systemic.

A disease many times arises in particular location only some times it is occurred in many locations, extremely remote location then the source,some times it makes local disease some times systemic disease ? why is this ?

A micro chemical distracted from inflammation will be readily mix within the blood and makes the disease where ever it is getting stimulation. Usually makes the disease anywhere within the body when they attracted and activated.

Many time a inflammation products carried along with lympatics will produce a local or regional disease of the same site of the inflammation distracted (example if the inflammation / skin disease distuerbed in the hands then the confused inflammation cells will be carried via lympatics will produce disease within the fore arm or arm of the same hands,if the confused inflammation is minutes chemical then that will spread along the blood stream where ever it goes then it will produce disease (systemic or anywhere within body or even a local disease).

The triggering factors mostly decide the location of the disease

21. Alternating disease :

The confused inflammatory cells shift between organ or body parts and produce alternating disease.

- Between skin and lungs
- Between joint and heart
- Rectum to skin
- Mind disease to colon disorders ,,,,,,,,etc. either it interplays and shifted by the strong medicine or due to climatic changes like in summer gastric complaints and in winter skin disease. This is typically seen when the use of allopathic local acting medicines inhalers or nasal drops to respiratory ailments so that the confused inflammatory

cells pushed away from nose to skin or to brain. When apply-ing ointments to the skin rush to lungs this will happen in the earlier days afterward this happens even without any local applications.

•   Mood swings period of melancholy and de-pression alternate with joyful energetic excited states

22. Associated diseases :

sinus or nasal congestion gives respiratory disease as the day progress but it gives a variety of local disease like pimples in the face, psoriasis of the scalp, many rashes in the face and neck associated with long standing nasal con-gestion .THE DESCRIPTION UNDER ASSOCIATED DISEASES IS NOT SAME WHICH IS TILL DATE OBSERVED LIKE ASSO-CIATED SYMPTOMS OR ASSOCIATED DISEASE OF PRESENT DISEASE. THEY ARE MORE ARE LESS SINGLE DISEASE BUT WIDE RANGE OF SYMPTOMS LIKE RHUOMATOID ARTHIR-ITS with its associated symptoms OR MULTIPLE SCLEROSIS and related symptoms sinus and related disease.

what I am saying is something different I found there are many diseases with multi-system involvement but with one source. Relevant and irrelevant to the disease.

Chronic pelvic congestion due to chronic inflam-mation gives rise to a variety of local disease irrelevant to PID.

23 . Migratory in nature :

Confused inflammation is not like a real inflamma-tion ,the real inflammation focused on small target. But the the confused inflammation is slowly migrating and covers almost major portion of the skin or internal body parts.

Spreads via lymphatics, spreads via blood,

spreads local migration example from nose to adenoid to throat and then to Eustachian tube and then to ear,etc.

Shifts from place to place especially after strong heavy local applications continually for long time.

- IT SPREADS along the course tract or lymphatics and blood vessel [if spread along with tract course expectable predictable like nose to throat throat to lungs - respiratory tract.

urethra to bladder bladder to ureter to kidney- urinary tract.

This migration will damage all the body parts along its path and slowly damage initially the mi- gration causes sensory and physiological symptoms then slow pathological and irreversible pathological changes.

Luckily it may shift from place to place then the Orgon damage is stopped temporarily.

To produce Slow spreading and damaging of the body parts need strong and repeated allopathic drugs especially external application produce this change undoubtedly.

Unpredictable run along the blood vassals stuck somewhere and produce disease.

- shift totally from one place to other place and produce disease according to the trigger or attracting factor or due to strong medi- cine pushes away [dangerous and unpredictable it may shift to any part of the body and produce the disease skin to brain or joint to heart or skin to lungs].

- interplay between two areas.

[predictable like skin allergy and nasal allergy]

This character help in trace the metastatic cancer foci and study the nature of the diseases and disorders.

Flare up and sudden rapid troughing of the eruptions all over the body decided by exposure to heavy cold or hot summer so total skin is dilated or constricted due to temperature change this will trigger the confused inflammation to all over the body usually happen via blood vassals.

Why it has to flare up and shift and migrate? since it was the warier cells it will move based on strong triggering factors. so that this migration or shifts. But even when there are no triggers the confused inflammation carried along the lymphatics and blood vassals passivly so that it will produce the disease along this way.

The confused inflammation has highest attraction towards skin,mouth,hands and foot .then how the internal body parts are getting disease that is due to Strong allopathic drugs,alcohol,smoking,harming food additives some invasive procedures,etc.

(18.shifting nature of the disease also considered here)

24.Good soil for best yield:

Generalized similar disease nature depends upon the presence of confused inflammation all over the body with same inflammatory cells or chemicals this usually happens after stopping systemic generalized illness.If a person get minor abrasions in different locations makes same eruptions.

Example :

Scratch in the scalp -- psoriasis

Scratch in the chest -- psoriasis

Cracks in the palms and soles – psoriasis

But majority of the occasion's disease nature is different in different locations it represents basic nature of the confused inflammation at the present body parts.

But here irritation in the soles --- corn in the soles for pressure

In the hands --- pressure makes urticaria

In the chest wound heals normally without any marks (no confused inflammation), In the face heal with elevated scar (presence of fibroblast excess in the face region).Here human body parts act as a soil for different confused inflammation chemical and cells.

This local expression of confused inflammation happens due to external applications and so that the confused inflammation chemicals and cells are accumulated within the particular site sometimes minimally spreads   to adjacent body parts and tissues. But are not spreaded much due to the presence of high attractive power in the same place itself [usually hands , mouth , soles].

(read along with 20. location of the confused inflammation disease)

25. The MASK :

The confused inflammation present in the patient produce lots of disease diagnosis thorught the life time,with that even nearly half of the diagnosis where ignored both by patient and doctors due to insignificant and non harming. During the course of the time many diseases looks like cured but it just changes the place, So gives the another disease but with same confused inflammation cells or chemical.

we may feel happy that we are cured few symptoms of the disease in one time and then patient come with another disease so we diagnose as different disease but this is the same which we are treated but here we give different diagnosis and we will treat that. Then it shifts to some other part and produce different disease.

Why single disease subsides in one place and starts as a new disease in different parts of the body ?

■ Due to shifting and migratory and metastatic nature of the disease.

■ Strong chemicals and medicines forcibly shift the disease so it moves and find some other place to settles produce disease.

■ Evnthough same blood cells and inflammatory chemicals will produce the disease doctors name this as different disease and considered as different origin.

Chemicals and cells in the sinuses will produce the pimples. Pimples treated with strong ointments shifts from them to thyroid or ovary or testis from their it shifts to some other body parts.

The allergic rhinitis if we treated with anti inflammatory and anti allergic produce the asthma if we treat asthma, then atopic dermatitis then if we treat that then it goes to increases asthma.

MASK

Every time doctors consider as different disease. The one department which is very clearly gives the clue that I am the one but giving different disease but even though they never realize that.

In ENT disease starts with rhinitis then adenoid then tonsillitis then ear infection and asthma and bronchitis and then eczema all the diseases in front of his eyes progress into worse but he considers everything he name in different disease diagnosis and expecting different cause and prescribe medicine for help growth of disease.

But surprisingly he diagnosis precisely accurately right diagnosis that is in cancer here only he diagnoses and conclude everything right I don't know how this miracle happen to the QUACK MIND.

He found in the cancer particle in the stomach then he accept it spreaded to lymph node he says it is not lymph adenitis it is cancer and then it is spread to liver he is not saying it is liver tumor , he is not waiting to diagnose different name he rightly diagnosing this is also cancer this cells are migrated from the stomach and he even believe that this cancer cells are reach to testis and he accept and believe that cancer cells reached to the brain and he concluded and start the treatment he judges rightly here the mask is teared by allopathy but in all other situation he is not accepting that.

Allopathy rightly judge the spreading and metastatic nature of the disease [THE TEARED MASK].The multi face of the same disease is rightly captured by allopathy. The migration or shifting or jumping, do what ever it may be but I know you are the only one doing much damage to the patient [He take right decision only in cancer]

He has to understand this every time he treats the disease it is not cured or vanished it is remaining inside the testis and remain inside the liver; it goes to the brain produce different psychological disease and shift to joint and bone produce different disease try to understand this. THE CANCER IS THE TOP MOST EVIDENCE OF SPREADING, SHI-FITNG NATURE OF THE DISEASE, BELIVE ME THE CANCER IS NOT SPREADED NOW YOU ARE SEEING TODAY BRAIN METASTATIC CANCER WAS SPREADED 5 YEARS BEFORE THE LIVER METASTASIS WAS HAPPEN AS HEPATITIS 10 YEARS BEFORE, SHIFTED TO BONE 3 YEARS BEFORE BUT ALL ARE TURNINING INTO CANCER CURRENTLY.

Use the standard law when curing the disease, wheather we are curing or helping in metastasis judge yourself.[HERING LAW OF CURE DISCUSED UNDER CHAPTER ASSESMENT OF CURE].

The top most mask is skin disease to internal body parts disease, they never accept that skin diseases metastasis to lungs and heart and liver. But recently they started accept atopy shifts to lungs as an asthma but they dont know exactly what is the cause for that.

(shifiting and migratory nature of the disease and alternating disease chercters has to be consider here)

26. Cause of the disease :

All chemicals or cells of confused inflammation Responding, reacting to varies external , internal stimuli so diseases arise due to this stimulus. Here we consider this stimulai as a risk factor or cause or the triggering factor.

What is risk factor what is the cause what you mean by triggering factor ?

A cause is the one realy produces the disease but we have no idea why the inflammation without the germs so eventhough the disease created now by a cold air exposure we connot consider this is as a cause since there is no germ. So, we call the cold air as trigger or risk factor , and we say we have not detected the cause yet.

But after the discovery of the confused inflammation the cause for the disease is confused inflammation again the cold air, hot sun, food, medicines ,hormones all are triggering of this confused inflammation so the triggering factor or risk factor is in the same place as triggering factor but we found the cause is confused inflammation.

But we can use the triggering factor as a cause (pseudo cause) since this pseudo cause act and replace the place of germs exactly.

Air, dust, fumes induce the athma we can call this is as a pseudo cause.

If you remove the cause the person will be in good health. But if you remove the risk factor or triggering factor then most of the time the confused inflammation will triggered by another triggering factors so it is tough to prevent. So, this is the reason a diabetes and hypertension and many more non communicable diseases is not preventable by means avoiding salt, reducing sugar doing regular exercise. More this physical measure fails more the current allopathy doctors thinking these diseases are genetic and hereditary base. But that is not true.

Even the germs (bacteria, virus also play a duel role like it could be cause if it is developed without any confused inflammation. it could be psuedo cause or triggering factor of the confused inflammation since here germs induce and produce inflammation).

In simple words when bacteria enter inside only good inflammation is there then the cause is bacteria and removing the cause (bacteria) the person will become healthy. But when bacteria enter in this situation confused inflammation present in the person health then killing the germ may not produce the health need to remove the confused inflammation also is consider as a cure.

27. Modality (worse or better) :

Once the diseases developed, now if the

person exposing to the same stimuli or different stimuli causes either further spread of diseases or disease condition worse (worse). Patient feel more pain or suffering.But some stimuli other then causative agent,reduce the disease intensity or make comfort to the disease (better).

Example - Joint stiffness Feel better by slow walking, joint pain better by massage. shivering worse in open aire, comfortable in closed warm room.

If the C inflammation is attracted to a particular site then the disease will be produced then further trigger of the same stimulai worse the disease and helps in keep the disease in the same site this stimulai needed for continuation of the disease in the particular site. confused inflammation chemicals respond to varies external stimulai then confused immunity.

Why the disease is worse when expose to same stimulai ?

Simple answere is confused inflammation chemicals more or less once again clubbed together by this triggering factors so the disease condition worse.

But touching the inflamed surface , wounded area,annoying inflamed surface give just a usual worse it does not have any power to invite the confused inflammation cells to this site (simple modality).

In a single disease some times so many factors will increase the disease more or less help to spread or just increase the disease.

PSORIYASIS – COLD WINTER CLAIMATE PRODUCE PSORIYASIS

(Causative modality) the same act as worse factor like if the person suffers severely again when he is exposing winter or ac room.

Asthma worse in winter

Wheezing better by stay in closed warm room

Asthma worse when walking

Stomach pain better by bending double

Back pain worse when sneezing

Joint pain worse when walking

Joint pain better when pressure

In the same way there are many external and internal factors reduce the intensity of the disease and sometime helps in complete disappearance of the disease from the particular location (curative modality). The factor which is makes comfort to the disease is some time opposite to the causative factor of the disease, but not all the time.

But there are many situations it does not help in cure the disease but just give the amelioration.

In some rare situation the destroying, damaging factor also gives amilioration a drunkard feels worse and nervouse when not drinking feel comfortable drinking (amelioration by drinking alcohol)

Example:

Like winter produce psoriyais. (cold air produces the eruption – causative modality)

Summer heals the psoriyasis. (sun heat ameliorates and psoriyasis disappear in summer – curative modality) Drinking cold water worse the wheezing Warm water relives the wheezing.

IN SHORT A FACTOR WHICH MAKES DISEASE WORSE, SUPPORT AND HELPS IN CONFUSED INFLAMMA-TION TO SPREAD THE DISEASE. IN THE CONTRARY SOME FACTORS WHICH IS DOES NOT SUPPORT TO DEVELOP THE DISEASE and TRY TO ELIMINATE THE DISEASE FROM THE THERE. It looks like a cure but not . The factors eliminate the disease from particular body parts but the disease will choose to locate in some other parts, it is not a cure just giving temporary relief.

So, it is better to give importance to give modifying factor of the disease here after. it can be easily obtained from the patient.

Examples :

Walking , day and night, sun exposure,claimatic changes , varies body posture sitting , standing,,,,,,etc. like that all this modality yet to up-date [extremely a smaller number of modalities has been added] in the pathology text and general medicine.all this modality is not something related only to Homeopaths this has to be added as importand in all medical field.

Significance of modality :

Modality is used in homeopathy for many years. Homeopathy giving highest importance to modality and occupied maximum disease pathophysiology as well as most valuable, considered in the prescription of medicine. So, that homeopaths aimed to clear confused inflammation without his knowledge and every patient seeking homeo treatment get free from this confused inflammatory cell.

Allopathy gives more importand and indepth study of the germs like virus and bacteria since he considers they are causing the disease so he study that and prepare medicine to kill the germs and prepare vaccine from protecting the virus.

Homeopathy consider miasm is the cause the miasm has to be cleared from the person so they collect all the minute details of the miasm and trying to remove that miasm by preparing a similar power medicine (homeopathy vaccine).

In simple words germ is the cause for communicable disease so to remove and kill the germ we study that and succeeding in that. But confused inflammation is the cause means we have to study the minute details of the confused inflammation.

When the confused inflammation formed it is not easy to remove that. Maybe I am saying and writing very simple this chemical or that chemical causing disease. What chemical and cells making sickeness we have to know then only we can remove them. Modality is one of the importand cherecter of the confused inflammation.

Ok I am having asthma every time I am drenched in the rain what is the significance ? how you will remove the confused inflammation.

Here the histamine or other chemical mediaters are triggerd by cold and produce more confused inflammation and produce broncho constriction. This person mostly relived by good sun heat more or less comfortbale in summer. In this way we can collect the unique cherecter of the confused inflammation.

This modality define the nature of the C inflammation and helps in finding the remedy for removing this c inflammation.

We have to select homeopathy medicine which is having power to produce same modality. It means asthma after drenched in rain – nat sulph or asrsenicum , rhus tox .

Homeopathy has mega index for modality in the repertory. This reportry is collected from artificial disease (Drug proving – giving drugs to human being and observing signs and symptoms including modality).

General modality helps in clearing the confused inflammation in genral and totally then local modality .local modality may not clearly comprise the true nature of the confused inflammation in total so prescription based on this will cause just disappearance of the disease in one location only but the confused inflammation will remain and produce disease again.

MODALITY GIVES THE CHARACTER OF CONFUSED INFLAMMATION. THIS CHARACTER IS USED FOR PRESCRIPTION.THIS TRIGGER IS SPECIFY THE DISEASE. IF THE TRIGGER IS COMMON WORSE OR BETTER FACTOR THEN THAT SCORE LESS MARKS. IF THIS WORSE OR BETTER FACTOR IS SOMETHING UNIQUE OR DIFFERENT OR UNUSUAL THEN THAT SCORES HIGH MARKS BECAUSE THAT IS VERY PRECISLY IDENTIFY THE CONFUSED INFLAMMATION REDUCE THE BURDEN OF CHOOSING SINGLE REMEDY IN A GROUP OF MANY MEDICINES.

28. Mixture of confused inflammations

In one single disease there are group of confused inflammation cells present, which was pushed away from regular normal inflammation functions in different time period, Throught the patient life time is inevitable in the current allopathic era so that painless old tumor (produced by confused inflammation) now painful because of the new wandering confused inflammation chemicals , so we can expect more number of erratic irrelevant disease (considered as new disease or comprehended as variety in old disease). if new confused inflammation cells reached to the old neuralgic site will build tumors or ulcers. This site was just painfull but the new confused inflammation cells produce the tumor or ulcer in the just neuralgic site.

But eventhough the troubles going in a regular course but doctor will be excited since they will think that they found something new disease.

So, when we treating such multi level complicated cases, prescribing homeopathic medicine will clear the current predominant disease symptoms produced by confused inflammations so we have to wait for another confused inflammation group of cells to surface and active and now prescribe for that.

In the same way we have to harvest all the confused inflammation cells.

Consider cherecter of how the c inflammation get augmented.

29.The confused inflammation remain silent (Latent Disease)

The confused inflammation remains silent without producing any diagnosable disease but it will do changes , we are unable to see that, it is micro level ,like some discoloration in the skin and mild dandruff and sub clinical changes within body parts like that. We start see the hairloss but we can see the real baldness nearly 5 - 6 years later is a simple example of confused inflammation changes. Similarly, the confused inflammation does microlevel changes within the body (sub clinical) not a showing any signs and symptoms visibly or clinically or even laboratory.

THE LATENCY CAN BE TRACED EASILY IF THE TREATMENT HISTORY IS WELL KNOWN.

30. confused inflammation increases the chance of infection:

Even though it is an inflammation and their basic character is to destroy the germs here it is not doing that activity. Infact this confused inflammation is favoring the infections.

Since the confused inflammation lost all its destructive power and locating the enemy and targeting the infectiuse germs to clear from the circulation.instead of that damagaing normal tissuse so the losing protective power and damaging the normal tissue together make a great space for source of infections eventhiugh it mimics like a inflammation.

It has been discussed under tendency and diathesis ,under infections chapter.

5. HOW BAD INFLAMMATION CREATED ?

Unscientific allopathic system

.

(**A**llopathic doctors having highest confidence that what they are doing is highly right, who ever it may be opposing, they may not think or realise that they are doing mistakes. This confidence is coming from their medical books, its necessary to prove this book are not right.

This chapter explains how allopathy devites from science).

Our body has enough protective mechanism. If the person is infected with any germs then body will clear that by using this mechanism. If any wound is happening, that wound will be healed automatically. Then how this many diseases happens to humans ? it may be caused by failure of above mechanism ? or something else ? ok then the treatment aimed to recover this failed mechanism ?

First of all, the doctors do not allow the body to heal themselves and almost many systems doctors are egar to prescribe medicines almost all doctors do not know where to prescribe ? where to observe ? how to plan the treatment ?

According to my observations /research almost all the disease to the humans is happened only by wrong treatment alone [allopathy is the topper in doing this]. They consider, they teach, they practice treatment for stop inflammation and reduce the immunity. Why ? they believe inflammation and immunity is harming the humans. The hypersensitivity theory says one strong information to the allopathic doctors, according to this theory allowing inflammation and immunity will cause harm to the patient. So, they decide to terminate this process as early as possible for that they discovered anti-inflammatory, anti-allergic , they not satisfied they found more powerful then that that is called steroid.

Hypersensitivity theory is taking the right path of allopathy into wrong path. I have disproved this theory in the whole book here and there. In a single line explanation of the hypersensitivity " inflammation is good no dought but if the inflammation occurs again for the same triggering factor then the inflammation doing harm to the humans " this is the hypersensitivity theory so allopathy doctors start prescribing the anti inflammatory. Why the inflammation doing favor in one time and harm to another time ? they say it is genetic ? or abnormal sensitivity (truly they do not know what it is ? why it is happening. They guess it could be genetic abnormality). Inflammation is good but it is turned into bad inflammation by allopathic medicine itself (how will discuss in detail in next chapter). From the day when they directly or indirectly stop the inflammation a greater number of new diseases arising to the humans.

Every doctor attending the fever patient , will try to arrest the fever so they encurage multiplication of germs. Why we have to stop inflammation ? allopath prescription is compulsorily having the anti-pyretic (in India).

Almost every fever patient will receive one anti-biotic (90 % in India, I am not sure about other country). Whether the person is having bacterial infection or any-thing else or fever is caused by what type of germ is not necessary. One antipyretic, one anti biotic, one anti aller-gic and one antacid is the common combination for acute febrile condition with cold. Most of the febrile conditions will have viral infections then what is the point in prescrib-ing anti-pyretic, anti-biotic and anti-histamine to the pa-tient. In what sense doctors prescribing this drug. What is the aim this treatment ? why we have to stop the fever. Then who kill the virus. What is the aim of anti-histamine then who kill the germs ? allopathic doctors studying almost 6 years of basic medical but still they prescribe medicine to terminate the inflammation process ?

Whether the medicine is needed or not to the given febrile case , no waiting they prescribe some medi-cine. If the person says running nose and head ache anti-allergic is an additional medicine ? joint pain with fever means strong painkiller other then [anti-pyretic] also pre-scribed still the pain is not subsided mild sedation with pain killers ? if the fever with loose stool or vomiting then anti diarrheal anti emetics and in addition compulsory anti-biotics. Allopathy doctors in India is doing Guinness record in creating lots of new disease to Indians.

It is not happening in every febrile case but in most of the cases this symptom will be there this symptomatic treatment collapse the basic functions of the human inflammation and immune system. Causing great many new disease.

If there is any abrasion or injury then we must use antibiotic creams or else wound will get septic and then you will end with severe complications this is the allopathic training to the public medically speaking it is the foolish Rumer created by allopath and applying ointments creates lots of complications including tumor and disease related with induration, infiltration.

If you prescribe medicine for stop basic functions and trying to prescribe some medicine, where actually that will take care naturally, then what you are studying in the medical college under the inflammation and immunity chapters. All above prescriptions 100 % against the human body functions. Then what science you are following ?.

The primary effect of the medicine itself poisonous to the human protective mechanism .I am not discussing side effects. I am discussing about only the first basic effect of the allopathy medicine alone.

The aim of anti pyretic, anti-allergic, painkillers, anti-diarrhea, anti-emetics, cough syrup, steroids all will aimed to stop basic functions of the body so now no fever, no pain, no loose stool, no vomiting, no cough so the patient is feeling better. But patient does not know that fever/pain/redness/loss of functions is actually a Treatment given by body through immune system. Fever is a treatment, Vomiting is a treatment , diarrhea is treatment but what you are doing you are stopping all these treatments ?

- stopping the fever, the pain
- stopping the vomiting
- stopping the cough
- Arresting diarrhea

- Stopping running nose, sneezing
- Trying to stop inflammation by eye drops
- Trying to stop inflammation by ear drops, Trying to stop inflammation by varies ointments.

So, patient felt better by fever and pain and cough and sneezing but who is going to kill the virus. This is not ideal prescription. No one is aware this prescription is not curative.

When I am having fever if I take the allopathic medicine, I am getting absolute relief from the fever, no body pain, no head ache.

So, I am thinking A PARACETAMOL IS CURED MY FEVER.

When I was having viral fever with nasal congestion, I take anti-inflammatory and anti-allergic. Now I am not having running nose, no fever, no sick feeling I am relived.

So, I BELIVE CETRIZEN CURED ME.

When I have stomach pain and vomiting, I am taking emesis and ranitidine or gelucil and some pain killer. Now I am not having vomiting

I feel my GASTRITIS CURED BY GELUSIL AND EMESET.

This is something cheating. Because you are killing the patient but patient believing you are the HIGHLY EDUCATED AMONG THE DOCTORS and he takes the medicine with the belief.since the complaints and symptoms are stopped, he thinks that he is cured.

My dear doctor its your duty to educate the world this is not a treatment. Explain to the public,this is against the medical profession. Advise the patient not to consume this drug. Advertise this to the media and online SAVE THE LIFE OF THE PATIENT. Childrens, elders all are consuming this drug. pediatrician, Prescribing full of anti-allergic, anti-inflammatory, Anti diarrheal, etc. all this fraud products.

THE INDICATED REMEDY HERE IS NOTHING YOU HAVE TO KEEP QUIT AND THIS IS DOCTOR FREE ZONE YOU ARE NOT ALLOWED TO PRESCRIPE MEDI-CINE.DONT DISTURB INFLAMMATION OBSERVE THE CONDITION, IF NEEDED SUPPORT THE INFLAMMA-TION. you are allowed to prescribe medicine only if you have the medicine to correct the or repair the inflammation malformation. allopathy is not having any medicine for recover or repair the inflammation-oriented disease so please avoid prescribing to just satisfy the patient.

You are writing your own indications. Under paracetamol, under cetirizine, you are writting the indications so, without your conscious you are prescribing. Not mentioning anywhere that it is wrong to stop the fever and colds. stopping inflammation is Contra indication except if it really going to severe life-threatening complications.

Homeopathy is slow and allopathy medicine is fast ?

IF ANYONE STOPPING INFLAMMATION IT REVEALS THEY ARE A QUACK. THEY ARE NOT ELI-GIBLE TO HOLD DOCTOR DEGREE ANYMORE.

The anti inflammatory and anti allergic

prescription in inflammation considered as CRIMINAL PRESCRIPTION. India is rich in qualified quacks; they overtake the non medical quacks by prescribing foolish medicine.

DOCTOR, PATIENT ASKING ME, "WHEN ALO-PATHIC MEDICINE STOP THE FEVER WITHIN HALF AN HOUR WHY DON'T YOU HAVE THAT MEDICINE ? he says ,YOUR SYTEM MEDICINES ARE SLOW, so I WANT TO TAKE ONLY ALLOPATHY.

IF ANYONE STOPPING INFLAMMATION IT REVEALS THEY ARE A QUACK. THEY ARE NOT ELIGIBLE TO HOLD DOCTOR DEGREE ANY-MORE.

TEM MEDICINES ARE SLOW, so I WANT TO TAKE ONLY ALLOPATHY.

Stopping the fever fast, stopping the vomiting fast, stopping the runining nose fast. So, I am not having such fast medicine to stop inflammation. can you teach me how to do this fraud activity, because people are not believing me ? THEY STAMP ME AS A SLOW SYSTEM ?

BY DOING THIS YOU ARE SCIENTIST AND HOMEOPATHY IS A PSUEDO SCIENTIST ? GO ONE MORE STEP PRESCRIBE MEDICINE FOR STOP BREATHING FIND MEDICINE FOR STOP PULSE.THEN GET THE NAME AS SUPER, DUPPER SCIENTIST.

Indian doctors are trained to prescribe anti inflammatory and anti-allergic. They train the public to take that medicines. The pharma company is adver-tising their medicine in the online and medias to con-sume with or without doctor advice. So, the patient buying and consuming medicine on the majority of the ailment (self medications).

Surgen role in breaking immunity

Surgeons taking another part of doing collapsing and destroying to the patient immune system.

Removing the tonsil (immune which act as guard which will prevent the entry of germs from mouth to atomach and intestine).

Removing the adenoid (immune gland protects the throat by destroy the germs).

Removing the appendix (immune gland destroys the germs in the intestine and colon).

Removing the lymph node (immune cells producer and kill the germs).

Removing the spleen (Blood purifier, immune gland). Spleen is the good germ killer.

WHY HE IS REMOVING THIS BECAUSE THEY DON'T HAVE MEDICINE TO RECOVER OR CURE THESE IMMUNE ORGANS. INFACT THEY ONLY DESTROYED THIS ORGANS AND MADE PERMANENT INFLAMMATION DUE TO STOPPING ACUTE INFLAMMATION.

• Stopping acute tonsillitis by allopathy, turn into chronic tonsillitis.Stopping acute rhinitis by anti allergic causes chronic adenoid infection but there is no medicine to cure allopathy so he recommends surgery.

There is very good effective treatment in homeopathy to recover. Tonsil,adenoid,lymph node functions consult homeopath.

At first, he stops the inflammation so he collapses the entire inflammation process so the person getting the sickness now he recommends sugen to remove the immune organ this will increase further infection chance.HE IS NOT RECOVERING FROM SICK-NESS, HE IS MAKING YOU SICK IN A STRONG BASE-MENT, YOU ARE GOING TO BE SICK LIFE LONG. HE IS STOPPING THE TREATMENT GIVEN BY BRAIN AND HE IS TEACHING THE PUBLIC IN WRONG WAY THAT HE IS RECOVERING, EDUCATING SOCIETY IN WRONG WAY AND SO THERE BY HE CREATES LOTS OF DISEASE AND HE IS BECOME RICH BY ACTING AS IF HE IS GIVING TREATMENT. So, allopathy in patient ward and ICU is always full of patient.

Allopathy doctors are disease producer and helps in infection support germ multiplications, so that is the reason the allopathy doctors and hospitals are top most profitable business.

So, the person now need continues allopathy medicine for survival, since his system collapsed it does not react normally to the germs or any other foreign body HE IS CONVINCED IN THE MEDICAL COLLEGE IN THE NAME HYPERSENTIVE THEORY-THIS THEORY STRONGLY OBJECTS THE INFLAMMATION AND IMMUNNITY AND FA-VORES PRESCRIPTION OF ANTI INFLAMMATORY AND ANTI IMMUNE DRUGS.I AM NOT SURE HOW HE IS CONVINCED TO PRESCRIBBING OTHER DRUGS AGAINST THE BASIC THE NUERO IMMUNE FUNCTIONS OF THE BODY FOR PROTECT-ING AND CURING FUNCTIONS OF THE BODY.

any scientist other then allopathy will not accept this is as a treatment.

*What is the scientific approach
to cure the patient ?*

Scientific approach is allowing the inflammation to continue and if there is any failure in continueing the inflammation or if the inflammation is hypersensitive then we have to make that into normo sensitive. Inflammation is good but hypersensitivity is bad so to avoid complications of hypersensitivity prescribing medicine for stopping the inflammation is not good not scientific.

Identify what is the cherecteristics of inflammation allow it to happen. At the same time identify what is the cherecteristic of the hypersensitivity and discover the medicine to handle the type 1, type 2 ,type 3 and type 4 hypersensitive and prescribe medicine to recover these 4 hypersensitivities to normal sensitivity. Till now you are discovered 4 hypersensitivity but you have not discovered any medicine to cure this condition to become normal.

And you are not diagnosing the present condition is normal inflammation or hypersensitivity. Prescribing medicine for all the inflammation and diverting the normal community to sick community ? how long I have to think that everything is happening without your conscitous ?.

Send the cases to homeopathy don't create the diseased community . What hemeopathy is doing we are allowing the normal inflammation and immunity and we have medicine for all 4 types of hypersensitivity we are not stopping inflammation and we are creating healthy community from sick and diseased patient. That medicine is a curative medicine not having any side effects and we make the people to face the germs with their own body immunity medicine support only if they failing in facing this infection, we support we does not have any medicine to stop or distract the inflammation and immunity.

How I can belive you are good doctor you are discovered 4 hypersensitivity but you are managing these 4 hypersensitivities with steroid and anti inflammatory. You know very well this is not a curative medicine for this hypersensitive. I am wondering that why you are managing every disease. Public visiting to the hospital has to be there with your life long.

Why surgery ? because no medicine, surgery is recomended.

When you are not having any medicine for one disease then you have to send the cases to someone has the treatment for that. *removing the spleen is not a right treatment since you do not have the medicine you are removing the organ. Removing the lymph node is not a right treatment since you does not have medicine to cure the swollen indolent, indurated lymph node you are removing the lymph node You know very well lymph node and spleen and tonsil is good for health but you are removing because you does not have medicine to recover.* But the right way is to send the cases to homeopaths. Since you are dominant now to the whole medical field you are keeping your own court and your own judgement.

Recover the spoiled system. Recover the hypersensitive to normal sensitive, don't make under sensitive or collapse further.

When the inflammation may damage more due to past history of anti-inflammatory drugs now you have to set right otherwise it will cause damage but you do not have right medicine work along with physiology so you are terminating the inflammation. Either you should not spoil the inflammation or you should send the cases to homeopathy to recover the spoiled system to recover.

Then what is right treatment ? how we have to treat patients ?

Allow the fever to run, if the child never received any allopathy medicine previous to admission or call a homeopath to handle the case. Interrupt and prescribe the allopathy medicine if the vital parameters for recovery goes in opposite direction or he is inefficient to handle the case. But sure after the allopathy medicine his immune system will collapsed, he need proper homeo treatment to recover that.

Allopathy is a best manager but he is not a doctor since he is best damager of the human protective system and he send the patient with collapsed system but the patient has to be educated to go and meet homeopathy after taking allopathy drugs.

During hospitalization iv fluids ,vitamins are allowed to prescribe non of the medicine needed during the course of treatment if the situation demands homeopathy medicine can be allowed.

Anti bacterial medicines allowed only if the body is struggling to over come the infections and after proper laboratory test, culture and if the course of the recovery is delayed [and the delay is not because of the anti-inflammatory or steroids]

Need proper punishment for allopathy doctors if they simply prescribe steroids for the patient just for making money. every case demands for steroid has to be send to the homeopathy to cure. prescribing steroid is absolutely not necessary if the homeopathy doctors are there in the location.

A manger is called to manage the critical situation a doctor has to called for remaining time . An allopathy has to learn homeopathy for being a qualified doctor.

We read page by page that all the protective functions of body. but doctors never wait for to carry out the protective functions normally. He feels satisfied only after prescribing some medicine.He belive , then only patient will be fine.this is doctors' delusions. Because of this patient suffering from long time.

Now you have to read the question once again. If total body is fully protected from germs then how the disease comes ? is that protections is failed ? Then, the aim of allopathic treatment is recovering and repair the failed inflammation and immune system to become normal ?

The one-word answer is no. not only no , they only make the protection system to be fail their aim is not to recover the failed mechanism they aim completely collapse and remove that from body. *actually, there is no medicine to do what is right. so, they doing harm to people by prescribing what they have.*

All type of chronic ailment comes one by one by allopathic direct effect and side effects of medicine just after treatment with some minor ailment. They are surrounded with themselves so, no one is there to point out their fault if someone is raising voice, they really think that person is fool, and what he does is right.

We have to keep warn them, because he creates lots of disease without his conscious. His mistakes are too dangerous and irreparable and takes lots of time and lots of sufferings to bring back the original conditions in many situations its highly impossible to bring the advanced pathological diseased condition to normal .It is easy to make collapse but tough to repair and bring back normal.

It is highest importance to stop using anti inflammatory, steroids, anti histamine, cough syrups, pain killers. We have to ban this drug he will not stop this on his own. More then patient doctors are addicted to prescribing many unnecessary drugs. Allopathy doctors has to train use other system drugs as an alternate until he is doing this the problem will not solve.

Then what we have to do when acute infection or fever or cold is there ?.

- *Allow the fever to run its course so that it will kill the virus and germs and It will limit the multiplication of the germs. THERE IS NO MEDICINE FOR MANY VIRUSES AND MANY OTHER GERMS FEVER WILL CONTROLE THAT. CONSULT HOMEOPATH IF NECESSORY.*

- *Allow the running nose and sneezing and nose block this is not indication for prescribing anti-allergic. This is the inflammation process under this process the germs in the nose is going to be killed ANTI ALLERGICS stopping this, so through that in dust bin that will kill your immune system. Go to homeopathy if you troubled by that more.*

- *Don't stop vomiting, you are consumed some infected or spoiled food so that body trying to eliminate that. Vomiting will stop soon **give adequate liquid to rehydrate**. Consult Homeopath if the vomiting is not stopped and exhausting.*

- *Don't stop cough ,cough is good if it is annoying then consult homeopath to solve the issue.*

- *Don't go to allopathy if your tonsil is swellon,adenoid swellon go to homeopath and take medicine ,he has to recover the gland function.*

Don't go to allopathy and don't take STEROIDS ,Through STEROID in his face and ask him why steroid to my childrens.SINCE STEROID IS THE STRONG IMMUNE SUPPRESSOR. He prescribes that in the aim of keeping your child all the time within the hospital

ALL THIS COMPLAINTS WHEEZING AND ALLERGY IS THE ALLOPATHIC MEDICINE INDUCED, SO GO TO HOMEOPATHY, THEY WILL GIVE GOOD MEDICINE, this was the allopathic words long back, they said openly this is not good medicine to humans . most of ALLOPATH DOCTORS WAS SAID THIS.BUT THAT GOOD ALLOPATHY DOCTOR WAS DIED LONG BACK , WHAT WE ARE SEEING IS FRAUD. KEEP AWAY FROM HIM. Similar to public all the allopathy doctors belives they can do anything and they think they have excellent medicine.

Keeping the disease but selling their product

If patient say head ache then doctors will send you ophthalmologist and sell the specks.Then what you will do ? prescribing specks will give temprory relief to the patient but at the same time disease within the eye will damage the eye further will cause more pathological destruction we have to aim to cure the disease.This is important.Prescribbing specks will ease the symptoms not cure the disease.

If you say neck pain and hip pain, they prescribe the pain killers and sell the lumbar belt and neck belt all are going to reduce the pain temporarily disease will grow, what if the disease worse ? will go for surgery.

That painkillers will cure the complaints are eye glass will cure the inflammation within the eye and sinus or the neuralgia will be solved by wearing glass. Why specks for head ache ? why you are not trying to treat refractive error with medicine ? because no medicine. Why you are not trying to cure the chronic sinus ? because no medicine.

Ok if you find that a child is myopic what is cure for that why don't you even attempting to cure that ,you do not have an idea of curing .why the child has to wear a glass life long. if you don't have medicine send the case to homeopaths we have medicine for refractive errors ,all the refractive error and visual and ophthalmic ailments curable by homeopathic treatment.

If there is no severe irreversible pathology is happened . is there any remedy for cure myopia ? if I am saying that allopathic doctors may laugh at this. In many situation he thinks other alternative system cheating the public .He thinks that he only have the medicine, if he does not have any medicine then no medicine in the world [this thought destroys whole alternative system and public has been accepting to live with the suffering].unless until we break this thought we will not achieve disease free universe.

When I have vision complaints, I have to meet ophthalmologist and he will check my eye and he will give the glass to wear is 100 % todays normal. I am not forgetting that you did cataract operation and saved vision of million people but at the same time I am also noticing your unwanted activity of sales marketing and utilizing that good name for improving sales. THE PATH IS DIVERTING FROM SERVICE TO BUSINESS. Keep insight upon your diversion.

ALL OPTHALMIC DISORDERS CREATED BY usage of allopathic MEDICINE INCLUDING CATARACT. Confused inflammation created many diseases including all opthalimic disease.

Refractive errors curable, try with medicine. Send the cases to alternate system. If he fails, then your turn to earn. Glaucoma, iritis, iridocylitis, retinopathy all are curable and most importantly preventable.

When I have vision complaints, I have to meet ophthalmologist and he will chec

Is that back pain will be alright with pain killers or hip belt what is the remedy for cure that . if the pain is not relived then steroid injection directly to the spots along with sedation in the night for sleep .if all this measure is failed then call for surgery. Why for simple neuralgia you are calling for the people to do spinal surgery. Because you are not having any more solution for the complaints.

- Pain killer is not a curative medicine for back pain.
- Steroid injection is not a curative medicine.
- Operation is not necessary for the acute, sub-acute, chronic back pain without any structural changes.
- Providing belt to the patient is really supportive. But all the above steps are only IF THE HOMEOAPTHY or alternative system failed. There is no question if you cure the patient.

90 % of the cases curable by HOMEOPATHY ALONE. They recover without any main effect or side effect. Will you refer the case here after ? will you behave like a professional.

Your need is necessary in an emergency situation but in ordinary opd cases you are after the Homeopathy and AYUSH but you are Hiding them and erasing them. The current generations believing you.

THAT IS WHY I AM GOING IN DEPTH DOING RESEARCH AND EXPLAINING ALL TRUTH TO THE PUBLIC AND TO THE DOCTORS ALSO BY READING THIS BOOK ALOPATHIC DOCTORS WILL ACCEPT OTHERS ALSO HAVING BRAIN. And they are also a doctor.YOU WILL COME TO KNOW WHAT IS YOUR LIMIT. HOMEOPATHS READING WHAT IS THEIR LIMIT AND SCOPE.

All your texts not including other systems of medicine. No where it is mentioned there is the medicine in AYUSH SYSTEM or nothing in the 2000 pages of general medicine text books or in other books, about other system. I know you are reading, but how ? "alternative system is not having any science and they are bogus system ; they are pseudo scientist ". Good teaching keeps it up.

I am not sure how they treat thyroid disease globally as for as India is concerned ,if you have thyroid disease you need to take a life time medicine. This is the demand in allopathy. Every 3-6 months once you need to check the thyroid level.

Pregnant women are diagnosed as thyroid insufficiency when they undergo thyroid checkup. From then they demanded to take thyroid supliments life long.

This if temporary defect it will be solved after the birth of the child more or less , but non of the allopath or endocrinologist ask to stop medicine. I have come across patient himself stoping the medicine. If they going to regular check up, they give regular medicine till death.

Many young women forced to take thyroid tablets. When they undergo regular check up for obesity and menses irregularity. So they take pills regularly for years together and they drop the medicine as their own.

Again, when they have issue in conceiving this is another reason, they forced to take thyroid tablets and different other hormonal pills and injection during this time. Indian allopathy is focusing fully upon fertility treatment. There are many gynocological test , by weekly scanning, hysterscopy and hormonal study like test itself goes like many lakhs and then for IUI and IVF they charge many lakhs. This is tha top most business in india now and in particular major city in india. WHO targets to reduce the infections and non communicable disease Indian gynocologist targets to deliver a greater number of childrens and earn more? Single couples will pay nearly 5-25 lakh for all the expenses till delivery. When a young girl is prevented not to fall infertile, they loss many lakh businesses in future. so, allopathy plan not to prevent better spread disease. Indian gynocologist are totally deviates from medical service and plan only to earn this is an obsolute negligence.

Endocrinologist?

- Why they ask the patient to take life long thyroid tablets.
- Why thyroid insufficiency when we have adequate fortified iodine salt daily.
- Why are you asking to check up periodically? to check the level and adjust the dose of thyroid. Ok , if the thyroid is keep increasing then what will you do ? I will keep increasing the dose,this is right way of planning the treatment ?

Don't you feel this is not good. you don't have any medicine to cure the thyroid insufficiency. ELEVATED PARAMTERS indicates that disease is increasing and so thyroid gland fully under damage so this is the reason the thyroid gland struggle to give sufficient thyroid hormone to the need so deficiency increasing.

You are managing the case, that is not necessary in all cases. Patient need treatment and patient has to be cured then to manage. Management is needed in specific situation.

The patient thinking that allopathy doctors are curing the disease [few]. Patient thinking that no other way, we have to bear this [most of them].

We can consult alternate system so that we can get cure (few of them, but the percent is eroding now, since domination of allopathy and selling the medicine like grocery item, including door delivery, specilists domination).

What all the allopathy doctors doing they are managing the low-level thyroid to normal by prescribing hormone pills. This work was done in by MBBS and then, MD allopathy. To just manage the case they have created endocrinologist. I don't know who else is going to come. Just for management.

Non of the allopathy doctor referring the case to cure simultaneously. If they found difficulty, they refer themselves. Managers only know how to manage the case and how to damage the case what else you are going to do with the case ?

If you are a doctor you will think about the disease, you will conclude the disease first cured then we can give management or else simultaneous management and cure. You are not a doctor you are a damager and manager so you are doing your work that's all.

PLEASE THINK AND RETHINK WHAT YOU ARE DOING ?

YOU ARE DUMPING THE CASE.YOU NEVER AT-TEMPTED TO CURE THE CASE. MANAGER YOU ARE SPOILING THE PATIENT LIFE YOU ARE SIMPLY PLAY-ING WITH PATIENT LIFE.

What medicine you are having for auto immune thyroid ?

What medicine you are having for thyroid nodule ?

What medicine you are having for thyroid goiter ?

I am doctor because I am treating the thyroid disease not managing the case. I am succeeding and failing when attempting the case but I am failing as a doctor not as a manager. You are not even managing the case.

As for as the manager, part is over when they difficult to manage the case. You need to send the patient to homeopaths. When managing the case MBBS then MD and then by endocrinologist means how I can call an endocrinologist is a specialist that's is why I am Saying cheating.People are believing that you are really know everything ,what you say is right. But really you are not guiding the patient in right way.

What I am discussing in the whole text not a rare phenomenon, not some where some minor fault. All are very common disease day to day we are facing. Most popular diseases and allopathy doctor management.

More or less all the people can easily accept my point including you. Then come to a decision. You are educating the world to bear the disease after you are collapsing. you are educating the people to live with the disease since there is no medicine ? but if you asked to bear the the patient to bear the cold and self curing disease, they no need to bear the pain and suffering life long.

When the disease coming to nose you are said it is because of virus and because of bacteria so that you prescribed so many medicines. now the disease coming to thyroid slowly your voice is less now, you are struggling to give explanation how this disease coming ? no idea how to manage this case.

In the thyroid you are not even managing cases.But still you are not stopped selling the drugs you are asking to come for surgery.You are cheating a patient in the name of specialist . stop this.

You are retaining all the patient yourself just prescribing some medicine. Patient feel comfortable as for as we are taking some medicine.

A fake negligence law which is kept in forensic medicine ?

We have to give right treatment otherwise we have to refere the patient to right doctor. If you failing to do this called negligence, then you have to punished for that. This law is made dead by allopathy. It is not applied for any doctors. There is no single laws used for the basic consumer and health rights for patient in india.

you need to say this is not curative medicine this is just a management you need to meet some other alternate system to cure your disease. You are never going to say that. So, diseases will bulge patient end with complications and you will do surgery. Patient still believe you. This is the fate. I don't understand then what is the meaning of negligence ? we have to give some medicine that medicine will produce the disease but patient will keep consume the same medicine they will have complications we will prescribe same medicine for the complications finally patient will come for the organ failure then we will ask for again medicinal management but we will not have medicine for recover the organ failure then patient organ will faile then will do dialysis if then the organ failes we will do transplant . but you will read page by page what is negligence. If really the medical laws are working then you connot able to prescribe single paracetamol or painkillers or any allopathic drugs since all are fall under negligence. When I can cure without complications if you manage the case without medicine then your registration will be cancelled if the negligence act is working normally.

When a patient is getting liver failure or kidney failure by taking allopathic medicine why the patient has to bear the treatment cost. What kind of consumer or health rights patient getting in India ? How many pharma companies is paying their fault how many doctors repaying the money to the patient for their mistake? How many cases is filed against the doctors and pharma company in India, surpricingly too less since the doctos cheating and hiding all the truth they have many shields to escape and support pharma company by saying varies reason for development of liver failures and kidney failures.

1.food adultration

2.genetics

3.diabtes

4.hypertension.

They have many stories to tell to their patient to divert the cause from medicine to some thing else Indians are now watching genarations like they will watch tv and they will watch mobile and they watch computer they never a creater they never a analyst they never a reader. If you say something, they will belive if somebody else will say then they will belive that also, its like that. So Indian doctors utilizing this weaknes.

Indians will destroy the hospital and beat the doctors only when patient died (its happen in rare situation), for that they will go to the police station, but they will not do what they suppose to do. There are many instances where actually the doctors are attacked but they suppose not to do that since that is mostly emergency. But they have to file a complaint agains the chronic opd and acute ip admissions, they will not do that since they strongly belive that when criminalisam going on but attacking the doctor when really in-service duty so the patient in jeil doctor escapes from their mistake.

Allopathy doctors are having scientifically approved medicine ?   (scientifically ? not approving yourself in your circle ,with your group , the medicine is approved biologically or physiologically acceptable to the patient).

The pharma company or the pharmacology very clearly explains there are more then100 of side effects and advers reactions for 1 single medicine but when coming to clinical practice not even 1 % of cases recorded as specific medicine related complications so the pharma company is escapes from their mistakes and doctors also escape and keep prescribing the medicine.

The magic

You are not a magician to hide the skin disease. Ask them to wait or send the cases to homeopathy or learn homeopathy. Hiding the complaints from skin is not a treatment. Think logically and scientifically. Read carefully and give your valuable comments so that I have to understand what you understood with my writing. So, need to correct that until you are in right direction.

You are seeing a wart you are applying ointment or removing that. You are seeing psoriyasis prescribe steroid and anti-inflammatory hide it to under the skin. If you see the dermatitis prescribe anti allergic try to vanish. If you see any nodule operate and remove it. If you see lipoma operate and remove it. if you see any scabies apply ointment and hide it. What is pathology behind it why there is unnessory pathology in the skin what to do. All this case is incurable according to you. Psoriyasis is not curable , atopic dermatitis is not curable then why are you attempting to treat that. Why are you making drug addict ? . the aim of giving treatment to skin disease is hide it by doing so many external applications and varies surgical and cosmetic procedures.

By reading incurable disease few more extra years the incurable disease is become curable disease ? why I am using the word you are hiding since you know very well few doses of internal medicine is not working no idea what it is . most of the skin disease not fit into any classification not fit into a inflammation not fit into a auto immunity not fit into a tumor so you are trying varieys external application with aim of making skin clean. No idea who is your enemy. What exactly the problem. Dermatologist trained to hide the disease .try to learn to treat and cure not to hide it.

What are all the measures was taken to cure the disease ? is another aspect. Because there are many instances where allopathy knows the cause but still, they say no cure for that. Since they not having medicine to cure. In other situation medicines are there but it will not cure the disease since allopathic core concept is like that, they prescribe crude medicine opposite to disease nature so body will react to this medicine and increases the disease further worse, so need of medicine is increases when we use allopathy. [Discused in detail in the book]. Due to this reason allopathy medicine never cure . But it will give relief to the suffering.

ALLOPATHY DOCTORS ATTRACT THE PATIENT JUST GIVING RELIEF TO THE PATIENT , PATIENT EDU-

CATED BY DOCTORS AS IF THERE IS NO CURE AND THIS IS THE ONLY MEDICINE SO YOU HAVE TO TAKE THIS MEDICINE FOR LIFE LONG.This is something wrong. He found one disease and he try to give medicines,but it is not cured by allopathy medicine so he names that it is incurable.this is allopathy observation and only limited to allopathic medicine alone not applicable to other medicinal system. But he tries to impose this to all other field of medicine and educate the patient that disease is not curable. But any way he never refere the cases to others.

THE OBSTINACY which is followed by allopathy is - I WILL NEVER ACCEPT OTHERS VIEWS AND NEVER CONSIDER BASIC SCIENCE AND MEDICAL SCIENCE SO I WILL PRESCRIPE MEDICINE BLINDLY AND I OBSERVE, WHAT I DID, I CONCLUDE THAT IS THE TRUTH. IF I CONNOT DO ANYTHING THAT IS THE FINAL SO EVERYBODY HAS TO SAY THAT AND READ THAT.THE WHOLE WORLD FOLLOW THAT.I MAY DISCOVER THE CAUSE FOR DISEASE IN THE YEAR 3050 THAT'S SURE. but what is the point in discovering the cause , anyway I am not going to cure you. I will follow, what pharma industry says.

I WILL NOT CURE AND I WILL NOT SEND CASES TO ANY ONE AND I AM NOT BOTHERED ABOUT STATUS OF THE PATIENT. Till this obstinacy is not broken by allopathy you cannot get cure any patient, no eradication of any disease.

Suppose if the same case is handled by homeopathy then he will prescribe medicine similar to disease condition so they will get cured.

IT MEANS ALLOPATHY WILL NEVER CURE THEY CAN GIVE RELIEF UNTILL MEDICINE ACTION IS THERE.HOMEOPATHY WILL CURE SINCE THERE BASIC CONCEPT IS LIKE THAT. So, the cure is depending only upon the basic concept of treatment.

" *When the protective functions are stopped now, creating disease at present but allopathic texts saying that all the diseases are happen due to genetics (coming from genetics from many years befor). Allopathic text book beautifully hiding the truth,they say all the disease is caused by genetics so due to this misguiding , doctors are accepting this disease is incurable only. Beliving that the disease is something beyond our*

controle so its impossible to attempt cure and they beliving and searching cause from genetics "

5.B. MODE OF INTERUPTION

Mode of interruption of the inflammatory, immune system.

How the confused immune / inflammation disease occurs ?

1.Direct Prescription of medicine which stops the inflammation [anti inflammatory],steroids, antibiotics, anti allergics, anti pyretics.

The concept of anti inflammatory is totally wrong. Discussed already enough. Cauasing nearly 20-30 percent of disease and help in creating more number disease but ned more cells to produce the deep-seated worst disease that can be done maximum by external applications (they create nearly 70 and more percent of deep seated and more pathological diseases) discussed in detail below.

2. Trying to heal the skin disease or ulcers in a by external applications (medicated ointments, solutions, sprays, nebulizers, medicated soaps, medicated shampoos, washings) by allopathy and remaining all medical systems including homeopathy. If any one doing this will produce confused inflammation but the severity is too high in allopathy.

Negligible distraction is possible in other system and in homeopathy since the external preparations are not having any strong chemical enough to divert the inflammatory cells in other system.

(external application is may be necessary in some situation but anyway it will distract the inflammatory and immune cells).

Confused inflammation get attracted to environment and produce disease in the peripehery (skin) taking this disease to internal causes severe disease to internal parts. Most of the time skin diseases are having indurations and abrasions and ulcers so definetly there is regeneration and repairing of these ulcers and abarasion so more fibrin and elastin when you apply external application possibility of tumor and sclerosis and abnormal depositis all over the body is caused by external applications.

The skin infections usually give pus formation and serus or pus oozing and tenderness so patient will seek medical atension here doctors will prescribe the external applications and internal and external antibiotics. This is the worst mistake done by dermatologist and many allopathic phycisian. Now all type inflammation and immune cells is available will produce any disease to the humans.

1. Like antibody + germ complex, all type ac-

tivated blood cells allowed to roam and where ever they are going and produce the disease (neutrophil,macrophage,lympho-cytes and antibody).

2. The elastin and fibrin produce indurations and sclerosis and abnormal deposites all over the body.

3. Tumor due to regeneration of the body tis-sues where ever it goes.

4. All other diseases so simply will develop by this only one skin treatment.

a educated and qualified allopathy doctors can able to understand what is going on inside the skin while infection is happen. There is to kill the germ or destruct and clear the waste debris of the tissues by macrophage or neutrophil or NK cells or there is a regeneration of the tissues you are abruptly stopping and intruding with-out understanding anything about what happen-ing inside the body like a layman. So, you are given strong foundation to many deep-seated in-ternal diseases. Don't do this.

3. Try to removing the immune producing body parts like tonsil, appendicitis, thymus, spleen, liver, lymph nodes without curing and recovering the organs. So, low im-mune status favors poor recovery so that need to hospitalize and heavy drugs and medicines will produce confused in-flammation sure. Fall in sickness often. Written enough ex-planation regarding this in chapter 1 and 2.

4. Removing the inflamed organs or TUMOR AF-FECTED organs without treating and curing the disease of the organ. When removing the inflamed or tumor will help in more confused inflammation since the primary location or secondary locations are removed but source and cause

for the inflammation or tumor is not removed. So, that new tumor will starts in unwanted place may be the vital organ. If we remove the inflamed organ still the true inflammation and immunce cells produced is does not have targeted orgen so there is high possibility of self destruction by this true inflammation and immune organ in future.

5.Stoping / interrupting the feed back and reciprocating mechanism in the mid. like prescription of medicine for metabolic and hormonal dysfunctions like if the person prescribed thyroid tablets in the mid will break the feedback mechanisam. (discribbed in feed mechanisam disorders)

6.PREMATURE FORCIBLE MID INTERVENTION MEDICATION TERMINATE THE INFLAMMATION BY DOCTORS BEFORE THE BODY DECIDES SO THAT NERVE CONTROLED AND SUSPENDED FUNCTIONS HAS NOT BEEN RECOVERED.

7.Suppression of the abnormal discharge :

Suppression (stopping the normal or abnormal functions without treating it on right way) kind of hiding without clearing from the root cause.

Very worst complications will arise by doing this. Suppression like pus oozing from ear, leucorrhea, gonorrhea ,ophthalmic disease by local applications will lead to 2 major impacts one is the dead cells and damaged tissues recedes in side the circulation, newly forming pus cells do not have way to eliminate outside. This will go inside and act as foreign body and stuck somewhere inside the body and it will produce disease. Then the circulating distracted blood cells and regenerative and destructive tissues produce disease all over the body.

Abnormal leaucorrhea and veginal discharge is a sign of veginal or uterine disease when prescribing external

medicated solutions and antibiotic liquid or anti-inflammatory ointment causes the external open wounded part of
vegina or cervix is closed so there by the disease has to try to
go inside the uterus and produce life threatening complications.

Imagine you have ulcer which was got infected so
that there is a pus formation when you applying antibiotic
ointment upon the wound will close the possibility of eliminating wast and pus and all other product. Then where to
eliminate that pus . The idea of sealing the wound by other
bacterial entry is correct for that wash with saline and apply
plain sterile cotton cloth. The body has already sealed the
wound by crust formation. Still there is a pus indicating not
only yhe bacteria it also a dead tissue which is eliminated
out side. In this satge if you close that then the wound will
be closed without properly cleaning the dead tissues. All the
ointment what you are applying will confuse the accurasi
of the regeneration of new tissues in the ulcers so this led
to distraction of many fibrin and elastin and other regenerative tissues causes tumor and indurations and deposition
of abnormal material all over the body. A tiny mistake in
the preventing sepsis causes heavy burden to the patient. A
worst gift from allopathy to his patient those who follow
all the advice of the doctors are t great risk of developing
tumor and sclerosis of the soft tissues and induraions.This
is the acute injury related ulcer. But the compliacations are
worst if you do this to chonic ulcers related with confused
inflammation. yes, the ulcer is developed due to confused
inflammation it means already this is secondary disease if
you through inside this ulcer will if it goes inside then sure
destructive disease of the colon and rapid destruction of the
parenchyma of the deepest organs.

Then he will do the surgery of the diseased part
send to the lab and found there is a neutrophil,macrophage
cell ,lymphocytes over here and there is an antigen anti-

body complex over here and then he will confuse how this cell came here and why ? will not consider he only did that. When the body tried to pour the garbage waste product to out side doctors take lots effort to take them inside patient body will give raise lot many disorders.

Draining the pus is not contra indicated but applying local dressing to that drained abscess is hyper foolishness due to there is a bacterial entry so that inflammation and pus discharge to make patient satisfaction and feel that arresting pus discharge is a treatment , doctors applying local anti-inflammatory ,it may cause inward intrusion of the waste cells and dead cells and it will greatly disturb the inflammation process so that confused inflammation will arises.

Trying to suppress the pus discharge from the vegina / penis by applying external applications and ointments makes life long chronic confused inflammation disease in the genital organs and urinary tract and pelvis.

Trying to suppress ear discharge causes many inner ear and brain disorders in future. applying ear drops will produce this impact.

Trying to suppress nasal discharge by nasal inhalers makes speedy formation of the confused inflammation to whole of the upper and lower respiratory chronic confused inflammation disorders.

In simple the highest possible way to create antibody, antigen complex ,confused inflammation, tumor possibility, allowing dead cells and inflammatory waste cells into the circulation is more powerful in external applications and stopping abnormal discharge then oral and iv medications.

Pus discharge or inflammatory or infectious oozing will be followed by wound healing or repairing the inflammatory /infectious site, so possibility of rich in gelatin, fibrous tissues as well as lots of nerve stimulus to repair the broken blood vassals as well as damaged tissues all the inflammatory signals will be collapsed by external applications which is used to stop the abnormal discharge.

Ihave found exact match of many disease after using anti inflammatory and anti allergics but this will cause only few inflammation disease but there is no much possibility to induce a tumor and less possibility of immune complex distraction and lymphocyte and macrophage activation all are question mark it means most of the series and complicated disease are happening more then just anti inflammation but how immunity is getting distracted there is no medicine is invented to interfere immunity steroid actually many not allow to produce immune cells even that will also never distract the iimune complex never able to produce tumor then who is the cause for all this remaining disease so I am fed up and then only I was re analysed and found externala applications and skin disease treatment sure will possibly produce remaining disease like tumor and indurations and sclerosis and all other disease and more or less frame by frame shot in the movie each time at what time you are using the external application will exactly produce the disease (that is described in the 7 th chapeter) suppose if you use the external applications immdiatly after injury then bleeding disorder will affected so you will have the possibility of blleding disease if you apply oinment or external applications during the time of wound closing almost going to heal then possibility of tumor will come. Why I am explaining this story is be carefull when prescribing external application this is very worst and very dangerus then anti pyretic and anti allergic. All the external applications has great power to distract inflammation and immunity more powerfully. External applications which include all ointments all lotions and all the eye and ear and nose drops and inhelers.

8. Normal but taking medications for more healthy

The current trend is many people are scared of future disease so there are many commercial preparations of allopathy and herbal product for preventing disease (But this medicine never prevents any disease). Cholestrol prevention and reducing, skin glowing, sugar reducing herbals and allopathic medicines. Patient is not having any complaints in sexual problems but need to have extra sexual power so trying to take many medicines for improve the sexual power more the urban and moderd city more the sales of this drugs there was a time herbs was used for this purpose but now a days all allopathy pharma company almost fully replaced all herbs into allopathy drugs for increasing male sexual power. Unnessory medications but damges liver and kidney and heart is increasing now a days. Ever youth formula there are concept of young look , people like to stay young so taking medicine for preventing aging , anti aging creams and medications. Most of the time patient hide this story to the doctor not purposefully but think that never cause any harm and they are not having any illness just took medicine for better health. But this is not true these medicines create many complications.

Cosmetic surgery a person absolutely not having any illness but doing surgery for looking buety is the trend now. Any surgery and anesthesia and pre and post medications like anti inflammatory and anti biotics have its own side effects. So better not to damage your body with kniff keep away from surgens kniff. Many tooth alignment prosthetics gives tha possibility of germ multiplications inside the mouth and cleaning the tooth and many dental related procedures like removing the stain in the tooth and all are unnessary post antibotics and anti inflammatory will spoil the health and give the way to many disease. Men and women are equally exposing such dental buety prsthetics and cleaning and procedures.

(The surgery for cleft palate never considered as a cosmetic surgery. But is advertised as acosmetic surgery government has to allocate a funcd for doing cleft palate surgery. Really the sufferer will loss the normal human facial normal looking and find difficulty in speech and masticating the food and swallowing. All the insurance company has to pay the money for doing this surgery. It should not be kept under exclusion). A person doing surgery for reducing the handihapped is not considered as cosmetic surgery insurance department has to pay the money especially more the handicapped and more the benefit to improve the normal from handicapped better need to be paid from insurance. Insurance can deni if the surgery never going to help the patient – the surgen role is very importand in accident and rehabilation related with birth anomaly and accident no one is replace his service my support always goes in this aspect, but be away from phycisian zone don't try to remove the organs without ayush phycision opinion before removing any organ especially other then accident)

9. not just cosmetic its importand disease.

As soon as we distract the confused inflammation immediately those confused inflammation will give raise to minor ailment like pimples and dandruff and hair loss so this is a early open warning sign we can easily see and luckily patient now a days seeking immediate treatment. So, removing confused inflammation will prevent major disease in future.

Treating hair loss, skin discoloration and other minor ailments looking like cosmetic ailment but they are actually reflecting confused inflammation so it needs proper treatment to eliminate the confused inflammation so that the affected person will be prevented so many diseases in future. not only that. White hair, hair loss, dandruff everything is happen not just aging or a scattered inflammation (confused) is the cause for that. When attempt to treat that condition may shift the inflammation to other vital organs and create the complaints over there. AIMING TO CLEAR THE CONFUSED INFLAMMATION FROM THE BODY IS THE RIGHT ANSWERE. This is again going towards like looking like minor trival ailments and most top cosmetic disease but it is a confused inflammation disorder. At present there are many more spa and hair specialiast and non medical professions are treating this disease since there is great marketing trichology clinics are so famous in the urban locality creating many fold suppression like many medicated shampoo and many herbal intake and so many allopathic remedies for treating skin and hair in the scalp and face altogether heavy and many fold suppression definetly lead on to more psychological and brain related disease.

10. Suppression of natural discharges

The word suppression often used in the homeopaths then rest of doctors. but basically, this word is common word for all doctors. Just preventing and blocking the natural elimination like perspiration, stool, urine , menses ,emotion ,,,,,,, etc.

Suppress the natural discharge like perspiration, menses happen in some clinical practice or some times patient himself do this by some medicated powders and tablets strongly contra indicated. Inducing abortion has the side effects. All the hormones which is ready for pregnancy is continuing to the women but we terminated the pregnancy?

Patient feel uncomfortable when they have excess perspiration in hands and soles so it is mandatory to identify the cause and solve that. Suppression may lead to diseases. doing surgery like innervations is hyper foolishness and unnecessary.

When coming to homeopathy they should also don't attempt to treat as a single symptom trace the history and treat in general. Using deodorant for offensive perspiration is superficial this is advisable but applying medicines or medicated powders in the axilla or genitals will cause suppression of the sweats lead to some other unwanted diseases like itchy papules and adenitis, retention cyst ,,,etc.

This in turn become source of infections if it is long running.

Suppressing menses by giving hormonal pills makes many diseases. How ? and why ? from starting of the ovulation and menses and cessation of menses or continuing as pregnancy everything under control of hormones all this function sequentially maintained by pituitary-adrenal-ovarian axis. when we try to solve the complaints without knowing this make the disease .it means the body get confused or body natural functions interrupted so that it may not do their actions again so hormonal disturbance will happen.

Similarly bringing menses by prescribing hormonal pills give raise to diseases.Prescribing medicines for some other ailment but it causes suppression of sweat may give raise to disorder in the skin.

Strong medicated shampoo or oil to scalp will cause so many diseases due to interruption in the natural perspiration and oil glands and take the confused inflammation cells in the scalp to other parts.

Applying chemical mosquito killing oil upon the skin is not good the skin will absorb the toxin in the mosquito liquid.

Trying to stop the excess oiliness in the face by medicated ointments or powders in the similar way trying to solve the dryness by medicated oils or ointments contra indicated. IN HOMEOPATHY THIS TAKEN ALONG WITH GENRAL COMPLAINTS AND TRYING TO RECOVER BRING THE NORMAL FUNCTION OF SWEAT AND OILY GLANDS. Either abnormal excess functions of the sweat glands or under functions of the sweat glands has to be treated properly then giving some external applications.

Applying cosmetic paste and powders which prevent the natural functions of sweat and oily glands will make the complaints. When patient having odor in the sweat then they take medicine to stop sweat (hear using non irritating deodorant in the shirt is enough.)

Suppressing natural desires like hunger, sex, sleep deprivation causes diseases. similarly, too much of the same is causes ailments. Trying to take medicine for improving or decreesing of the above cause's illness (when it is normal). means even though normal patient or attender thinking it is less so they taking medicine causes illness.

Trying to take vitamins, minerals more then requirement causes illness similarly deficiency will cause ailments. Correction and advise of proper diet is the first choice. there are many confused inflammation disorders mimic like vitamin and mineral deficiency and again that will also give some results when taking supplements but it is important to assess the real deficiency from confused inflammation, if it is confused inflammation related then need a treatment.

Vitamin deficiency and mineral deficiency again happen due to confused inflammation of colon and intestine so that absorption is hindered need proper treatment for confused inflammation. anyway, prescribing vitamin and mineral orally will be safe then iv transfusion.

Trying to gain the weight or loss the weight by forceful medication causes ailments (The primary aim is treating the cause) do regular exercise to maintain your weight. This is often missed in the regular past history of the patient since patient think that is their regular activity not fall under any disease and treatment. Ask a specific question to the patient, are you under any weight reducing plan ?. For reducing weight there are many clinics and many herbs patient using to loss weight. This is ideally not good.

This tiny dysfunction may not go to cause any series illness .But this disruption allows the weakness of the particular part either they stop functions and produce disease or sub normal functions allow the possibility of the disease like that.

Taking any medicine by anypathy just for improving general health status is contra indicated unless otherwise there is a clear-cut indication.[homeopathy never encourages that].

6.CAUSE AND EFFECT

C onfused inflammation is not like diseases produced by infections. They produce damage. The difference is here the healing power distracted to produce sickness and destruction. This is something new , we have to understa nd this to treat that, present we read the pathological changes and trying to treat that pathological changes homeopathy largely ignores this pathological change but consider the cause. ALLMOST ALL THE DISEASES ARE PRODUCED BY THIS CONFUSED INFLAMMATION ALONE. If this confused inflammation is prevented then there is no disease at all. Again, the confused inflammation is produced by strong allopathic medicine. as for as allopathic medicine is there there is large number of diseases will be produced every day. So, that ban allopathic pharmacology and ask them to use any other scientifically accepted medicine.

CONSIDER THE CAUSE IGNORE/GIVE LESS IMPORTAND TO THE EFFECT [homeopathy] , CONSIDER THE EFFECT IGNORE THE CAUSE [ALOPATHY] CONSEQUNCE SINCE THE CAUSE IS IGNORED IT WILL KEEP PRODUCE THE DISEASE ONE AFTER ANOTHER AND MAINTAIN THE

DISEASE TO RUN LIFE LONG IS THE REASON BEHIND WHY DISEASES REMAIN LONGER PERIOD. When we find the cause and set right the cause then body will heal the effect. Actually, speaking there is no medicines to recover the effect. But in real understanding why we need medicine when everything readily available within body. Just remove the cause and just regulate the altered system to do their work.

This is the important aspects of 2 school of people. But it is not simple stand point just read we have to discuss this in depth. Whatever it may be the cause we no need to worry just solve some major discomfort to the patient and aim to discover the medicine for the effect total and mass ignorance of the cause is the key point of the allopathy. Since the cause is remain still will keep produce the disease.

If they spend bit more time to find the cause they may be find the treatment so effective and their aspect must be preventive.

Why surgery is occupying most of the allopathy treatment ? ,their aim is to harvest the yield not preventing the disease, seed to implant within the body. The surgery often says final part of the treatment it actually announces the world that the doctors are failed to recover the person.

No one will study and spend their life to fail, to participate loser side but allopathy does this because money decides everything, failing makes more money. The top most their fundamental take them to this level its highest foolishness but thye feel proud to be a surgeon [the exception is emergency]. they start reading anatomy as a basic then again studying disease anatomy so they finally decide remove the diseased body parts [surgery] as a treatment choice. Then definitely you will choose the knife you will not use your brain for treatment.

The judgment is considering the cause don't give too much importance to effect. Giving importance to effect is taking you to more particular then considering general view. Without our conscious we focus and search cause within the particular locality. Our medicines and directions always have to work longer time to harvest rather then quick short relief.

We can simply say a tiny inflammation cells distracted from throat can make any changes anywhere within body.so this is the cause, we should not allow this to roam but the effect is pathological changes which was made by the inflammation cells.alopathy spends their whole life to name the effect and more focus upon the effect they never considered about the cause initially their ignorance due to the cause is not logically fit into the category of disease cause which was identified till date, but over the period of they stopped searching the cause itself.

Confused inflammation cells present in the particular patient decide the next disease example :

> The available confused inflammation able to produce congestive stage it will produce vasodilatation and heavy congestion after sun exposure [acne rosacea] or after expose to heavy cold in winter [psoriasis].

> if the available confused inflammation is fibroblast and wound healing cells, it may produce tumor or tumor like pathological changes and again it may produce the same changes anywhere in the body it could be lung or kidney or liver or brain or hands or legs.

The highest easiest way is to finding the cause and removing it, then trying to treat pathological changes. Since disease producing agent is our own body cells we know very well their characters so it is simple to withdraw the cells and we can prevent the disease before it makes the disease then why we are going to wait till its going to make irreversible pathological changes why we are going to take surgery. The surgery department is largly depand upon the effect.

A cause [confused inflammation] takes few months to many years to produce severe pathological changes. It gives lots of time to develop fully matured disease so, we can prevent the disease.

THE TOP MOST CAUSE FOR ALL THE DISEASE IS STOPPING THE INFLAMMATION AND IMMUNITY AND DISTRACTING THE WOUND HEALING IN THE NAME OF EXTERNAL APPLICATION STOP THIS UNSCIENTIFIC TREATMENT PREVENT CHANCE FOR MAKING NEW DISEASE ALLOW THE PERSONS LIVING HEALTHILY DON'T PRODUCE DISEASE DON'T ACT LIKE YOU ARE SAVING THE LIFE.YOU ARE CREATING AND YOU ARE STRUGGLING IN GIVE CURE.YOU ARE NO MORE ALLOWED TO DO THIS NONSENSE IN THE NAME OF DOCTOR.

Otherwise you decide what can be done in this situation. We will listen that and will follow. Like prescription of antipyretic to stop the natural cure and will get the sickness and then we will suffer then again will take antipyretic and steroids and anti-allergic again we will have lots of new disease and we will take the medicine for that lets this cycle continue the problem is not ended here read the whole text what are all the confused collapse you made here and decide at last don't go for haste judgment.

GIVE IMPORTANCE TO CAUSE, THE CAUSE OF ALL THE DISEASE IS YOUR MEDICINE SO REMOVE THE CAUSE. PEOPLE WILL BE SAFE.Dont say you are researching and finding the remedy for cancer or HIV. No need of any New for cure liver damage or no need to invent some new approach to organ transplant. STOP YOUR MEDICINE EVERYHING WILL BE ALRIGHT. No need to invent or do research on the effect of the disease, remove the cause. Remove the confused inflammation this is the cause and remove the allopathic remedy which causing that.

The inflammation and immunity are the best gifted power of human being. We should not afraid of inflammation and immunity, the allergy, auto immunity, self destruction all is happened due to interference with medicine and importantly induced by prescription of allopathy medicines [IATROGENIC] and interruption of the inflammation, so allow the inflammation and immunity to continue their work don't interfere because interfering causes the allergy , auto immunity ,and lots of disease. Be very clear inflammation (good protection) to confused inflammation (bad destructive).

A writer has to read his article once and twice that aim of the text is completed or not and again he makes sure that he is not misguiding or diverting the realism into something else then what needed.

since the inflammation and immunity chapters in the textbook of physiology and pathology not appreciated the excellent function of the body and they directly blame the inflammation is not good for health, now and then they come to the conclusion that auto immune disease and self destruction and enormous explanation of the self destructions in great depth (actually speaking the auto immunity is the rare part of the inflammation and immunity) but this is occupy maximum portion of the immunology and inflammation so when anyone [student or doctor] reading this chapters will definitely think that allowing inflammation/immunity will cause danger is not something strange , so an allopath will take anti inflammatory and steroid for controlling this effect .so this in turn really increases the immune disorder so now rare immune disorders is become more immune disorder due to wrong impressions.

All hypersensitive disease from type I to type IV is developed due to continues strong anti inflammatory and steroid and antipyretics and anti allergies not because of any inborn error [it is highly negligible] but I am seeing almost maximum patient is coming with hypersensitive disorders. This happened because doctors are misguided by medical texts.

rarely accepting the immunity saves ,very rarely in the viral fevers they mentioned like it's a self-limiting, disease will heal themselves due to immunity so its not self limiting its **self curing power**.

THE TEXT BOOK OF PHYSIOLOGY,PATHOLOGY AND GENERAL MEDICINE HAS TO WRITE IN SUCH WAY WHERE TO INTERFERE WHERE TO KEEP QUIT AND EXPLAIN WHAT IS RIGHT CHOICE HERE [SO IT WILL HAVE AN IMPACT TO A DOCTOR HE HAS TO PRESCRIBE LESS AND INVENT MORE FOR CONVINIANT AND RIGHT PRESCRIPTION].IF AT ALL THE HYPERSENSITIVE DISEASE IS MAKING GREAT TROUBLE,CORRECTING THE HYPERSENTIVE TO NORMOSENTIVE IS THE RIGHT ANSWERE.DISTRACTING, DIVERTING, COLLAPSING OR TOTTALLY MAKING ABSENT OF THE inflammation / IMMUNE SYSTEM IS NOT A EDUCATED MAN WORK , it is absolutely criminal treatment since it makes life long danger to the patient.

7.CONSEQUENCES OF INTERRUPTION OF INFLAMMATION.

Are you going to treat patient ? yes, ok then treat the disease, don't stop the physiological treatment process in the name of treatment. Treat the disease don't stop the normal functions. Keep this in your mind. Recover the repaired system. Don't make the healthy system into collapsed system. So first define and differentiate the disease and healthy function.

Allopathic medicine having intension to stop the healthy protective function they say that is the treatment. the patient get sickness due to the treatment. So the patient get sickness due to the treatment but there is no treatment for the sickness, he created. They never understand the disease arising because of their treatment. So, they keep all the disease as unknown etiology.

allopathy understanding about the disease makes

the confusion about the treatment, we understand that all the suffering (pain, fever during inflammation) is the disease, so doctors decide to relive the sufferings, but not worried about consequences.

Not all DIS EASE (DISCOMFORT) demanding medicine, actually collapsed system demanding correction. DIS EASE [discomfort] may happen in healthy physiological process also, DIS EASE will be there in protecting febrile condition, DIS EASE happen in healthy physiological function like vomiting ,cough, Rhinitis so dis ease not demanding medicines.

Bear a discomfort, it leaves you soon or choose the medicine which give the comfort without stopping natural protective action. Homeopathy is the best medicine which relive the suffering without stopping the natural process like fever, running nose, cold, head ache, vomiting and diarrhea ,,,, etc. this is the very common complaints we are addicted to take allopathic medicine which causes severe disease .

BUT DIS EASE CONTINUING UNUSUALLY LONGER TIME, DIS EASE NOT KILLING THE GERMS, DIS EASE NOT ELIMINATING THE POISON , DIS EASE NOT CURING THE PERSON, DIS EASE NOT HAVING THE PURPOSE IS NEED TO BE IDENTIFIED AND CORRECTED. SO, MAKE THE CORRECTION MAKE ALTERED SYTEM INTO RIGHT SYTEM. IT MEANS WE NO NEED TO BEAR DIS EASE OR DIS COMFORT WHEN THIS HAPPEN FOR HELP US BUT IF IT IS NOT GOING TO HELP US ITS SPOILING THEN ? WE HAVE TO ELIMINATE THAT AND RECOVER THE SYSTEM.

Unfortunately, allopathy not having any such medicine to recover the spoiled system.

They want that to happen they expect it must damage further then we will remove it finally (surgery) or we prescribe something to satisfy patient but the disease matures inside then we will call for organ transplant is the fundamental of allopathy. THEY NEVER TRY TO CURE ANY DISEASE.

EDUCATE THE SOCIETY TO BEAR THE DIS EASE IF THE DIS EASE IS PRODUCED BY HEALTHY SYSTEM AND FIGHING AGAINST THE ENEMY. *But allopathy asks the patient to bear the disease only if they spoil it and produce severe disease, they ask you to bear the disease lifelong no single day. Each and every system they keep lots of incurable disease everything you have to bear no medicine no cure.*

Accept the fault and get ready for recover the patient, open your eye see how many suffering individuals you are created. Homeopathy is not only for heomeopath, allopathy is not made for allopathy doctors so don't hesitate to choose right system to give cure. A doctor duty is giving the cure , don't make the sickness any more.

Entire general medicine text and all other specialty medicine text books fully discussed only about this immunity and inflammatory diseases . All the diseases happen directly, indirectly related with inflammation and immunity interrupted consequences. He will read page by page many numbers of disease in different text as pathology, general medicine and systemic medicines and specialty medicines, regional medicine all disease he only made it he reads many texts. He worried about complications and how the people are getting this many numbers of diseases. He forgot that he did one small change in the system that is order to disorder, organized good curing power to disorganized destruction power. He did extremely mild changes without knowing the consequences, the universe crying for that. he does not realize that even now is good treatment. Diseases, everywhere disease, every person in the world is having fear of disease. For giving treatment so many doctors, they prescribe again illogically and produce many diseases . Its, happen endless disease cycle.

So many researches so many useless medicine discoveries everything is for controlling this collapsed inflammation. But he was made it from just 1 week or 10 days of allopathic medicines. It is enough to collapse the automatic self-curing power, afterwards the body will start disobey it will become the room for multiple germs. Then the patient will fall many illnesses one after another with different names, endless.

The doctors of different school attempt to solve it or cure it again life long since the inflammation and immune system is repaired the disease may mimic like disappear but comes in different organs or body due to inflammation process is remain repaired. All one thing you have to do is repair the inflammation or immune system [homeopathy has the medicine at present] then remaining thinks body will take care.

The pathology could be beginning in many ways, as for as body take care of self curing it is fall under physiology. When this self curing is not working then pathology starts.

The confused inflammation produce disease by interacting with varies environmental stimuli and day to day activity.

•   Either due to uninterrupted dumping of chemicals or blood cells of inflammation produce the new disease. [histamine, cyclooxygenase, etc.].

•   Distracted orders from brain to carry out inflammation has not been withdrawn due to interruption with medicine. so that work is completed by doctors but feedback not received by body. So, there by inflammation is remain incomplete will produce number diseases.

•   Due to non-clearance of the inflammatory waste cells and immune complex this was produced, dead tissues as result of interruption of the inflammation this waste products not cleared so many micro vasculatures blocked and creating disease, they deposit and stuck in the within the organ and damage produce the disease.

Now we will see what will happen if the inflammation interrupted just immediately after beginning:

The given example is too less , I am giving only major interruption and their consequences. because the cause for all the disease is there within the inflammation and immunity itself, when we do complete micro and macro analysis of inflammation we will surprise from where disease originates.

I am finding out more and more diseases in relation with inflammation like treasure. suppose if you stuck up and clueless to find the cause of disease read inflammation, immunity chapter thoroughly you will get the idea how the disease originates.

Applying varies external applications produce number of varieties of confused inflammation cells then rest of the procedure , it   will produce many diseases to the humans.

From entry of germs inside to end with complete recovery there are many chemicals and inflammation, immune cells involved so if you know all of them well then it is easy to understand where we stopped inflammation what are all the chemicals and cells are involved in that particular functions then we conclude what kind of disease we can observe in future or we can judge the disease by understanding the present pathology and pathophysiology to past inflammation interruption.

Confused inflammation arises due to stopping the

normal inflammation and immunity so in this chapters (7) explains how confused inflammation formed when we interrupt the inflammation in different stages of inflammation and immunity.

All this 7 th chapters and its sub headings fall under new pathology nothing is old all is based on new discovery.this 7th chapter is replacing the general pathology of old pathology textbook.

7.A.INFLAMMATION INTERRUPTED AT THE BEGINNING.

• Diseases with excessive neutrophil, eosinophil but without infection.

• Diseases due to histamine and leukotrienes and other chemicals which is Involved in the early stage of inflammation.

• Diseases due to excess prostaglandins and other consequences of interference in cyclooxygenase metabolism.

• Diseases due to bleeding disorders and clotting disorders without obvious cause.

• Vaso constriction and vaso dilatation diseases.

All this disease happens when we interrupt the inflammation or wound healing in the early stage.

When the injuries agents [chemical or germs] enter

inside the body then the inflammation begins by moving the basophil and must cells near the noxious agents. Now it liberates histamine, bradykinin, serotonin (chemotactic). If we prescribe **anti histamine**, it will block the histamine sensor .The histamine has been blocked ,but not removed. So, there by this

histamine not allowed to work, inflammation is not completed .but the germs still present will attract the eosinophil must cells it will again release the histamine if we continue taking anti allergic for few days the eosinophil will be dumped in the site and excess accumulation histamine will be there it spreads all over the skin, nasal cavity and bronchus and including lungs and skin near the nose and ready for life long respiratory disease and eosinophil dominant disorders like asthma ,allergy , skin diseases , hyper activity, sleeplessness etc.

it will also make the local disease into systemic disease since widespread histamine now signals to the inflammation process.so the local disease now become systemic disorder.

but **anti-inflammatory** block the whole inflammation process by preventing cyclooxygenase conversion into prostaglandin so that no inflammation at all. This cyclooxygenase again and again formed due to injury in the tissues happened by the germs but anti-inflammatory prevent the cyclooxygenase to prostaglandin so that excess accumulation of this chemical will be circulated all over the body this histamine and cyclooxygenase will be hyper active since we have enough chemical in the body without any injury and germs so in future if you sitting long time you will have the pain cause now the readymade cyclooxygenase easily converted into prostaglandin and produce the back pain. You go to the sun head ache will come if you drink cold then cold will come because you have readymade Histamine. This is the way the diseases are produced.

Basic body mechanism is we have to have cut injury or fall and erosion then only inflammation starts. similarly, the inflammation has to start only after any germs entry any virus or bacteria enter inside the body then the disease starts by step by step by process but we have already enough number of readymade inflammatory chemicals more than sufficient, here we are not only have inflammation it will make a destructive violent inflammation, this is called HYPERSENSITIVITY.

But allopathy doctors read hypersensitivity in different way it means once the body is undergoes inflammation everything is going normal but the second time the inflammation happen violently, dangerously ? because they will give so many story like complement fixing to IGE or this on that, but they never mention any single word that we prescribed first some medicine that medicine stopped that that's why the hypersensitivity we are facing when enemy is entering second time. They satisfy themselves prescribing steroid is the only choice for handling this hypersensitivity. It is better to manage the hypersensitivity in an emergency with steroid but what is the cure for this hypersensitivity because it is not one time process it may not go once if it is formed. The hypersensitivity nature of the human inflammation and immune system is curable and revert to normal by proper employment of homeopathy medicine.

May be the bacteria or virus killed by immune system by producing antibody or the germs multiply inside the body without any resistance will produce disease but without any fever or pain or malaise since we stopped all by anti histamine and anti inflammatory.

The chemo tactic chemicals [histamine] spread all

over the body invites the body to send neutrophil / monocytes so that after we stop anti histamine and anti pyretic then all inflammation process but vigorously since the
dumped eosinophil invite massive neutrophil this happen
rarely. Mostly the inflammation process is abolished and
excess histamine will roam in the circulation - confused inflammatory chemicals. But this chemical when come in contact with any minimal changes then it identifies that as an
enemy then initiate the pseudo [chronic inflammation].

Usually a germ entry will initiate inflammation
by releasing chemo tactic chemicals, but here chemotactic chemicals (HISTAMINE) already there abundant all over
the body especially within the respiratory tract. If any new
germ or noxious agents entered, then inflammation begins
so abrupt and violent like sneezes or running nose or
itching or heavy wheezing immediately after entering the
germs or any irritating agents (TYPE-1 HYPERSENSITIVE
REACTION). Due to heavy histamine stimulation massive
neutrophil will come and initiate inflammation. usually
histamine helps in choosing the site of germs to engulf but
here the histamine is there almost all over the respiratory
tract and even to the skin so the inflammation is starts all
over the respiratory tract and all over the skin (where ever
histamine is there). So severe itchy dermatitis with worst
asthma is started now (atopic asthma/dermatitis).anaphy-
laxis.

(But what allopath text says about type 1 hypersensitivity the mast cells and basophils play an exceedingly
important role in some types of allergic reactions because
the type of antibody that causes allergic reactions. the
immunoglobulin E (IgE) type, has a special propensity to become attached to mast cells and basophils. Then, when the
specific antigen for the specific IgE antibody subsequently
reacts with the antibody, the resulting attachment of antigen to antibody causes the mast cell or basophil to rupture

and release exceedingly large quantities of *histamine, brady-kinin , serotonin , heparin, slow-reacting substance of anaphylaxis,* and a number of *lysosomal enzymes* —

a LOVELY STORY BETTER SCREEN PLAY NO ONE CAN WRITE SUCH A WONDERFUL STORY but story missed Villon role anti histamine and anti-inflammatory in this, OK WE WILL WRIGHT A ANOTHER GOOD STORY AND WILL GIVE A CHANCE FOR THEM.

The monocytes and esonophil not releasing the histamine and serotonine and other chemokines due to IGE presence they all are already present in the circulation due to prescription of the anti histamine so this proinflammatory chemicals triggered by cold air and so they now accentuate and induce the inflammation. IgE also present in the circulation they come and join to this inflammation.

Here the histamine and pro inflammatory chemicals spreads across the respiratory tract and skin misguide the real neutrophil to attack the entire respiratory tract and skin but actually there is no germs or noxious agents present in those site [Auto Inflammation].

Here after the histamine where ever sticks and touches, when it will react to that chemical products and react to sun, cold, pressure, new bacteria and virus, ornaments, foods and send the signals to deliver neutrophil and initiate confused inflammation without any real antigen.

Due to interruptions many cells and chemicals of inflammation is there in the body which is I named it CONFUSED INFLAMMATORY CELLS / IMMUNE CELLS Which makes so many diseases alone or in combination with new inflammation process.

Wound healing distracted in the early stage causes receding of the bleeding and clotting factors inside the circulation and vasoconstrictive and vaso dialting factors also enters inside the circulation these chemicals get accentuated and produce the internal bleeding or clotting or vaso-constriction or dialatation etc

7.B. EFFUSIVE DISORDERS

DISTRACTING THE INFLAMMATION AT THE TIME OF EFFUSION.

E very inflammation will follow order like pain, redness, fever and swelling of the affected parts. The
swelling is happening due to more fluid accumulation with collection of fighting cells.

Here actually the blood vassals are broken and
allowed to leak more amount of serous fluid to the extra-
cellular space causing swelling. When you arresting this inflammation by applying external medications in the skin or
in the mucus membrane will lead on to inward receding of
the active inflammatory chemicals and inflammatory cells
involved in this stage so that we feel happy that we stopped
inflammation. But hereafter if the inflammation is starts

then the effusion will be marked.

We helped to spray the confused inflammation cells which is involved in the inflammation.

This chemical sprayed all over the body produce diseases with marked exudation with serous effusion or diseases with blisters formation, excess edema without kidney, cardiac or liver involvement and without disorder in the fluid balance.it means a swelling or edema is a confused inflammation irrespective of pitting or non pitting.

It is not because there is an imbalance in the secretion and absorption in the cavities.

- weeping eczema,
- pemphigus diseases
- effusion within the plural cavity and pericardial cavity and peritoneal cavity.
- meningeal effusion is enhanced. Hydrocephalus.
- Hydrocele (inflammatory origin).
- Elephantiasis.
- Swollen joint space.
- Severe dengue
- Septicemia related inflammation changes within the human body is similar to this effusive stage lead on to severe damage in the blood vessels so lead on to ascites , plural effusion, effusion into the brain, etc in most of the cases the condition improves in many situation so patient will improve but in many condition patient will die ,since the effusion is not reabsorbed. (allopathic doctors believe that it happens due to cytokine storm).

(this is not related with secondary edema due to liver failure or congestive cardiac failure. Again, the body will not recall the effusion mostly need homeopathic medicine or surgery need to remove the effusion).

The problem with this abnormal effusion is patient will experience only effusion that will going to stay life long. A normal inflammation related effusive fluid and material will be reabsorbed so the swelling of inflammation parts will move to next stage, but here swelling will remain same or swelling will be absorbed partially or swelling re absorbed but unusually late. Patient may feel satisfied since his swelling is subsided but a physician has to observe this slow and tardy recovery and has to solve this before another effusive disease happen.

If the effusion is happening along with inflammation or infections, we can easily trace the effusion is related with inflammation but most of the time the effusion alone will happen ,so the doctors does not have possibility to suspect this effusion as a part of inflammation so consider this is as a new disease. most of the confused inflammation will produce disease like that but most of effusive disease happen along with inflammation or in connection with inflammation.

Effusion and septicemia

Broken blood vessals and effusion is paly import-and role septicemia. Yes, every infection if it is going to be a genaralised septecemic conditions then the blood vessals all over the body including lungs and heart and brain is broken and causing fluid leaking into the lungs and kidney and liver exatra. Eventually the blood volume is too low so the bp is again low. Since the low bp and low blood volume causes significant reduction oxygen and nutrition supply to the brain,kidney and heart so this will lead on to a great emergency.

In one hand the blood vessals broken and causes leaking of the blood or plasma fluid into the heart and brain and liver. In other hand fresh fluid has to pass through this major organ is too less due to low bp and plasma leakage so over a period of time the organs functions slowly detoriarate and causes permanent organ failure. But many patients recover despite this effusion. This is achived by effusion stage followed by recovery stage of our vital power (our body). The septecemia causes great many numbers of death rate.

We can prevent this septecemic state by preventing the confused inflammation. yes this excess blood vessal destroying pro and inflammatory chemicals and complement and cytokines produce sever damage so the effucion stage is prolonged and unusual causes organ failure and death. If we not interfere in the effusion stage of any inflammation then there is no possibility of septecemia in the patient. Septecemia it does not mean you are dead by a bacteria it is caused by excess destruction of blood vessal but it just triggered by bacteria and virus. Even though the excess germs is there in the blood the way to control in other meadiam can be easily kill the germs and effusion can be done minimum not excess and unusual, like upto death this is not a function of inflammation and immunity this is pure confused inflammation cytokines and compliments and other inflammatory chemicals jointly makes this life threatening complications. Globally many crores of the people die because of the septecemia. We can prevent just keepin our hand quit.

(dengue,ebola,typhoid,sars (corana). Allmost all the virus and bacteria can go to the septecemia but with ex-

cess confused inflammation presence need to induce septecemic death and orgon failure).

7. C.
IMMUNOGLOBULIN DISORDERS

Suppose if the inflammation is interrupted when about to deliver the IMMUNOGLOBULINS (By antibiotics):

The immunoglobulins will come to circulation but now they don't have any bacteria all destroyed by antibiotics but not cleared from the circulation . This immune cell is not having work but they are special cells prepared to destroy that virus or bacteria's but the bacteria's killed by antibiotic. So, these immunoglobulins will circulate within the body and throughout the life and will produce auto immune diseases.

Possibility 1 : now anti body inside the circulation but there is no bacteria, So the anti - body (immunoglobulins) will recognize the antigen chemical still present in the blood so they start eating the human cells which is having even minimal antigenic property or where ever the antigen scattered in the body is there, Sure the digested bacterial wall antigens chemical will grasped by adjacent cells so all this will be destroyed by the antibody AUTOLYSIS (TYPE 2 HYPERSENTIVITY OR IMMUNE MEDIATED). But when this process is happening severe form of anemia , thrombocytopenia and other cells deficiency will happen.

Possibility 2 : The distracted immune cells and lymph cells and neutrophil circulate within the body and do the damage to the human body parts these cells wander around the circulation and produce the disease (confused inflammation cells and confused immune cells now ready). This immunoglobulin will join to create the disease without any real bacteria or germs.it is difficult to differentiate these cells from normal cells. Immune complex disease (Type 3 hypersensitivity). The inflammation initiates the disease and then immunity join over there. After the partial destruction by the inflammation. Due to excess accumulation of the chemo tactic chemicals and circulate in the body may attract (mis direct) the antibody against the human body parts and tissues so there by antibody will destroy the human organs and tissues (autoimmune disease). This auto immune disease so weak and slow and long duration due to initiation and continuation is done by the confused inflammation.

Suppose if the germs entered is a virus, not a bacterium, then the virus is killed by antibody then inflammation subsides normal way. The antibiotic prescribed here is not worked due to entered organism is not a bacteria so this is the reason type 2 hypersensitivity is happening rarely then type – 1 hypersensitivity. EVENTHOUGH HEAVY ANTI BIOTIC PRESCRIPTION OF ALL THE CASE the entering organism mostly virus, so antibody formed against the virus kills the virus so patient escape from immunoglobulin disease,just to promote sales they prescribe antibiotic.

(Discussion in viral hepatitis virus is present and

antibody against the virus also there but the disease is run longer duration without clearing the virus ? like hepatitis B and HIV this is could be the immunoglobulin present over there is not a immunoglobulin against the particular virus it is misinterpreted as antibody against the Hepatitis or HIV. The antibody is confused antibody it is joining to the liver inflammation or HIV related inflammation Not a true specific immunoglobulin to the particular virus if the immunoglobulin is a true immunoglobulin sure it will kill the virus.)

Lymphoma and Luekemia (blood cancer)

The immunoglobulins keep coming to the circulation and no reciprocation or feedback to stop immunoglobulin production causes more than excess immunoglobulin in the circulation will create immune globulin disorders and excess cell proliferation similar to myeloma, leukemia , lymphoma (blood malignancy). All proliferative disorders have been simple induced by medicine itself. This hyper function of the bone marrow and lymphnodes sure will attract the confused inflammation so now the bone marrow is inflamed and will produce abnormal cells and then produce lymphoma .

When the bone marrow recive the input to produce excess blood cells and bone marrow making excess blood cells but the inflammation disturbed by prescription of the antipyretic and anti allergics or prescribed anti biotic the bacteria cleared from the circulation so now there is no enemy but the excess blood cell production order is not withdrawn so neutrophil monocytes lymphocytes everything is produced unusually longer period causes either bone marrow failure or the confused infllamtion will also attack the bone marrow inflammation lead to production malfunction . the demand to excess cell production and confused inflammation disease in the bone marrow causes blood cencer (lukamia)

SO NOW THE DOCTORS WILL RECOMMEND YOU TO GO FOR BONE MARROW TRANSPLANT for bone marrow failure or will recommend for radiotherapy pr chemo therapy.

Inflammatory disease or immune disease ?

Since the confused inflammation not cleared in the circulation, no feedback or reciprocation mechanism, the process may not complete endless (CHRONIC INFLAMMATORY DISEASE). Since the inflammation is continues and long lasting, they slowly damage many adjacent tissues by chronic passive inflammation. (INFLAMMATION OR THE IMMUNITY IS GOOD PROTECTIVE MECANISAM BUT IT HAS SIGNIFICANT REVERSIBLE PATHOLOGY IF IT IS RECOVERED NORMALLAY within short period] BUT IF IT IS DELAYED UNUSUALLY LONGER PERIOD DEFINETELY DAMAGE THE AREA ADJUSCENT TO THE CONFUSED INFLAMMATION) . Most of the chronic inflammation will induce the significant pathology yet lack of any antibody, It happens not due to purposeful destruction by inflammation chemicals but damage due to chronic stagnation of the confused inflammation in the particular site. Many numbers of this type of chronic disease waiting to add up into the autoimmune disease yet lack of sufficient proof. Of course, this is also technically called autoinflammatory but ALOPATHIC DOCTOR MADE AUTO INFLAMMATORY DISEASE.

Why above paragraph it may be bore to read again and again similar writing. Doctors identified auto immune disease since there is a immunoglobulin in the particular pathological process but they does not have any sufficient proof or idea what is happening in many disease. So not only auto immunity auto inflammation too is happening you no need to look for any proof in any usual way but we have another way to trace it learn it by reading this book and understand missing to identify this fact alone causing huge loss to humans and heavy suffering with disease. Auto inflammation making more disease then auto immunity. In many places it makes disease but without any clue that inflammation byproduct is doing this. Auto immune disease also happens but it is too less then auto inflammation.

7.   D. AUTO
IMMUNE DISEASE

In current medical belief auto-immune disease con-sidered as some special immune cells is started attack-ing the human body and again thinking that ,this cell is prepared to attack their own body parts and tissues.

The confused inflammation is attracted by min-imal over stress of the human body so that it is initi-ating the confused inflammation (auto inflammation) and confused immune cells available within the human body is attracted in similar way and produce confused auto im-mune disorders (auto immune disease). The explanation is the immunoglobulin is not produced for destroy our body but it is distracted from their functions of killing enemy so the excess immunoglobulin makes the disease.

BASIC TRUTH IS OUR BODY NEVER PRODUCE ANY CELLS OR IMMUNOGLOBULIN AGAINST THE OWN BODY. The problem is immuno-globulin is taking special training in the thymus not to attack our body but kill enemy. So this is a confusion to the doctor how this special trained cells will attack our body so they come to conclusion, the production itself wrong the thymus gland is doing some malfunctions due to this malfunction the immunoglobulin loss the (not to self attack coding) basic funciont and start attacking our own body cells. allopathy doctors research is in this direction. all you know then why you are prescribing antibiotic to a healthy human, wait and watch if bacteria not killed then prescribe antibiotic. Necessity of prescribing antibiotic to the humans is when the person not able to produce immunoglobulin against the bacteria. But most of the allopathy doctors violating, respect body functions and rules and act accordingly we have to save the people and at the same time we have to do that in right way. Prescribing something because we have medicine is not helping to the public it's a sales technic. So, do research and search the cause where you did the mistake don't blame the human natural protective mechanism and don't distract by some other useless research.

THIS RULES HAS BEEN BROKEN NICELY BY PRESCRIBBING ALOPATHIC MEDICINES. WHEN YOU DO GOOD WHEN YOU OBEY THE RULES YOU CAN ALSO EXPECT EVERYTHING NORMALLY BUT AFTER COLLPSING ALL THE NORMAL SYSTEM HOW CAN YOU EXPECT EVERYTHING SHOULD WORK NORMALLY.

HUGE COLLECTION OF HISTMINE IN THE BODY THIS WILL SEND A SIGNALS TO HUMAN TISSUES IS THE MASSIVE ENEMY BUT THE PARTICIPENT IS THE HYPERSENSITIVE ULTRAFAST EXISTING CONFUSED INFLAMMATION / IMMUNE CELLS THEN REAL INFLAMMATION.

There are many situations actually the same autoinflammation happen but there may not be any auto immune cells but in few disease only immune cells present the reason behind this is if the confused immune cells present in the body ,then it will come and participate in the inflammation so we name this c auto inflammation disease into auto immune disease due to presence of immune cells.so we make great story behind that and we see the immune cells with great fear.

Mostly this confused immune cells will not have enough natural power of the true immune cells so that difficulty in killing the germs and also destroying our body parts so that it run chronic course of eroding the parts slowly along with confused inflammation cells (HEPATITIS B).

If there are no available confused immune cells, then the confused inflammation produces the disease but this disease make confusion to the doctors what is the cause for inflammation here ? there are huge category left, unknown etiology due to this reason. So, keeping all the confused inflammation disease in the unknown etiology group (not only unknown etiology not even know that is inflammation related disease).

vitiligo -cause -confused inflammation,

atopic dermatitis — cause confused inflammation.

Thyroiditis --- Cause confused inflammation

Confused inflammation (with ESR elevated)

Confused inflammation [with auto antibody present]named as auto immune disease.

Hepatitis --- cause confused inflammation without antibody, C inflammation with anti body present.

Antibody, antigen complex disease

when the immune process is interrupted at the time of clearing the immune complex , then immune complex allowed to roam in the circulation and this causes many diseases. Type III hypersensitivity. Systemic lupus erythmetosis, glomerular nephritis, rheumatoid arthritis, vasculitis etc.

OTHER IMMUNE DISORDERS

• **Normal immunity**: no need of medicine.IF You allow the body to heal themselves many diseases will recover themselves .There is no self-limiting disease it is actually a self healing disease. All the diseases curable by body itself if body struggle to heal themselves need a support but that support must follow the true science. Immunoglubulins is a protein in the blood which is converted in to a special protective cell in the lymphnodes.

• **Hypo immune status** : Identify the cause why low immunity and try to recover the hypo or nil immune status to normal. Need more diet and healthy living environment and more protein supplements and medicine to improve the immunity prescribing steroid is highly contradictory and makes the situation greatly worse, homeo medicine is good to prevent recurrent infection due to low immunity [hard indurated lymph nodes recovered by suitable homeo medicines , hard indurate non functioning tonsil, spleen recovered by medicines .bone disorders and bone marrow dysfunctions recovered by homeo medicines SO A HYPO IMMUNE STATUS NEED A MEDICINE TO RECOVER FROM HYPO STATUS NORMAL IMMUNE STATUS AND GET READY FOR RECOVER THE DIS-EASE.

• **Hyper immune status** : Need to identify the cause and then eliminating the cause. prescribe the medicine to recover the immune system to be normal. Homeopathy medicine is good in set right the hyper immunity , since the hyper immunity is again a altered immunity it happened due to repeated interruption in the inflammatory and immune system functions by steroid and anti inflammatory so prescribing the will further worse but can be prescribed as a life saving but homeopathy act as a curative here. (the underlying basic pathology for hyper inflammation and hyper immunity is confused inflammation that has to be cleared).(discussed above)

• **Altered immune status** : neither high nor low but not normal is fall under altered immune status need medicine to regulate the altered immunity to normal . Due to confused inflammatory cells and chemicals it happens ;Homeopathy medicine is the medicine of choice to recover this.(discussed above)

Our aim is to recover the natural immune power of the humans and nothing else then that. so, we need to worry about then .if any infections occur,the affected person immunity is good then inflammation and immunity will take care of that.

I AM NOT PURPOSEFULLY INTRUDING HOMEOPATHY AS A MEDICINE OF CHOICE PRACTICALLY NO MEDICINE FOR THE ABOVE CONDITION IN ALOPATHY .ALL ALOPATHS ARE TEACHED TO REMOVE THE ORGANS OR SUPPRESS TOTTAL IMMUNITY FOR PREVENTING CURRENT SEVERITY OF THE DISEASE EVEN IN WORSE POOR IMMUNE STATUS,SO I AM UNABLE TO SUGGEST ALOPATHY HERE.

But other then normal immunity all are consider as an altered immune status.[but low immunity partly altered but mainly born with deficient of tissues which making proper protecting cells or acquired due to long time immune suppressants].

7.E. ULCERS

Very important process in the inflammation is destroying the waste cells and clearing the waste cells from the circulation. Anyone is interrupting the inflammation at the time then the destruction process is distracted and allowed to spread so this distracted destructive process is starting in an unnessaory healthy parts.

Usually body send the signal to destroy all the cells which is broken then the cells will destroy themselves (apoptosis) and then send other signal to regenerate the same cells. Ok what will happen if the destructing signal diverted or distracted then the signal, go to good cells and destroys that so that ulcers can come in un unnecessary region. We are clueless why ulcers here. It may not look like frank ulcers it may reflect sudden and massive destruction of cells and tissues of nerves,blood vessal muscles, orgon anything , but destruction is marked.

Most of the time the diverted apoptosis signals may not withdrawn since it is may not get the reciprocation of completing the task. So, the destruction continues. Suppose if the new fresh inflammation happens now then this destructive process will join together and causes congestion plus destruction, swelling plus destruction, its like that. In homeopathy we call this prominent stage as syphilis miasm. According to syphilis miasm destruction is marked, ulceration is marked and necrosis marked.

programmed mass death of the cells (apoptosis). A destruction is a finest process of the inflammatory process of course many cells and tissues are involved in the inflammations are broken and damaged severely has to be cleared from the circulation so body select the cells which is damaged and then ordering to suicide [apoptosis] so all the cells are going to destroy themselves.

Natural killer cells are also used to utilized in clearing the waste and damaged products in the inflammation. This natural killer cell is identifying the cells which is marked for destruction and then it will clear that cells.

Not that the cells which is suicided and self-destroyed is the body own tissues and natural killer cells clear the abnormal damaged body cells as well as foreign invaders (germs).

A massive chemical used for treating humans either antibiotic or anti-inflammatory or other drugs especially external applications distract the accuracy of the natural planned purposeful clearing of the abnormal cells in the body.so that the destruction part easily turned / distracted towards good and normal cells causes sudden destruction of the purely normal cells or tissues causes ulcers or destruction lead to many diseases.

Here there is another drawback is in the inflammation process a destruction followed by building of the new cells and almost all the abnormal cells are cleared and we will get the fresh new cells. But the distracted apoptosis totally loss in control of the real inflammation so that the distracted apoptosis or order of cell destruction is not going to be replace normal cells example non healing ulcers, delay in wound healing, chonic inflammation (it means the inflammation also has the micro ulcers and need to be cleared if apotosis not happen that will stay here and produce chronic disease and then on day turn into cancer.

THE DISTRACTED INFLAMMATION TO THE PARTICULAR PART DOES NOT HAVE ANY POWER TO REBUILD THE DAMAGE.BUT ONCE THE DESTRUCTING ORDER IS MOVED SOMEWHERE ELSE THEN THIS NON INFLAMMATORY YET FALL IN INFLAMMATION PROCESS DUE TO DISTRACTION IS REBUILD THEIR BODY TISSUES AND CELLS BUT THIS IS HAPPEN LIKE A INJURY IS ORDERING A NEW INFLAMMATION PROCESS AND REPAIRING THEMSELVES BUT THIS PROCESS ALMOST ALWAYS IS INCOMPLETE AND NOT A SUCCESFULL AND COMPLETE RECOVERY. A COMPLETE RECOVERY IS POSSIBLE IN ALL OTHER MINIMAL DESTRUCTION DUE TO STAGNATION OF THE INFLAMMATION IS POSSIBLE [IF THAT IS MOVE TO OTHER PARTS].

BUT THE DESTRUCTION OF THE NORMAL TISSUE IS SOME THING DEEP AND MOST OF THE TIME IRREVERSIBLE SO THAT RECOVERY WILL BE HIGHLY INCOMPLETE AND PERMANENT IT MEANS SURE THAT DISTRACTED DESTRUCTIVE INFLAMMATION PART NOT GOING TO REGENARATE IT AND AGAIN SELF CURING AND REPAIRING MAY NOT BE POSSIBLE FOR DEEP DESTRUCTION [BODY CODING]

ULCEARTIVE COLITIS,CHRONS DISEASE,,,,,,,,,ETC.

Parkinson disease only destruction or apoptosis of the brain cells.

(THE DESTRUCTION IS ALMOST ALWAYS LESS IN AND INFLAMMATION SINCE BODY HAS ENOUGH POWER TO KILL THE GERMS IN SO MANY OTHER TECHNIQ.IF ALL THAT PROCESS WORKING PERFECT THEN THERE IS NO GREAT MANY BURDEN TO DESTROY greater NUMBER

OF DAMGED CELLS SINCE NO HEAVY DESTRUTED CELLS DURING THE INFLAMMATION. so, there is no deep and heavy destruction, for this good and superficial inflammation is possible only you understand the value of immune glands and not removeing that for your financial need and allowing the fever to controle the germs and many more interruption and precisely no confused inflammation and especially no destructive confused inflammation if that is there then heavy and deep destruction will happen then and that may not recover) reading biology and physiology is not hobby it has to be applied when ever need to save the sufferer.

Negative Impact

- if the destruction and apoptosis of the abnormal cells are not happening what will happen. The abnormal cells will be allowed to stay in the body and this cell will be turn into *cancer in future*.

- The abnormal cells asked to regenerate so that whole inflamed surface regenerated with abnormal cells itself. So that this cells again does not close the wound properly and again excess sloughing will be there may not be healthy granulations. This site is going to be the future source of infections and great deep abscess inside. Bleeding and oozing may not be properly revascularized so bleeding will be there or oozing of serous fluid or frank blood not fixed properly. The most important drawback is regenerating abnormal cells is in abundance is nothing but cancer.

- Evan though functions recovered the cells and tissues will underperform due to regeneration is abnormal cells.
- *All the immune complex and waste products are allowed to roam in the circulation. causes so many new disease-like indurations. Produce a condition called hypersensitivity (III). Blocking the microcirculation and produces the disease. This dead bacteria's, damaged tissues and antibody antigen complex produces variety of the diseases.*

simple stagnation of the confused inflammation cells and chemical can also produce ulcerations and destruction of the tissues but this ulcer heal if the confused inflammation withdrawn from the site or even wound healing will happen even if the confused inflammation present in the site.

So, the wound making and wound healing is again depending upon the presence of confused inflammation it is absolutely not depend upon the level of sugar in the blood.

7.F. DEPOSITS IN THE INTERSTITIAL SPACE AND BLOOD VESSELS.

It is not only the confused inflammation produce the disease actively. The presence of confused inflammation along with dead cells will deposits in the interstitial cells just a deposit itself causes a disease. This roaming confused inflammatory cells when circulating via blood vessels along with dead and damaged tissues deposited invariably all over the body make passive slow obstruction of blood vessels and also make the slow passive inflammation inside the blood vessels or deposits within interstitial space causes thickening of the epidermis [indurations]. This will produce again disease due to vascular insufficiency or indurations itself consider as a disease.(callosity, cataract, atherosclerosis, arcuate senilis,baldness,,,,,,etc.) and recurrent infection due to loss of basic protection cellulites and if the obstruction is severe then gangrene infarct.

Micro deposits within the soft tissues of human body parts before attaining real indurations or thickening will reduce the functions of many sensors in the body so the hearing will be slowly low due to deposits in the bones of the hearing. bp will be low or high due to micro deposits in the baro and chemoreceptor's and carotid and aortic body. It affects many receptors and sensor in the minute structures of the organ and produce severe disability and doctors are clueless about this effect. Similar deposits in the brain makes lots of diseases and disorders of brain and **psychological disease.** Most accurate body functions losts its function due to slow micro deposites and micro destruction of the minute structure within the circulations.

The deposites include just deposites like a gelatin matrix so that it will have minimal indurations nothing more then that, but mostly it has other chemicals and cells of the inflammation so that the deposits do many inflammation functions where ever it deposites (so the deposits may have inflammation signs and symptoms rather then just deposits) deposites within the fingers and joints causes swelling and indurations along with inflammation signs and symtoms, so over a period of time the joint will become stiff and fibrosed lost its functions,here deposites + marked inflammation signs and symptoms will be there.

Eventhough the deposites are simple but if the deposited site is importand organ then the impact is severe like this micro deposit makes the closure of pores of sweat and oily glands (acne pilaris, sebaceous cyst, acne, pimples, retention cyst).

Deposites within the endocrine or exocrine glands causes initially changes in the secretion the course of the disease may changes either simple enlargement or particular part of the gland is swellon or whole or particular part of the gland is inflamed for a longer period and do changes , so the gland will have either hypo or hyper or nil secretions along with some inflammation signs and symptoms. The top most gland fall in inflammation (named auto immune thyroiditis) is thyroid gland then rest of the endocrine glands.

Most of the lymphnodes loses its functions due to this simple microdeposites of inflammatory remanands.

Deposites along with mucus membrane of the particular tract causes initially changes in the secretion of the mucus glands and sensations and functions slowly detoriarate.like the secretions is altered its colore and consistency changes their nature like it may corrode or itches ,,,,etc.this deposites react with the substance passing via the same (if the mucus membrane is mouth then it will react all the food substances and produce inflammation signs and symptoms produce tumor if they have increadiants it's a potential site for development of all type of cancers).

Atherosclerosis is one of the importand disease of the abnormal deposit plus proliferation and deposites of fibrin and elastin and cholesterol and matrix causes sclerosis and thickening of the blood vessals.

MOSTLY PRODUCE SLOW, INSIDIUS ONSET DISORDERS.

7.G.CANCER

C ancer is most dangerous disease in the world. People having better knowledge about the disease, but this knowledge is not helped to improve the cancer prevention. Instead of that people are more scared about the disease so repeated tests and scans whole body checkups going on. Some people help to quit the smoking and other cancer producing agents.

Most of the disease we can prevent so easily when people educated about the disease. But here it does not work out since we teach them risk factor prevention rather than prevent the cause of the cancer. And again, the failure is happening due to cause of the cancer is not fully known to the medical field.

The most prevalence, rapid spread, more people is having risk of getting cancer is due to stopping and interfering healthy natural healing power by allopathic medicines.

When the person stop smoking may not get the cancer in the lungs and mouth but get the cancer in the stomach due to allopathic medicine ,it means we identify the risk factor but missed to identify very common cause of the cancer (allopathic medicines directly and indirectly cause the cancer). Some time they say the cause for the cancer is genetic and radiation so people cannot do anything on this part including doctors. But the true cause for cancer inappropriate usage of the allopathic medicine. Some of the virus and bacteria causes cancer but again most of the virus is not curable by allopathic medicine no medicine for HIV. But vaccination for human papilloma virus and hepatitis B virus playa better role in preventing cancer too some extend.

WHO says since there is change in culture ,world is adapting western culture causes great change in cancer occurrence like infectious cancers are reducing but the cancer of breast and prostate and lung is increased. the indication is cancer prevalence remain same but the place of cancer has shifted from one place to another place.

Ok the suffering related with cancer is more then why the doctors are not discovered some good medicine for cancer. Medicines are there but the cost is too much and again so many new medicines are coming to the medical field. But the suffering is remains in the same level.

My view upon the cancer is different from regular concept. I am not showing interest in finding the remedy for the cancer. Why cancer to the humans ? it is not acceptable ,but anyway some reasons people or having cancer . I need to find the real cause for the cancer and prevent that and I have to create the cancer free world. The aim is before 2050 I have to make sure no one in the world is having cancer. I am not looking for good remedy for cure the cancer ,when you do that you are accepting the cancer, when you accept the cancer occurrence you have to ready for accept the consequence of the cancer burden . no I am not going to accept the cancer.

I am very clear that human protective system is build in such a to prevent the cancer. I am accepting this factor. I am going to reboot this natural cancer preventing system and I break the cancer possibility so no cancer to the people. Be relax and be cool. It is not simply foolish stubbornness and it is sensible scientific stubbornness YES , CANCER IS POSSIBLE TO PREVENT EFFECTIVELY MASSIVELY AND TOTTALLY.it is not to just few people, cancer prevention in general to the whole world.

Problem statement :

Cancer is diagnosed earlier or late is not much beneficial in many cancers. It means in many diseases early detection helps in cure the disease easily and there may not be any destruction in the body tissues so no severe morbidity, no mortality and no handicap . But this is not applicable in the most of the cancer case since the disease progress rapidly and the disease makes handicap or surgical removal of the affected organ makes the handicap and severe pain, bleeding, emaciation severe loss of function of the affected parts causes severe morbidity , running rapid deterioration of the health due to cancer and eventual death. Need more money to take treatment for cancers. The decision maker for the surgery in most of the cases by patient but not in case of cancer, here doctor will decide and fix the date of cancer. patient have one option alone that is to pay the money for surgery. Many people scared of going for surgery. So, they delay or postpone not having adequate money

but this option is not there in cancer. Testing (diagnostic as well as prognostic) cost more money. Cancer medications (chemotherapy) and other remedy level treatment like radiotherapy all costs more money. Cancer makes fear and panic and depression of the suffering individual and family members and neighbor , so, the people rush to the hospital and frequent whole-body checkups .

Nearly 80 lac – 1.5 crore people dying globally every year. Most of the cancer death rate is more than 50 % and more then that 5 years survival rate is less and further increase in every more 5 years survival rate is too less.

Every year nearly 1.4 crore new cancer cases is diagnosed this cancer incidence increase slowly to 2.2 crore per year.in 2018 there are 96 lac cancer death globally.

20 lac lung cancer / yr

20 lac breast cancer / yr

18 lac colon cancer.

12 lac prostate cancer

10 lac skin cancer

10 lac stomach cancer

70 % cancer deaths are occurring to the poor and middle class family.

Obesity, alcoholism, cigarette smoking, eating rich animal foods no exercise these are all some of risk factor for cancer.

Human papilloma virus and hepatitis virus produce cancer and we have vaccines to prevent this cancer.

Increasing age is considered as cancer risk as the age progress the cancer possibility is increasing since the repairing the damaged cells is decreasing as the age advances.

Some important preventive measures for prevent cancer :

1.Reducing house smoke (in the rural villagers use the wood and coal for cooking instead of gas so this house fumes encourages cancer risk for those people).

2. Reducing smoking and tobacco, pan parag chewing, betel nut usage.

3.Reducing air pollution by using electrical vehicles.

4.eating healthy fresh vegetables , fruits, nuts like that.

5.maintaining ideal weight. doing regular exercise.

6.taking vaccines for Hepatitis -B and human papilloma virus

7. NO alcohol drinks.

8.Reducing excess radiation from specific industry and proper preventive measures for the workers. reduce the chemical exposure to the labor by using proper precautions so that preventing chemical carcinogens.

9.Dedecting cancer earlier and giving immediate treatment.

These are all some common preventive measures practiced in the current medical field.

New perception about cancer and its cause and prevention.

Carcinogens [cancer producing agents Chemicals , smoking, virus,,, etc.] maybe or may not produce cancer. But if the immune , inflammatory systems are active to destroy the cancer cells then no cancer. But when the confused inflammation presents then the cancer possibility is high. Carcinogens are ineffective if there is no confused inflammation and if there is no chronic inflammation.

- a person having poor immunity having risk of developing cancer.

- under Allopathic steroid [making direct low immunity - causes cancer risk. anti-inflammatory drugs prevent and collapse the possibility of cancer killing cells to form. natural cancer killing cells will not destroy the cancer cells. if the cancer or tumor develops now by any cause does not have objection.

Due to low or nil production of lymphocytes, phagocytes, natural killer cells due to suppressor effects of steroids or the confused inflammatory cells are not identified as this cells has to clear from circulation since it is not completed its functions and lost control from brain.

• But in clinical practice not only the low immunity or no immunity patients having cancer, all persons are developing cancer. Believed that some error in tumor destroying cell production itself, lacking capability to destroy due to inborn error and also believed cancer cells formed in such way that it is lacking antigenic property (if the antigenic property is there then only all cancer killing cell will come and destroy that) and lack in some identifying marker for binding the cancer cell with killing cell. But this is not true.

• CANCER IS A NOT FOREIGN INVADER / NOT an EXTERNAL NOXIUSE AGENTS (In most of the case), if it is a foreign body or external injuries agents of course it will have an antigenic property so that the cancer cells will be cleared by immune cells.

• There is no inborn error in the cancer killing cell formation if at all it is there it could be extremely rare. Because cancer is now is more general and widespread.

• A Truth is cancer cells are our own body cells. old body tissues, inflammation cells or immune cells . This waste body cells have to be cleared from the body earlier during the inflammation process but we stopped it by anti-inflammatory so that now that cells undergo severe changes and turn into cancer cells.

Explanation:

I will give a new clue which is most beneficial to understand how the cancer cells are originating. In contrast to popular medical belief cancer is not something coming from externally as carcinogen. It is formed by a confused inflammatory cell. this cell is allowed to roam by wrong treatment of allopath. it happens in every treatment given by allopath, so, there are numerous blood cells, body tissues are allowed to stay in the body. It is not that cancer, tumor cells alone left unclear, many killed virus, bacteria and a virus + antibody complex allowed to roam or remain inside the body which is not normal.

This cells usually engulfed by natural immune cells then that immune cells cleared from the circulation immediately after the inflammation by apoptosis. Here it is scattered in the circulation before it completing the functions so this cell will not be killed or engulfed even after the life span is over.

If the brain decides the body tissues are damaged partially, fully or decided to remove that from the body then it happens in many ways like self-destruction [apoptosis].

Some of the cells which is still present in the body but need to be cleared from the circulation is removed by Natural Killer cells, but before doing that the body cells have to be destroyed identified and given a marker by the brain order. Now the NK cells will destroy that marked cells. [But all this clearing of waste and damaged cells will happen at the end of the inflammation] But since we prescribe the medicine in the beginning of the inflammation itself so that the inflammation process totally collapsed now so that damaged tissue identification and requesting apoptosis or ordering NK cells everything is not going to happen. So, even though adequate natural killer cells is there in the body it does not kill the dead tissues and antigen antibody complex and even if the cells undergoing cancer that time also body will not attempt to clear it. This roaming inflammatory cells and antigen antibody complex, dead tissues will produce varies Chronic Disease. [SLE,PSORIYASIS,ASTHMA, HEPATITIS,,,,,etc.] will not respond to anti-inflammatory now and need massive dose of steroids, steroid will again suppress the natural production of healthy blood cells in general will cause low blood cells and low cancer killing cells. Here low immunity helps in getting more infections. more infections need more steroid anti-inflammatory anti-biotics and steroid, this cycle will be repeated.

The damaged cells has to cleared from the body, is allowed to stay inside along with confused inflammatory cells will produce the chronic diseases and to control it prescribing huge medications all this procedure along with carcinogenic agents will give severe stress to the damaged tissue , so this tissues and cells undergoes further damage repeatedly for many years so that tissues DNA alteration happened and turn into cancer. When discussing carcinogenic agents or chemicals ,it will not produce any effect upon the healthy tissues but the carcinogenic agents can able to turn the damaged dead tissues and damaged cells to cancer. Or the growth stimulation by regenerative cells causes severe proliferation of this severely damaged tissues.

The confused inflammatory chemicals make the body cells to react to the sun. Now the body gets the impression that sun heat is like bacteria, rain is like virus, dust is like a fungus in that way all the external stimulus considered like enemy (germs) and produce pseudo inflammation. The confused inflammation makes sensitivity to normal tissue with external environment as well as sensitive to carcinogenic agents. Due to this confused inflammation this damaged cell also undergoes chronic confused inflammation changes so that, this tissues initially undergoing stress so that morphological changes and structural alterations will be there due to long living without destructions, so sensitive to carcinogenic agents now turn into cancer.

Misinterpretation of cancer tissues

It is not that cancer is spreading via lymphatic's and blood vessels you are reading upside down actually in the similar way only the acute disease formed you are interrupted and then it turned in to chronic disease and now turned into cancer.

It means a chronic disease with organ damage (Tumor) so there by the infections cleared and controlled by lymphatic's (Nodular involvements) , This disease spread from place to place according to the (negative magnetism) a smoker invite the disease to mouth ,a drinker invite the disease into stomach / liver, sexually active person invite that into genitals heat and cold invite this cells to skin [Metastasis via blood or bone marrow or local induration] so all this is happening many years before now all these cells turn into cancer after this many year.

Metastasis a cancer spreads from one place to another place via lymphatics, blood vassals or local erosion. BUT TRUE UNDERSTANDING IS A chronic damaged tissues undergoes cancer changes where ever the chronic confused inflammation was spread already now turned into cancer cells we can predict the cancer in the regional lymph node and along the lymphatic drainage and blood vessel supply. THIS TIME MOST OF THE ORIGINAL SOURCE OF INFLAMMATION ALSO TURNED INTO CANCER.

Example : a duodenal diseases and germs carried to liver to clear it [to hepatic lymphatic's] so in this way the cancer cells metastasis to liver. further spread and metastasis is identified as circulating confused inflammation chemicals or dead cells or antibody , antigen complex etc.

whatever it maybe we are GRADING the stage of the cancer [TNM] now, has been formed as a benign chronic disease in the same route many years before. A CANCER ACT AS GREAT EVIDENCE OR PROOF FOR THE CHRONIC CONFUSED INFLAMMATION.CANCER IS HELPING TO TRACE AND STUDY THE NATURE OF Confused INFLAMMATION.

We are interested only to detect the cancer, so now only tracing this. but here after either we are not going to violet the body rules so no cancer possibility or if the chronic disease formed anyway, we will detect it earlier we can prevent it. Now it is very clear how the cancer is forming.

Harvesting our fault :

What we see as a cancer today has been formed many years before, we assume that when we suppress and interfere the inflammation really but feel that we are cleared it. The inflammatory remnants now turn into cancer.

The first and very important question here is why we have to stop inflammation ? a trillion-worth question. Its just after all we assume that inflammation is a hypersensitive reaction and more ever we are not identified any impact due to diverting the inflammation. We feel we gave relive to the patient suffering (pain, fever, breathlessness ,, etc).

We assume that we only protecting the wound by anti-bacterial cream so we forget the micro chemical automatic process happen in wound healing and it may interfere the wound healing process here and we never observed any impact after this treatment so we are doing what we feel and what we do is right.

But now I am explaining what is happening and blaming you with evidence. You have come with a unsolvable question and I solved it with reason. So, don't repeat the mistake again. I SAY WHAT WE FEEL PROUD WHAT WE THINK WE DID GREAT SERVICE TO THE PATIENT IS NOTHING BUT OUR OWN DELUSION ON THE CONTRARY WE ARE SLOWLY SEEDING THE DISEASE TO THE PATIENT. This is not treatment ; this is our innocence. Don't give such foolish treatment. Do service relive the suffering but without doing harm to the natural protective system.

we use strong chemicals to interfering the inflammation. inflammation is a basic body protective functions, I hope I am mentioning here more then 50 times so don't interfere inflammation and wound healing. The hypersensitivity is the cause for prescription of anti-histamine and steroid you (allopathy) don't have any other medicine so you are not having any other option then closing the inflammation, either it is normal inflammation or confused inflammation.

But I am clearly explaining one better idea to tackle this hypersensitivity. So , stopping inflammation first time causes hypersensitivity then when you repeating the same every time the hypersensitivity is not cleared but your managing. But you are absolutely unaware that you are the cause for hypersensitivity. Why you are managing the hypersensitivity with the medicine that's again the same medicine which caused the hypersensitivity because that is giving relief and you does not tried to cure it because you are in a delusional world here you believe that the asthma is incurable and allergic rhinitis is incurable and everything is incurable. Its all again and again mistakes. Don't do that. Use the word in the book prevent and cure it is possible.

it is danger to the human body this is how disease are seeding. The first step doesn't interfere inflammation suppose if you did that allopathy does not work out to clear the hypersensitivity (confused inflammation) we have to choose homeopathy if you do that or sending the case to homeopathy but clear the hypersensitivity (clear the confused inflammation). Managing here after will be consider as a crime. Because that will take to a high cancer possibility. long standing chronic inflammation with heavy allopathic medicines turn the damaged cells so easily to a cancer. there are many chemical carcinogens but here we saw a common day to day using chemical carcinogen is simply allopathic drugs. (but allopathic books explain accidental micro chemical ingestion will cause cancer but taking every day heavy allopathic drugs for many years consider as a good food not a chemical it does not cause cancer and it is not classified as chemical carcinogen). It is a great surprise that under many allopathic drugs written as this medicine will cause cancer but non of these medicines diagnosed as a cause for the present cancer not even suspected.

we are not cared about it, now we find it as a cancer because it is giving life threatening prominent symptoms and still believe that cancer is something coming from genetics so we again search for what is the cause for cancer. Even though we accept some chronic diseases are turning into cancer. we know that even a sun heat can induce cancer. The sun is a fault or we are doing the fault. We have to realize that. We make the healthy individual become unhealthy and vulnerable to sick and we make all his enjoyable things to be dangerous once he had food with happily now we restrict it once he enjoyed in the rain we warn it not to go out in the rain, once he was enjoyed the sun we asked not to go out without sunscreen ,don't you realize we make all his healthy environments become sensitive .now he is anxious and apprehensive to go out and live itself without many medical aid .all this notorious things we do in the name of profession .we never make life as easy and enjoyable we make it miserable.

THIS IS THE FUNDAMENTAL CAUSE FOR MANY

CHRONIC DISEASES INCLUDING CANCER.

Don't prescribe unscientifically and don't prescribe without the basic understanding of the Human physiology and pathology. Think once and twice before prescribing anti-inflammatory/anti-allergic, for fever, cold, running nose, and other acute inflammatory condition. don't use external application for chronic diseases.

Decide What is harmful ? Fever ? running nose ? or cancer is harmful ?.

7.H.NEOPLASM (TUMOR)

The Inflammation Is Interrupted At The Time Of Reconstruction :

now more fibrin and elastin cells will come and revascularization will happen new body cells will be generated to fulfill the ulcers , tissue damages, after this process whole damaged tissues reconstructed and tissue damages repaired.

Suppose if anti-inflammatory drugs, steroids , ointments or external application used to stop the inflammation at the end of inflammation process, especially when regeneration of the tissues happens, there is few basic effects will come.

If you use the ointment for treating skin disease then sure high possibility of getting of more confused inflammation cells (skin disease itself is a confused inflammation disorder, this again distracted to produce a confused inflammation)

- Regeneration will be stopped so ulcer formation [POSSIBLE SOURCE SITE FOR FUTURE INFECTIONS,FREQUANT INFECTIONS, HEMARRHAGES IN CASE VESSAL NOT CLOSED FULLY,DELAYED WOUND HEALING,,,,,,, ETC] or &

- Reconstruction may complete normally (or) &

- Keloid : over growth in the same site [due to poor feed-back reciprocation stop signal not received from the regeneration site [TUMOR WITH MARKED INFLAMMATION CELLS TOO]. Or

- Tumor : The regeneration shifted to other then inflammation site (healthy site) so the new mass or extra growth formed in the body (TUMOR). SINGLE OR MULTIBLE GROWTH IS STATIC AT ONE POINT or KEEP GROWING, tumor with damage tissue as a basic cells or tumor with new site tissues ,,,, etc. all probability is decided by when we interrupt how strong chemicals, we use that decide the choice.

- Hypertrophy : when the organ is over function this over functions get accentuation of the regeneration stimuli so that the organ tissues are hypertrophy (cardio myopathy , goiter ,,,, etc).

Tumor is a 6 th finger

•   Generalized proliferation of many cells and organs may take place this is because the stimulation or order for proliferation only just distracted so that distracted orders makes the new growth of the organ or tissues which is getting the stimuli everywhere proliferation (neuro fibroma).

will gives raise to construct the keloid or tumor all over the body inappropriately and continuously [but this is ideally benign tumors mostly keloid or lipoma, but it is the cause for tumors in general].

Say for example when the body ready to give order to regenerate new body cells now we apply strong chemical in the wound so there by the body confused, where to order a regeneration of cells or where to close the wound so if the chemical or cells involved in the inflammation or wound healing is speeded somewhere else then excess fibrous deposits over there [KELOID , LIPOMA] and demand to regenerate the body tissues is happen [BENIGN Tumor].

Try to applying antibiotic and anti-inflammatory in the ulcers will distract the wound healing/regeneration of new cells and develop the possibility of tumor inside the body. Due to spraying of the fibrinogen and other constructive cells used for regeneration .[EVANTHOUGH THIS TUMOURS ARE FORMED INSIDE THE BODY BUT THE TNF WILL NOT TRY TO ENGULF THIS BECAUSE IT IS BUILDED BY BODY ORDER BUT PLACE IS MISGUIDED by using some medicines].

A Tumor is a new body part even though it is unwanted and placed in on unusual place ,that's why I give the new name to tumor as 6 th finger (this name simply explain tumor is not a pathology) . So cure by medicine is more or less equal to giving medicine for removing one finger or toes or taking treatment for vanishing the some body parts. It means tumor especially regeneration of new cells to build a tumor is almost identical with body parts. A 6 th finger is a extra growth but normal growth it does not help us , and at the same time it does not hurt us it is just there with us. But some tumor may give some pain and pressure symptoms.

A Tumor may not change into cancer until the tumor has some confused inflammation cells within. trauma or other secondary changes the possibility of cancer is high as well as possibility of regression when right remedy chosen is there.

Treatment to a growing tumor is allowed to carry out and it is possible to stop and similarly a constructing tumor we can expect possibility of shrink this is because the body has the mechanism to readjust and fit the regeneration and wound healing during the process of building the tissues.

a corn , callosity, indurations, keloid possibly able to revert to normal if we use proper medicine since they abnormal cells and body has the regulatory mechanism to withdraw the excess blood cells and wound healing cells.

SO, AVOID EXTERNAL APPLICATIONS FOR WOUNDS WHICH IS NATURALLY HEALS AS FOR POSSIBLE.

A tumor necrosing factor will destroy sure cancerous waste cells but not the healthy tumor cells yes, a tumor is healthy new tissue body is builder of that.

So benign tumor and malignant tumor is the older

name. now excess body tissue construction (ETC) and tumor proper is the new name. so the tumor proper signify the cancer or confused inflammation cells rich excess growth. The etc signify that excess cell growth (6 th finger) lipoma is a 6 th finger (older benign tumor).

We don't want that 6th finger to appear all over the body so don't try to stop the inflammation. Don't apply external application for ulcers, wound, skin diseases.

Tumor

Tumor is classified into benign (not having heavy destruction or in simple understanding, it is not harmful like cancer). Malignant tumor is harmful and gives trouble and destruction leads to severe morbidity and mortality mostly related to cancer.

Even though benign tumor is not producing any harm but the people are scared to tumor in general, they look all the tumor fearfully and consider all tumor as a cancer this fear is worse when coming to know if there is any internal tumors so people now days do whole body checkups regularly due to fear of cancer.

The lipoma is the one where many people are commonly seeing in their life it is not doing any harm to the people so they are bit relaxed and seeing practically there are different tumors and they understood now, there is harmless tumors (benign tumor) also.

Lipoma I am seeing to many peoples now days, lipoma is very simple example of harmless tumor.it will be there mostly in the abdomen, hands and legs and in the back commonly . freely movable in the skin .slowly grows bigger in size and many new lipoma occurs in most of the people suffering with that. *We can simply prevent the lipoma by allowing the wounds to heal normally and don't apply ointments and any other herbal or homoeopathic ointments. just wash the wounds with sterilized water then allow it to heal naturally if the wound is having possible to get infections seek medical attention doctors clean the wounds by saline water or sterilized water then close the wound by sterilized cotton cloth allow the wound healing. Any external application which is having any chemical or herbal will confuse and distract the wound healing material and produce the tumor. These ointments are So explaining this tumor possibility so patient will not attempt to applying ointments. Surrounding areas in the house must be washed with phenol and other disinfected and washing the hands with soap all will prevent the wound getting the infections possibility.*

Most of the females having tumors either that in the thyroid or uterine, mammary (breast) or ovarian tumor now days a tumor chance is increasing its like almost all the women is having tumor one of the other of the above organs or some of their body parts. Since women are now targeted by allopathy, they invite the female to the hospitals and provide many useless unnecessary treatments and heavy hormone supplements so female now days targeted for potential customer for earning money by the allopathy doctors field. Fibroid tumor ,tumor in the breast are fall in surgery. most of the women in the India losing their uterus since allopathy is not having any medicine for control the bleeding and no effective treatment for many uterine ailments including fibroids. So, educate the women and educate gynecologist that how the tumor forms so that a woman may not loss their organ so simple for preventable cause.

A cyst may not be tumor in the classification tumor cyst is kept under tumor. A cyst is not a tumor .in most of the case cyst is formed as a effusive disorder like hydrocele, plural effusion ,,, etc. in that way a cyst in the kidney is fall in the same classification but ovarian cyst is not a tumor not from effusion and again in the same way hydatid cyst and cysticercosis is origin is not like tumor origin not fall in effusive disorder they are parasitic fluid filled wall that's all. So tumor is proliferation of cells all other simple space occupying lesions may not be classified as tumor. They must have cell proliferation in its tissue composition. When you use right terminology based on some core future then that will be easy to understand and helpful to trace the history and treat well.

But when coming to brain tumors most tiny tumor or swelling causes great trouble and morbidity so here there is no point in classifying benign and malignant growth of tumor. A benign tumor also causes severe harm like pain, convulsion, paralysis and area specific symptoms, but most of the benign tumors withing body other then brain never causes much trouble and even many tumors are asymptomatic. Millimeter level blood leakage within the blood vessels of cerebrum causes stroke and paralysis of the extremity.so how the big tumor will grow without doing harm, all this is because there is no space for any substance which occupy the skull space which is fully occupied brain and cerebrospinal fluid.

Most of the benign brain tumor arises in the meninge (meningioma) which is covers the brain this is most common tumor of the brain. Tumors arising many glial cells in the brain and then tumors arise in the pituitary gland and blood vessels of the brain. More then distress even in benign tumor it is not simple to remove the tumor so please be aware we can prevent the tumor better we can prevent the tumor don't look for treatment option after getting the tumor. Brain surgery is more expensive and having lots of risk in doing that surgery, prevent brain tumors.

Tumors which is compressing the nerve produce the pain and paralysis if it is severe tumor compressing the blood vessels causes reduced blood supply to the particular body parts ,the tumors causing great cosmetic discomfort if the tumor present in the exposed parts especially in the face and neck.

Hunting : the surgeon in India searching a tumor patient for the purpose of removing the tumor. So, they money and commission those who are referring the tumor case and paying money to scanning centers to inform the tumor patients they are waiting to get the tumor patient for hunt. This approach is not only in the egarness in earning money but basically no idea what to do like no one teaching what is right way in surgery. Moralism in the profession is lacking because no clear-cut guidelines to do better treatment.

The right way of handling the patient is train the patient to prevent the tumor and you will be paid for prevention of the tumors in future. You will get negative remarks when your areas are having more tumor cases you might temporarily suspended from medical practice if any one is died due to cancer or tumors. This will be implemented in future. at present there is no law and moral practice to the allopathy but homeopathy all those thinks in Organon of the medicine written by Dr.Hahnemann, this book guides what is right and what is wrong in the medical practice it is not encouraging any punishment but it taches what is right way in practice.

In olden days tonsil swelling is considered as a tumor so the people are scared of hearing tumor in the throat and rush to the hospitals for removing the tonsil. Some of the ENT doctors educate the people to undergo for turbinate swelling these again makes the panic so people undergo surgery. Polyp is another tumor in the nasal cavity so people undergoing for surgery of the polyp.

All this ENT tumors are preventable and curable by homeopathy medicine but its always better to prevent tumor or tumor like lesions not to surface again and again. Allowing the inflammation of the nose is the simple way to prevention of the tumor.

8. CAUSE OF DISEASE

(PSUEDO CAUSE)

A true cause of the disease is a substance which is distracting the inflammation (allopathic medicine and the distracted confused inflammation and immunity). But here we are going to see other factors which supports and reduce or cancel the diseases.

Triggering factors for confused inflammation : it is not the real cause of the disease but it will mimic like a cause. A virus or infection has to make a disease but exposing to cold and drinking ice water bringing the disease is just a trigger which stimulate the confeused inflammation and produce the disease. They are not the cause since the cause is confused inflammation. a virus or bacteria alsos trigger only if the confused inflammation is formed already.

NEGATIVE MAGNATISAM-Like magnet attracts the iron, many environmental and other day to day activity , food ,,, etc. all will stimulate the confused inflammation and create the inflammation or worse the inflammation so I name this as negative magnetism (when we attract the confused inflammation for cure I name positive magnetisam,but here attracting confused inflammation for creating disease, so this is negative inflammation).

The roaming confused inflammatory cells will be attracted in many ways. a normal inflammation can be triggered only by real microbes like bacteria, virus ,, etc or injury or similar strong triggers. But this confused inflammation will behave differently, it is hyper active, hyper responsive to any / many stimulus.

A confused inflammation roaming all over the body will get attracted by minimal pressure of the body , cigarette smoking, alcohol, extreme heat, extreme cold, bodily strong chemicals like HCL in the stomach, strong continues pressure , industrial and chemical exposures , fumes and dust , Metal rings or ornaments , rubber ornaments ,long standing ,long sitting , strong emotions like fear, shock, stress, pressure and friction in the joints, all can attract the confused inflammatory cells and chemicals and produce confused inflammatory disorders so there by thousands and thousands of new sufferings or diseases. The response hyper and abnormal.

So ? so diseases caused by just a external and internal stimulus itself.I mean to say there is no need to wait for or search for some bacteria or virus causing disease.a confused inflammation cells and chemicals will react to the external and internal factors and produce diseases.THE GREAT JOURNEY OF SEARCHING FOR THE CAUSE OF DISEASE END HERE.yes all the diseases caused by confused inflammation alone by reactigin to this factors.The cause of the diseases is discovered from the route how ? why ? when ? all are explained.

We name this is as allergy or hypersensitivity. A normal person will slowly start experience unplesancy and uncomfortable to the external environment in general he connot able to welcome the summer or winter or rainy season as a normal person he is slowly panick about winter or rainy season or he expsose winter with panick and welcome the rainy by anxitiuse and started worry long before the winter starts.

- A normal person can sneeze when he exposes to **dust** but not abnormally, continually and he will not initiate the rhinitis [nasal inflammation], he will not invite the inflammation but a person having confused inflammatory cells will induce the rhinitis and inflammation in the nose by exposing **ac room** , by exposing dust environment, by drinking **cold drinks**.

- A woman having confused inflammatory cells in her body is greatly troubled by exposing **sun heat** [SLE] , Greatly troubled by ac room and chill weather her joint will swell and become tender connote able to walk in winter cold [Rheumatoid arthritis] . A normal inflammation will never give joint pain and inflammation in the joints by just exposing cold weather itself ,here a cold weather is act as a cause for triggering the confused inflammation

- Walking bare foot or **pressure** in the soles invite the confused inflammatory cells all over body towards the foot [sole] and produce heal pain [plantar fascitis , callosity formations. (POSTIVE MAGNATISAM here the confused inflammation cells invited to the foot from vital organs).here the pressure is the cause for the inflammation to the soles.

•   Since this confused inflammatory cell are living more then their usual life time, they easily fragile and respond very quickly even when roaming inside the blood vessels by trapped and get **little more then usual pressure** then they start inflammation process over there [vasculitis / lymph node enlargement without real inflammation or infection or strong antigenic or injuries agents]

•   Severe   myalgia   after   over work / even **normal work**

•   A sun exposure with normal temperature will also bring the severe tanning or ulceration or skin disease to the extreme even cancer is absolutely not a normal inflammatory response.[cancer is again confused inflammation].

•   A **stagnation** of milk causes mastitis , an induration in the breast will turn into cancer is not a normal inflammation all are induced only by chronic confused inflammations. A normal response to stagnation of milk is, to reabsorb it not to produce an abscess. Indurations is tackled by clearing and destroying the cells and healing repairing and recovering the part to be normal is a normal inflammation work not to produce cancer in it.So a normal lactation process of a women invites all the confused inflammation towards the breast and produce diseases within the breast.

A development of breast during the pubertal life causes excess blood circulation and heavy new cell formation to construct the breast all this hyper function invites the confused inflammation cells all over the body and produce breast disease (Especially if they have confused inflammation cells witin their body).

A child who is under allopathy may not have a healthy pubertal life or healthy women anymore.since the confused inflammation cells will attract in the same way towards uterus when they develop and again every monthly period. So the uterus will start produce disese in the unusually earlier life and they will suffer rest of their life many gynecological diseases.ALLOP-ATHY SYSTEM IS A MEGA DISEASE PRODUCING SYS-TEM. KEEP AWARE THAT. manipulating your mistakes towards genetics or environmental pollution or other system of doctors may not workout anymore.accept and try not to produce disease to public.

• A mucosa in the stomach can bear the **HCL secretions** will not cause any harm but when the confused inflammatory cells are passed inside will respond to HCL and help in erode the gastric mucosa and causes gastric or duodenal ulcers.

• Eating warm foods, cold drinks, spices, pan masala , tobacco attract the confused inflammatory cells from sinus or all over the body to mouth and tooth to cause cavity and caries.

• I was had a great doubt in the early days that why confused inflammatory cells are often chooses skin as a first choice ?

[yes, it chooses the skin initially] and come to brain and heart bit late then expected. but now I am clear that sun heat and **weather changes** will act as stimulation for confused inflammation so this chemical will come to skin and produce dermatitis or any of the skin related ailments so that less possibility of internal organ damage. but those who resides as Indore person keep their confused inflammatory cells inside the body so they will come with quick internal organ damage then those who are expose themselves to varies climatic changes.

•   A woman will suffer numerous uterine complaints due to **hormonal changes** and uterine monthly vascular changes attract this confused inflammatory cell towards uterus and start giving long standing trouble in the uterus . once the uterus is filled with enough confused inflammatory cells this cell now moves [non menstruating period] from uterus to vegina and fallopian tube and ovaries causes series disease over there .

•   a normal inflammation never accentuated by normal physiological hormonal changes during menses .many women have lots of trouble during menses pain, weakness other many organ symptoms like vomiting and diarrhea, migraine, visual disturbance so many symptoms [named as premenstrual tension ,,etc.] but this are not physiological but not a true inflammation also ,it is all confused inflammatory disorders.

•   A men or women will have piles or fissure due to **sitting** longer time (pressure) or **travelling** long distance or hard stool may invite the inflammation in the anal and rectal region. The normal inflammation will not come here to induce the inflammation for sitting long time.

•   Accentuation of **hyper function** of sweat glands will not induce inflammation (acne/pimples) all the pimples and acne are caused by confused inflammation . **Excess secretions** in any gland will not close the pores in any way. but in the chronic confused inflammation may cause closing the pores of the sweat and oily glands [comedones].yes of course the confused inflammatory cells will reach to the site where hyper functions of the body parts are happening since it is so sensitive because it is a fired cracker always just waiting for burst. A normal inflammatory cell is also a cracker but not get fired [it means not called for work in inflammation it happens only when real germ enters or injury entered then brain orders to involve in germ killing even now the cells are not allowed to work then another confused inflammatory cells arises [fired crackers].

•   A **pregnant** woman will have variety of disorders if she has confused inflammation cells and also this cell will damage the conceptual product and causes abortion or genetic/ hereditary disorder induced by this confused inflammatory cells .if a woman consult homeopath taking treatment for her diseases before pregnancy will reduce the possibility of hereditary disorders.

What is the use in studying in depth analysis of this confused inflammation nature ? This is the specific nature of the confused inflammation we have to consider this is as a NEW DIAGNOSTIC TOOL since laboratory test shows negative but patient will be in suffering due to this C inflammation so we have to clear the confused inflammation completely from the body by prescribing homeopathic medicine.

HOMEOPATHY DOCTOR USE THE REPORTORY WHICH WILL ASSIST TO SELECT THE MEDICINE IN FINEST AND MINUTE DETAILS ALSO.

Patient complain pain the little finger only in winter season – we can search in repertory and get the medicine.

According to my observation homeopathy doctors almost discovered confused inflammation already and they are having all tools to remove the confused inflammation from very longer time. BUT TRULY SPEAKING I DON'T GET ANY CLEAR-CUT EXPLANATION AND WHY WE HAVE TO DO THIS ? IS UNCLEAR AND THE ANSWERE IS NOT ACCEPTABLE BUT NOW I AM UNDERSTANDING IT.

Repertory is a collection of symptoms and remedy for the symptoms we can say repertory is the great tool to select the indicated medicine quickly.no need to memories all the symptoms of confused inflammation, even half matured confused inflammation will have nearly 50 and more symptoms and each and every patient is having different symptoms according to the present confused inflammation.so no need to worry REPORTERY will help you to find symptoms and appropriate right remedy

Example : Complaints after sun exposure.

Or head ache after sun exposure [symptoms] –

Nat mur,glonoinum,nat carb [medicine].

9. TENDENCY, DIATHESIS , RECURRENT DISEASE .

(This tendency, diathesis is 30 or 31st cherecter of confused and distracted inflammation).

A inflammation eradicates the possibility of disease and recurring disease, but confused inflammation gives lots of disease in a single person trouble them by repetation now and then. Confused inflammation is the cause for tendency and diathesis.

Tendency (prone to get disease especially same disease again and again) a person often falling sick in typical similar way . like recurrent infection, recurrent, boils, recurrent ulcers, recurrent gastric upset,,,,,,etc.

Why it is happening ? how we can cure this ? How we can prevent this ?

When a person falling sick, he will be recovered by natural immune power so never going to get fall sick again or again and again .

Confused inflammation is usually producing disease life long with available same chemical composition and blood cells.

Example : if the available C Inflammation chemical is a blood vessel damaging histamine and leukotrienes, then this will produce hemorrhage in one location, when we treat by allopathy medicine then that same chemicals (histamine and leucotriens) increase more and it will shift to other location develop bleeding here then allopathy treatment and then it shifts this is like HIDE AND SEEK play but with same diseases again and again - Hemorrhagic tendency.

This tendency may be disrupted due to getting additional confused inflammation and cells while getting allopathic treatment.

We are belived these many days the cause of recurrent disease could be the following but the true is confused inflammation.

Cause For Recurrent Disease

- But the recurrent illness of same disease is happening due to broken barrier and protective system in typical way.
- Second factor may be residing in the particular locality which is provoking the typical disease often (unhygienic place).

- occupational hazards or residing in unhealthy admosphere.
- Sometime it may be due to poor immunity.
- It may be due to deficiency of some body part improper growth which helps in recurrent disease [anomaly] like DNS or hormone or chemical reduction.

BUT THE TENDENCY AND RECURENCY IS MORE POWERFULLY CREATED BY CONFUSED INFLAMMATION THEN REST OF THE ABOVE.

Tendency To Infection :

We are really expose lots of virus and bacteria's everyday and body is killing them (normal healthy immune status) with or without our conscious so we are healthy. The day when this protection is lost then only, we really suffering with heavy infection. A bacteria or virus has to come inside and has to multiply and then only disease will attack us. but our body is not a incubator to allow the viral and bacteria growth & multiplication inside the body without any resistance. The entry itself is tough for the germs and even if it is come inside, then high raise of temperature, heavy neutrophil accumulation to swallow that, eosinophil must cells attack and crores of antibody will swallow and digest bacteria's and germs in general (read more in chapter 2). All this cell will liberate the chemicals and acids which is really giving trouble to survive inside the body, then how it is multiply and producing disease and even again and again (tendency) sometimes it resides inside without our knowledge for many years ? carrier state or latent period.how all this happens ?.

Mechanisam Of Recurrent Diseases, Infections :

Allopathy medicines collapses our inflammation and immune system so due to this the body is dumping by large amount of waste confused inflammatory [INFL] / Immune [IMN] cells, damaged dead tissues abnormally all over the body parts .This deposits still produce mild chronic weak INFL cells so this chronic inflamed area helps in germ entry inside the body due to loss of basic protective mechanism [example chronic nasal congestion, chronic bronchial congestion].

a real inflammation will protect us but confused inflammation will not protect us so germ entry is so easy.

Major entry of germs is through nasal and upper respiratory tract. So, any germ or dust and other foreign body enter from hereafter may not produce the regular inflammations, it is totally altered. This altered inflammation, immune response is due to acute infection or inflammation in the base of chronic confused inflammation will produce totally different INF/IMN RESPONSE.

Now the germ or foreign body enter into the nose. The inflammation starts quickly as ultrafast due to excess histamine in the nasal mucosa (only when patient is having regular use of anti-allergic) as well as all over the body (normal inflammation is germ entry then eosinophil, must cells visit the germ site and then release the histamine now the inflammation starts by neutrophil entry).The inflammation is give high fever, heavy sneezing,wheezing,cough looks like normal ALLERGIC ATTACK OR ASTHMATIC ATTACK RATHER THEN GERM INFECTIONS [TYPE-1 HYPERSENSITIVITY] Since the patient is regular anti allergic user he know himself or he will rush to hospital admission and take anti allergic,steroid,anti pyeretic,bronchodialter,anti biotics.So all the sufferings like fever,runining nose,cough,wheezing, everything alright but the virus escaped and multiply.

And again, excess sneezing,wheezing,excess cough all not a normal symptom of infections since all this altered symptomatology is caused by confused inflammation. This confused inflammation favores infections never resist the infection busy in doing and damaging healthy tissues rather then protecting.so the direction of killing germs is distracted and healthy tissues also destroyed by the confused inflammation so this site is become source of infection .so recurrent disease is possible always.patient will be irritated because he or she is highly protecting themselves but how they catch cold or infections is something irrelevant. It is not only germs alone produce cold dust,fumes,smokes,ac, fan,open air ,some times excess perspiration the hypersensitive person will respond to everything and produce disease.

The excess histamine or the confused inflammation will be started responding to dust and ac, cold, rain, climatic changes, water changes so that patient has to visit the hospital often or he has to avoid many things to escape even then the person fall in sickness often. So the confused inflammation gives many tendencies with or without infection. But anyway, infection is secondry. unless this confused inflammation is not cleared from the circulation all the disease will come and all possible infection will come.

Example :

• TENDENCY TO RECURENT THROAT INFECTION,
• TENDENCY TO COMMON COLD,
• TENDENCY TO RESPIRATORY ATTACK.

- TENDANCY TO RECURENT FEVER.
- TENDENCY TO SINUSITIS, eye infection and facial eruptions and so an.

When we Stop the normal inflammation at the level excess histamine release itself by anti allergic. Then germ will grow without any resistance additional histamine related chronic disease *Tendency to itch*. Patient used to have only itching the excess dryness will cause itching, sweating causes itching, ac makes itching, emotion causes itching, what happen to me. The pruritus and itching without eruption is again takes lots of anti-allergic, the problem will be temporarily stopped the itch will worse now so by this time patient nail will be eroded half due to scratching. His money also will be eroded in the same way to do varies test for even simple skin itching patient do many tests and again he will bye a disease by taking anti histamine.

The histamine spread across the skin and produce varies skin disease and with severe itching, to control that again the same anti allergic and anti inflammatory drugs prescribed so the histamine and along with confused inflammatory chemicals develop severe skin disease is so common in day to practice eczema, lichen planus,,,,etc. [prone to skin disease].

Tendency to to develop auto immunity :

Prescribing antibiotic will kill if the bacteria is the cause, antibody came for destroy the bacteria will now don't have work due to all bacteria's cleared by antibiotic but this antibody has duel function will start destroy the human body parts or cells more powerfully and continues AGGRESSIVE AUTOIMMUNITY due to bacteria's are killed by antibiotic but the antibody productions may not be withdrawn so that heavy antibody production without need since the antibiotic destroyed the bacterias now the antibodies will destroy the body parts where ever they stuck and start produce auto immune disease.THE ANTI-BODY CONSIDER OUR HUMAN BODY PARTS AS A ENEMY THEY CHOOSE TO ATTACK USUALLY ONGOING INFLAM-MATION SITES.the usual way of entry of the immune cells only after the commencement of the inflammation almost second or 3rd day but here the immune cells will participate in the first day itself here it does not kill or swallow the bacteria or virus but rather then it will just eat the dead body tissues damaged by the inflammation over there and stay within the inflammation sites to further damage.

Truelly speaking every disease in the humans except true inflammation and true infections all others or either auto inflammation or auto immune disease.discussed later.

Once the inflammation is distracted from the normal site then it start produce many auto inflammatory disease to humans.then auto immune diseases.

Tendency To Tumor:

Ointment application for any open wound will distract the fibroblast from the circulation to all over the body,this confused fibroblast cells along with other waste materials produces many tumors all over the body.

More then all other inflammatory cells and immune cells, excess fibroblast and gelatin material deposited in the Sino-nasal pathways and bronchus site causes resistance to the action of allopathic medicine like the antibiotic resistance, post inflammatory fibrosis in this case is too high due to vascular endothelial damage due to excess histamine, auto inflammation and auto immunity all will welcome the huge fibrinogen . this increased fibrinogen will reduce the elastic power of the lungs severe wheezing irreversible asthma and chronic bronchitis [lungs will have possibility of developing abscess and tumor here after] and start giving hard swelling. *Tendency to Induration and tumor within the respiratory tract and lungs.*

Mucosal linings of nose, sinus - tendency to polyp, turbinate swelling, this excess fibrosis not only limited to respiratory tract this will happen all over.

The body causes generalized fibrine and gelatin excess disease.

Scleroderma, atherosclerosis, cataract, keloid, lichenoid eruptions, nodule, small tumors, indurations of the glands [goiter and swellon nodules in the thyroid], lymph node induration and swelling, blocking the openings of the glands and duct causes pimples & sebaceous cyst, glaucoma, all the bodily functions in total collapse if the fibrin, collagen deposits are not stopped. The fibrin and collagen deposit within bone marrow causes poor blood cells productions and prone to get infections. Deposits inside the brain causes series, many psychological as well as neurological complaints, etc. *Tendency to get multiple disease.*

This fibrinogen and gelatin deposits increases resistance to over all medicines due to poor blood supply to affected area this poor blood supply reduce the normal protective functions so more possibility of easy thriving and multiplications of germs. *Tendency to get infection.*

Regeneration help in rebuild the infected. Inflamed site somehow normally. But when this regeneration is distracted with external applications and ointments then the accuracy will be low so the regeneration with different shape permanent swelling of the inflamed organ or tumor within the inflamed organ and if the distraction heavy the regeneration may happen other then required site (Tumor)

tumor will develop anywhere in the body.

Rebuilding of the injury of the nerve here end up with neuroma since available constructive material here, rebuilding of the endothelium will turn into vascular tumor ,of soft tissues as a lipoma , Bony tissues as osteoma of different locations **Tendency to tumor.** It will also produce the tiny to big tumors where ever the auto immune, auto inflammation happened so lead to massive generalized tumors like neurofibroma or generalized lipomas in multiple sites . if the rebuilding is stopped after one point then the tumor will not grow further.

If the rebuilding is disturbed by means of any medicines or due to the current infection also then the rebuilding order is not withdrawn which is helpful for continues tumor growth. Most of the neurofibroma and lipoma is growing tumor but very slowly. The tumor is formed well by utilizing few materials send for inflammation/immunity like fibroblast,gelatin,dead tissues and finally the rebuilding material.

10. INTERUPTING SELF REGULATION (AUTONOMIC NERVOUS SYSTEM)

Actually speaking this self regulation disturbance and recovering the functions suspended during inflammation related disease all has to be kept under confused inflammation disease since all are happen during that time but it will confuse you since all this disease may not have much involvement of confused inflammation cells and chemicals or immune cells so I have kept this after clear study of the confused inflammation.

Inflammation process has many steps in that reducing the functions of the gastro intestinal system and reducing the mobility in general is also happen. After completion of the inflammation the reduced functions has to be recovered successfully, but if we stop inflammation then we cannot expect the functions will return normally. Example : the patient loss the appetite long time and will not get his bowel move normally ,,,, etc.

Before proceeding that we have to see one more importand aspect of the automatic self regulation and feed-back machanisam to understand self regulation of the body.

The most important other body's work is finding and address the issues so according to the need either increase or decrease the function or secreation so maintaining the balance.

• When the person needs macro nutrients like carbohydrate or protein or need excess water or need more hormones all will be assessed and it has been solved by supplying them from storage and reduce excess elimination temprorily and increase the absorption. Once the need is fulfilled then slowly the recovery functions withdrawn like absorption is normalized and elimination allowed by normal level.

• In some situation the glands or the body parts get stimulus to work more or less according to the need and according to the situation. If the thyroid hormone is less then the TSH will secrete more this TSH will stimulate the thyroid gland to secrete more. Similarly, more less all the hormones and secretions of other enzymes and all metabolism is regulated and body is kept in balance to run the normal day to activity.

The most important work here, is, these hyper or hypo functions rectified and once the situation is normal then the regulatory functions will be withdrawn.

If you prescribe some hormone pills or injection iv fluids without considering the regulatory mechanism and feedback mechanism then these mechanisms will collapse and Diseases arises due to that

- Another automatic function is carried out during inflammation and infections these times other then redness, pain, swelling there is one more work is loss of functions like loss of appetite,reduced or excess bowel habit, increased or decreased thirst , increased metabolic rate,increased heart rate etc. We should not forget this when we treat the patient abrupt cessation of the inflammation will damage all this automatic function.

a judicial or biologically accepted intervention [medicine / surgery] is limited up to the borderline of the automatic zone of the living being, you can intervene by any way, where actually there is no automatic self regulation is there. We [doctors] are not allowed to intervene the automatic power zone of the living body.

We can offer carbohydrate rich food to the person if the body is need more carbohydrate according to the brain order to receive or absorb more carbohydrate [this is advisable].But since we have iv fluids and we have vitamins and other minerals , So, that we will inject that [we saved many life's with that] but aware that it is violation. We violate to save the patient life is acceptable.so don't use the direct administration of any minerals or vitamins ask them to consume. Oral rehydration solution is advisable, it is good to administer that then giving iv fluid. Iv fluid collapses the feedback mechanism.

we should not violate for sale the medicines.

What we discuss is something and extremely minor defect or not fall under defect at all in the medical field, but giving an insight that how is that also creating the disease.

Body need just a water so self-regulating power will retain the water by reduced the kidney excretion, increase the thirst and lot many other measures by order by the brain and altering hormones secretions [ADH],vaso dilation to the vital organ like brain,kidney,vaso constriction in the periphery like that etc. and etc.

We have to remember always there is a great natural doctor and more powerful doctor sitting inside and he started his duty now we can offer or advise the patient to drink enough water is the medico legal or biological intervention. This is what our limit.

What will happen if we administer iv fluids ?

You have to tell me now. What will happen to already ordered vasomotor action [vaso constriction or vaso dilation] any idea ?

We assume that all thinks will be withdrawn when water deficit is solved . You forgot that you are entering and disturbing the natural doctor's duty without any basic sense and science, you are crossing the borderline.

We need to be a smarter doctor we need to be a more scientific doctor where this violation needs where it is not need. where the violation is unavoidable.

n the majority of the major hospitals almost all the clinics in rural and almost all quacks happy in IV fluid injection. People in the rural may not consider you as a doctor when you not giving iv fluid injections.

I HOPE NONE OF THE DOCTORS FROM ALOPATHY CONSIDER IV FLUID ADMISSION MAKES THE DISEASE,BUT THEY KNOW VERY WELL SUDDEN EXCESS FLUID WILL OVERLOAD THE HEART AND OTHER DISTURB THE WATER BASE MECHANISAM,YOU ARE VERY WELL EDUCATED NO CONTRADICTION ON THIS PART,BUT YOU ARE NOT IMPLEMENTING YOUR EDUCATION TO THE PRACTICE YOU ARE JUST FORGOTS PARTICULARLY BRAIN NATURAL RECOVERING MECHANISAM, ADAPTING MECHANISAM, FEEDBACK MECHANISAM, SELF CONTROLE,

SELF REGULATIONS AND SELF ADJUSTMENTS.

Don't prescribe food supplements when the person is able to eat well-don't prescribe hormonal supplements without solving the diseased gland and don't advise iv fluids where there is no emergency or ongoing surgery,,,,,,,etc.

We again assume that prescribing vitamin and mineral supplements good for health it may not cause any harm [100 %] in recent days there is a awareness in the doctors community regarding hypervitaminosis and its complications and some adverse reactions, but 100 % not on the basis of self regulation or feedback mechanism they consider this is not right, their idea is regarding complications by excess dose. But I am discussing about every single dose is a violation of the biological rules. EAT WELL I WILL TAKE IF IT IS NEED OR I WILL NOT TAKE THAT is the body rule, direct injections not giving the choice to body to decide what they need.

Example:1

If thyroid low then brain receive the signal and produce excess TSH .then the excess TSH stimulate the thyroid gland to secrete the thyroid hormon to meet the hormone imbalance.and now sensor will dedect that and singals the brain.Brain will withdraw the stimulation. Now all are in good control.

If the thyroid is given directly without considering the internal adjustment and self regulation then the Thyroid stimulating hormone will not functions so at present 2 basic defect is possible

Thyroid stimulating hormone will not work since thyroid hormone took that place. [most of the cases]

If TSH started then hormone injection also administered then possibility of hormone excess will happen [rare cases].

Example:2

When the person is fasting his sugar level is reducing, the brain receives signal that alarmingly low blood sugar so that brain reduce the insulin secretions [this will allow the blood sugar within the blood will not reduce rapidly], increase the glucagon secretion this hormone convert the stored protein and fat into glucose.by doing this basic steps patient blood sugar maintained as normal after doing this the brain withdraw this effect.

Self regulation of the body without any medicinal or other intervention.

When we increase the sugar level with direct glucose it will reduce and collapse the self regulation so that either excess sugar level [type 2 diabetes mellitus] or the insulin secretion will be low level always causes type 2 diabetes with normal liver and pancreases.

injecting iv fluid NS in case of low bp [hypotension] causes normal bp but the regulatory mechanism will not be able to come to normal so that the bp will be high due to nerve regulation to increase the low bp is not withdrawn . or the axis for self regulation of blood pressure will be in collapse.

Example 3:

The appetite, stool, urine, sweating, generalized malaise and body pain, so many internal metabolisms which is involved during the inflammation and immunity all will be withdrawn by brain alone [after the inflammation is success].but when we prescribe anti inflammatory all this systemic upset during inflammations will be left unrecovered.

Self recovery of the appetite.

See here the brain act as a self appointed as doctor it identifies the defect and take the decision and solve the problem and coming to the normal position.

feedback mechanism this mechanism is greatly interrupted by many medications and IV fluids and other medicines which aimed to overtake the feedback mechanism .like administering glucose in case of low sugar, administering sodium and potasium or stopping an inflammation may also interfere the feedback mechanism involved in the inflammation process.

Prescribing hormonal pills will break the axis of feedback mechanisms. What are the possible problems or diseases arise due to interruption of the feedback mechanism ?

When we allow the disease to recover themselves then the body order to recover all the changes which is happen during inflammation including feedback mechanism in the process. But when we interfere then the feedback mechanism allowed to continue their functions and loss the control over the same.[most of the time feedback mechanism is revert to normal on its own ?]

-       Metabolic disorders,
-       hormonal disorders,
-       fluid and electrolyte balance (edema,hypertension, diabetes).
-       Acid, base balance
-       Heart rate and respiratory rate.
-       Appetite, thirst, defecations,
-       intestinal motility,
-       sweating,
-       all sensations [pain, temperature, tactile,] ,,
-       anxiety, moods, depressions,
-       all the body function like loco motion, hearing ,smelling ,vision, taste ,,,,,etc. .All are under the control of feedback mechanism, regulatory mechanism Etc.

Deficiency and excess will be identified and body will take an action to balance situation .Like maintaining the basic chemicals, hormones and minerals and metals in the body .

Excess of these will attract the body sensor will send the signal so there by body will identify the fault and bring the situation balances by reduce the secretary signal by stimulation of the nerves.

Similarly, if hypo hormonal status or less salt or chemicals in the body then the body will induce the gland to secrete or retain the loss of the salt or chemical or making compensatory works.

When we prescribe without considering the

body basic functions so that chemical or hormones excess or low then body will not do their automatic regulation functions as well as feedback mechanism ,so the feedback mechanism axis is disturbed.

The chemical or hormonal imbalance has been made by the body continually , the automatic regulation may not be withdrawn in some situation.

• An adaptive mechanism of body keeping the hyper function or hypo function by default due to long lasting demand.

[example low sugar or high sugar long times without coming to normal]

• The imbalance is happening due to diseased target gland [it means when the hypo thyroid status is happening due to excess demand then body will understand that then demand to produce thyroid gland to more but when the gland is under function due to damage in the gland then there is no possibility of balancing by producing excess hormone.

[Example -- so TSH will be elevated but thyroid hormone level may not come to normal So treat diseased thyroid no hormone supplement]

• There is no actual demand but the particular hormone or chemical minerals nutrient is excess / low in the circulation due to PRESENCE OF THE WEAK ORDER STILL PERSIST IN THE CIRCULATION, whenever the body has taken action for either regulate or supply the demand related functions. interfering this will cause permanent hypo or hyper functions due to interruption when regulatory function is in the mid.due to allopathic medicine.

• THE AXIS OF THE CYCLE IS

MISSED TO REGULATE DUE TO CONFUSION MADE BY DRUGS.

•   a diseased [confusion for CONTORLLING SYSTEM WILL PRODUCE THE SIMILAR LOSS OF CONTROLE MECHANISAM.-diseased controlling system like sensor got inflammation or indurations or neurological disease.

Autonomic nervous system :

Autonomic nervous systems has 2 componenets sympathetic and parasympathetics. These 2 components carry out their functions opposite to each other but occarding to the need of the body requierement so the body has kept in auto regulation (homeostasis).

The sympathetic nervous system, also known as the "fight or flight" system, increases energy expenditure and inhibits digestion. The following changes take place on activation of the sympathetic nervous system:

- Heart rate and cardiac muscle contractility increase
- The ciliary muscle relaxes, and the pupil becomes dilated for the betterment of far vision
- Bronchodilation of the lungs
- Decreased GI motility
- Decreased urine output
- Relaxation of the detrusor muscle of the bladder and contraction of urethral sphincters
- Increased secretions from sweat glands
- Increased blood flow to muscles because of relaxation of arterioles
- Dilation of coronary arteries
- Constriction of large arteries and large veins

- Increased metabolism
- Increased glucose production and mobilization by the liver
- Increased lipolysis within fat tissue.
- ejaculation
- Suppression of the immune system

These changes function to increase movement and strength. Stressful situations that threaten survival; exercise or the moments just before wakening are just a few examples of increases in sympathetic nervous system activity.

The parasympathetic nervous system, also known as "rest and digest," can be thought of as functioning in opposition to the sympathetic nervous system. Its functions include:

- Decrease in heart rate and contractility of cardiac muscle
- Constriction of the ciliary muscle and the pupil for near vision
- Increased secretion by lacrimal glands and salivary glands
- Increased gut motility, bronchoconstriction of the lungs
- Contraction of the detrusor muscle with the relaxation of urethral sphincters
- Glycogen synthesis by the liver
- Swelling of the clitoris and erection of the penis

· Activation of the immune system

The parasympathetic nervous system does not appear to exert much control over vascular tone as the sympathetic nervous system does.

When the inflammation or other functions happen when we interrupt inflammation, then the suspended / accelerated or normally involved autonomic function left unrecovered in many cases.This will lead on two many diseases.

Appetite,digestion, fever ,sleep ,sex ,sweating ,heart rate ,blood pressure, endocrine secretions all this function are frequently affected , after many acute illnesses . But this symtoms either recover spontanuesly after few months to years but most of them suffering with that (I have classified this under (failure of loss of function in inflammation) . The autonomic nervous system falls in frequent trouble when interrupting inflammation,its functoin left unrecovered often .

The disease discussion under autonomic disease is very less then what we observe in day to day clinical practice and most of the symtoms like constipation and mild to moderate sleep disturbance and loss of hunger all or patient ignore to seek the medical attension except in childrens (parents are observing this complaints in childrens and seek the medical attension especillay in eating and toilet habbits) many autonomic symptoms are missed easily including sexual complaints. Hypo tension is considered and observed as autonomic dysfunction easily but hypertension is not been suspected as autonomic dysfunction.

Homeopathy prescription largly based on this

autonomic nervous system recovery.

11.TISSUE RESSISTANCE (OR) POOR UTILISATION ?

The confused inflammation circulating all over the body produce the tiny,subtle changes to the major destruction to the tissues in the body.In this process early functional change causing tissue utilization disorders and there by many disease (type-2 diabetes, peripheral neuropathy ,, etc).

Inflammation is there effectively but the result is not good as expected, need more and more powerful inflammatory cells for completing minor task. So, when completing the task, it gives lots of post inflammatory damage which is not normal (abcess and induration,granuloma ,,,etc). This is happening because the utilization of inflammation is not effective in fighting site, need massive dose and more powerful giant inflammatory cells. All is happening due to abnormal deposition as a continuation of the inflammation (papular amyladosis),deposition of the dead tissues and waste materials.

Micro or macro Indurations is happened due to poor clearance of previous inflammation so that collection of weak inflammatory cells and dead, damaged tissues, micro deposits in the vascular channels including lymphatic vessals, leads many subtle and majaor disease but we does not suspected this could be a disease until it causes severe damages then also it may be diagnosed as some other disease (the atheroma of blood vessal causes hypertension we diagnose that at the end even we have to fond bothe atherosclerosis and simultanues hepyertension and heart attack then this atherosed blood vessal has given lot many disease we never probed in that aspect), which hinders normal blood supply poor nerve conduction and poor signal perceptions of sensors and poor tissue utilization of insulin / antibiotic / all allopathic medicines / all body basic preventive measures like inflammation and immunity. All are delayed and underfunctions. especially periphery of the extremities.

The peripheral circulation is the ideal site for developing confused inflammation especially in the foot, hands causes poor wound healing this will happen irrespective of diabetes. Peripheral neuritis is the pure confused inflammation disease not due to vitamin deficiency but sure vitamin injection relives the pain temporarily and in early neuritis,similarly chronic silent vasculitis,chronic tissue inflammations ,,,, etc.

THE INSULIN RESISTANCE IS HAPPENINING IN THE SAME WAY. IT IS POOR UPTAKE OF INSULIN DUE TO INSULIN PATH TO TISSUE IS HINDERED THEN INSULIN RESSISTANCE MINOR. The nerves lost its sensor to to sening the glucose saturation and reply ,vessals and tissues is under slow,chronic confused inflammation so they have defect in precepting the real insulin and other tissues. The confused inflammation is making tissue damage but extremely minor but widespread (MODERATE CAUSE FOR INSULIN POOR UP-TAKE). So this abnormal but functioning cells loss some of the thir functions will slowly produce the disease it may produce any changes or any disease in future it may be poor utilization of the sugar and minerals and vitamins or poor bodily functions lack of producing pigmnets or loss of sensations or pains suppose if the confused inflammation chemicals too heavy to make maximum cell injury then it may be appear as ulcer or sloughing.

Not only poor insulin supply, poor inflammation utilisation, poor blood supply (micro vasculitis previus to the proper diagnostic vasculitis) to the cells leads to starving for basic nutrition too , hence prescribing VITAMIN B 12 OR other supplements will not help in improving the disease if the induration enough to block the whole blood supply then gangrene or cellulitis will come, numbness and tingling sensations precede this attack many years before. A gangrene is preventable many years before a cellulities preventable many years before.poly neuritis or mono neuritis is not a inflammation it is confused inflammation giving warning that I am spoiling the periphery nearly 10 or 15 years before tha gangrene and cellulitis going to develop. (EXCEPTION THERE IS A GANGRENE WHICH IS HAPPEN AFTER SUDDEN BLOCK IN THE ARTERY OR GANGRENE DUE TO ACCIDENT).

I was observed this fact. Not the guess work. you can also
easily observe this fact near the chronic inflammatory site or infectious sites.

a chronic nasal congestion and sinus will produce the micro indurations and there by poor blood supply and poor insulin uptake, poor inflammation response in the face and scalp. this is so simple to observe again to develop dia-

257

betes you need this local insulin poor uptake has to become generalized to develop diabetes mellitus type-2 (I am guessing that this poor insulin utilization in multiple sites is enough to develop diabetes then all the tissues in the body especially in few vital organs like brain and lungs, kidney). so, the sugar level in the blood will slowly increases despite anti diabetic, indicates tissue injury increases slowly.

So, diabetes is an adapting mechanism, if the poor utilization is the cause for raise of blood sugar but anyway the uptake may not go to solved then the raise of blood sugar will further increase due to cry of cells.prescribbing simply anti diabetic or INSULIN directly help in clear the sugar will increase peripheral tissue low sugar so the tissues hypoglycemia will in turn increase the sugar level more.

YOU NEED LOTS OF SKILL AND OBSERVING CAPACITY AND BROAD SENSE OF BASIC MEDICAL KNOWLEDGE TO COMPREHEND THAT REMOTE POOR INFLAMMATORY RESPONSE THEN NEAR INFLAMMATORY SITE DAMAGE. It means doctors understand and comprehend that inflammation related complications happening adjuscent to the inflammation site he is not yet aware that inflammation can travel along the circulation and produce genaralised and widespread changes to all over the body without having any signs and symptoms of inflammation, not even pain will happen to this tissueas it very and very minor subtle changes but everything comes obviyas and shows their presence initially by sensation (burnining pain in the soles or tingling sensation in the palms and soles) poor inflammation response like cellulitis and gangrene and poor wound healing . It the macro diagnosable disease occurs and we are treating again and creating more confused inflammation but all over the body micro inflammation is happening all over the body that is the cause for many diseases including diabtes.

Suppose if the inflammation happens with less inflammation signs then they consider this is something else then considering that this also an inflammation. This is also inflammation but completely lack of inflammatory signs.

you need great inquisitive and logic and reason-oriented person to comprehend that why few people having tiny prickly heat like rashes in the face as a pimple but some one is developing deep scared and keloid formation in the face ? if you raise this question why this difference then you will have the answer but you reading and remembering all are acne.then how ill you do research.

All caused by usage of anti-inflammatory drugs by allopath's and applications of lots of external ointments and medicinal preparations .the all this change are not happening within a day it may takes few months to few decades to develop.

The chronic nasal congestion is causing many diseases but this nasal congestion and sinus is again caused by misguided inflammation so sinus or nasal inflammation not caused by simply infections, misguided inflammation is the cause.

MY OBSERVATION -- The time when type 2 diabetes is develops simultaneously the nerve, kidney , eyes , blood vessels ,,,,,etc. damage is beginning in the same time.so diabetic complications are may be slightly exaggerated by excess sugar but even if the diabetes is not there these changes will come. All the diagnosis falls under type 2 diabetes complications is produced by or caused by modified, misguided, confused , passive inflammation not because of diabetes [including infections].

We can understand the poor utilization when the delayed wound healing as well as ulcers or gangrene formed in the toes and fingers.

12. DIAGNOSIS OF CONFUSED INFLAMMATORY CHEMICALS AND CELLS

Diagnosis of confused inflammation

The confused inflammation can be easily identifiable by clinical ground like based on signs and symptoms and past and treatment history. Since I have given clear cut explanation what is normal inflammation and what is confused inflammation cherecters (in the 4th chapter). So, it is easy to differentiate normal and confused inflammation easily. but how to detect the confused inflammation by lab test. What ever it may be the test we do till date for all chronic disease all the tests are helpful detec the confused inflammation but only thing we may not know that we are searching the confused inflammation. But very importand factor is as if now there is no clear-cut demarcation of some cells what is confused inflammation chemicals and which one is normal inflammation chemical.Like rust will mimic all the characters of iron but when coming to functional utility we will use iron is normal, rust is abnormal.

Laboratory will give the same report, there is no special reports like normal inflammation to confused inflammation.Infact the chemicals almost same only.

This mimicking in nature of inflammatory cells giving great trouble and confusion to the medical profession this many days.when doctors identifying neutrophil,lymphocytes in the healthy infectious site as well as non infectious site (auto immune disease) but the infectious site has true inflammation cells but the auto immune site is having confused inflammation cells ,immune cells but how we can differentiate this ?.Read the character of the confused inflammation cells/chemicals chapter then you will have an idea about how to solve this confusion.

WE SEARCHED AND FOUND THE CONFUSED INFLAMMATION EVEN WITHOUT KNOWING THAT. IT MEANS ALMOST ALL THE DISEASES ARE CONFUSED INFLAMMATION THEN ALL THE DIAGNOSTIC CRITERIA DEFINE THIS CONFUSED INFLAMMATION ALONE BUT WE ARE NAMING IT WRONGLY.ACTUALLY WE NO NEED SPECIAL TOOL FOR DETECT THE CONFUSED INFLAMMATION WE NEED TO UNDERSTAND THAT.

The confused inflammatory cells and chemicals are found already but it has been there in different names Type – 1 , Type – 2 ,Type 3 and type 4 .hypersensitivity and related inflammatory abnormalities is actually indirectly revealing of the presence of confused inflammation and causing disease there from. But Confused inflammation is the cause for all hypersensitivity.discused earlier in this book.

Autoimmune disease reveals that there are no external factors causing the disease. Diseases are caused by our own body cells [but the auto immune disease are not caused by auto killing its actually forced destruction due to improper clearing or spread of confused inflammation , so the proper name for auto immune disease is Doctors made auto immune disease.

- Crp elevation indicates the presence of confused inflammation.

- ESR elevation indicates the presence of confused inflammation.

- IGE elevation of other immunoglobulin elevations other than acute true inflammation indicates C inflammation.

- Abnormal blood cell count other than true inflammation is indicated confused inflammation presence.especially in chronic disease.

- All autoimmune disorder marker everything reveals presences of confused inflammation.

- Any marker which is indicates the presence of any chronic disease reveal the chronic confused inflammation.

- All the tumor marker indicates c inflammation in the body.

- The presence of the immune complex indicates confused inflammation.

- The presence of immune cells does not show confused immune dis order,since it may be normal immune protection but immune cells present in chronic disease confirm confused immune disease.

The presence of immune cells in the acute inflammation with severe destruction rather then protection indicated confused inflammation.

• All the chronic disease falls under confused inflammation so,the test which confirms that disease proves that confused inflammation.

Here the main issues are there is no difference between confused inflammation chemicals to normal inflammation chemicals and cells otherwise everything is ok.

There is no great struggle in identifying the presence of confused inflammation when reading characters of the inflammation. An only an extremely minor part of the disease falls under TRUE INFLAMMATION rest of all confused inflammation only.in future the rapidity and universal application of allopathic domination you will see only confused inflammation there is no true inflammation.

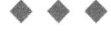

PART-3. General pathology continuation

13. Infection

14.genetics

15.vitamines and minerals

13. UNDERSTANDING ABOUT THE INFECTIONS

(also read book written by me – Prevention and homeopathic treatment for communicable disease)

Before going to read the infection disease first try to understand about the infection. The reality of infections is manipulated by current medical trend so they decide to panick us all time. This help to sale the medicines. They distract us to focusly clear the infection but direct us to buy medicine for every infection. This is a time to take a decision what exactly happeninig in and around us and how to tackle the infections. The one comfortbale news while we treat the infection atleast we know the cause of the disease and we can prevent it. But non-infectious disease the cause of the disease till date we don't know but I have solved that issues.

It is only the patient fault that we loss our life / our relative with infection. Yes, it is very clear that how the infection spread and cause the illness but unfortunately, we are not known that. Then what is the duty of the doctor other then save the patient. It is better to prevent the disease since we know the cause. But we do opposite every time when we get infection we rush to the hospital. In this way only patient trained in India and even most of the developed country. Either it is harmless virus or harmfull virus that is not true the truth is how you are going to handle this what is your body immunity is decides that say for example if you have weak immunity then the disease will shows it worst face and if you have best immunity then disease have very less clinical manifestation you will recover without any medicine. So, what ever it may be , would you like to take a risk of getting infection or you want to keep away from infection. Since every infection have some impacts upon the human body death or chronic disease risk is there and medicine complication and losing more money everything is there but what will do how to tackle this. You no need to study a medical course but try to understand how to keep your self away from infections. This is what my belief till today a mother is thinking that pneumonia is caused by some unknown reason for her but she does not know that she can prevent save her son life without any fever or infection by keeping their environment and surrounding is clean because we are all focused diabetes and hypertension and cancer meanwhile we suffer this communicable disease (this is also importand but you are learning something unnessory and you have less role here). Infection is preventable. If your family member is losing their life a patient attender and relatives and others are having major part , you can prevent the pneumonia and you can prevent any infection then why are you beliving doctors and others ,first give your part of saving the child and your relative life then also there is the possibility of infection in that case the responsibility is going to doctors. I am sure that we can prevent many numbers of infection by knowing how the disease arises. Try to learn how the infection spreads and how to protect and what is the source of the infection. What is the use of learnining about prevention aspect of the disease ? 1. We can prevent the infection.

2. We no need to loss the life of our loved one 3. We are safe from devolopping the drug related complications like side effects 4. We save the money (we are reducing hospital expencess 5. Very importantly when we treating the infection by allopathic drugs from that day onwards we are getting non infection diseases (this is importand research I have did) non infection disease created only when we go and to take the treatment to allopathy doctors or when we take self medicine (allopathy) then we have non infection disease.

So, by preventing infection disease you and your family members safe from non communicable disease and communicable disease.

(I have written a book about infections and how to prevent the infections and how to cure safely by homeopathy medicine – prevention and treatment of infectious disease.)

Infection prevention is many level first is prevent the infection source like (safe water, hygine food preparation , food storage godown hygine ,food and water preparation with hygiene , healthy unpolluted surrounding environment, neat and clean home environment, then personal neatness and cleanness, caring our relatives in sick with care and with best knowledge about how to take care without getting the sickness , helping our office and public property infection free , we have have to help in blocking the infection spread, we have to learn we should not spread the disease to others because when we have anu infection our family members are having first risk then anyone else. Sexually active couples spread the disease from one another so easily and rapidly and mother child bond will make so quickly infection from child to parent and parent to child and we all take the infection to spread to the public. So please help in break the infection chain it is very important)

Crowded living, crowded gathering, multi sexual partners, drug abuse, alcoholisam, chronic illness, organ failures, patient under steroids, orgon transplanated person all are having high risk of infection eventhough you do much precautions you may fail in escaping from infection and to-gether I am adding one more new addition that is confused inflammation when you have confused inflammation you will have high chance of dangerus complications of the disease. Since the body immunity is collapsed so the infection will spread faster .

So, if you have infection don't stop the fever ,don't stop the runining nose don't try to stop the inflammation because that will help the virus or bacterial multiply inside the body. Take help of homeopathy if you really suffering more and connot able to tolerate the infection symptoms. Try to do accessory way to reduce the suffering like sponging to reduce the fever, taking ORS to rhydrate ,like that. Try to learn some homeopathy remedy to take in an emergency situation.

After the invention of microscope and discovered microbial agents the allopathic doctor's world fully occupied with germ invention. The whole of the allopathic texts and their medicine everything is fully focused with bacteria and germs. They search the cause of unknown disease in the same aspect it means they expect even the non communicable diseases could be infection their search is in the same way. Based on this germ theory there are many evolution and revolution was happened in the medical field. Hygiene was given high priority, Germicide and antibacterials was discovered. This penicillin antibacterial was given effective results in the treatment. Vaccinations are prepared based on germ theory and homeopathy theory; this was given excellent results. The major killer diseases like small pox was eradicated and ugli and contaminated nature of leprosy is been eradicated many other killer diseases effectively controlled. Polio is nearing to say zero attack. But almost this story was been achived many decades before but we earn the money by repeted advirtisment of the same. Eventhough doctors reading the cause of the disease multi factorial they expect all the disease infectious. This is because allopathy trained and well equipped in becaterial hunt.

Failure In Killing Bacteria ?

Eventhough many bacteria controlled well ; patient recovered from illness but the patient still loss their life with bacterial infections. The antibacterial is not working the bacteria multiply inside and they loss their life. In septecemia why ? allopathy belvied that that is antibacterial resistance but I am saying this is because of the confused inflammation explaned in detail in the prevention of infection disease. So anti bacterial eventhough bacterial infection we canot able to save the life of the patient many crores of the patient die each year in septecemia.

No Medicine For Most Of The Virus ?

Doctors not reveling this factor to the public or they are not preparing the patient about how to prevent the disease.

Bacterial disease we have achived success what about virus ? . Doctors here in virus accepting one terminology like SELF LIMITING it means if we allow the disease then the patient recover. The patient cure himself with his natural immune power.

Why we have to allow the virus it may kill us please do something ? sorry we don't have any medicine for killing the virus. So, when we do not have medicine, we observe the diseases does not harm us. when we have medicines for the germ then we have to advirtise you will die if you not eat this medicine.In this world there are thousand virus this virus attacking us unfortunately there is no medicine at all for kill virus humans are still alive it means we have enough protection even after many folds destruction of immune system by allopathic medicine. This is what nature success story.

DR.Hahnemann says that germs creating disease due to weakness of vital force (failure of protecting system or immune system in the body) secondary to inflammation and immune failure. This theory is strongly supported and evidenced by living human being even after many viral attacks. It means we have better protective mechanisam it will kill them when our inflammation and immune system is in good condition. But when we do not have enough fighting system, we may fall illness,disease over come us make the chronic disease.

Many laks of doctors are there now, but still we have the same fear about virul illness and other infections even in the modern era. Allopathy is too busy in celebrating 1 or 2 viral disease elimination. No change even this many years. Why are you panic about hepatitis ? , why are you panic about the flu every year ? why are you panic about every minor ailment. I have appointed you to save me but

I am getting fear even when your presence. what you did to protect me ?. This many thousand of virus are you going to prepare vaccine for these thousand viruses.

Homeopathy gives the confidence that viral illness is easily over come by our body itself and at the same time when the virus is over come us, we can fight with homeopathy medicine sure you will recover safely, because homeopathy is highly accentuating the inflammation and immune system work along with natural healing power so no fear about the virus. The epidemics are so common and so easy so frequent but when we start fearing about this, we need to fear about this every year and even every month till death. But this fear is created by allopathy as if we will dye from virul illness or germ illness.

HOMEOPATHY SAYS NO FEAR ABOUT THE GERMS HOMEOPATHY SUPPORTS YOU AND SAVE YOU.

There are many other groups of worms and para-site homeopathy having limited scope in controlling the worms and parasite it means less effective, there are many ways to prevent the parasitic and worm infections but when we suffer with parasitic infection, I recommend take allopathic medicine. worm infestation is happening con-taminated food and drinks the preventing open defeca-tion and safe healthy food prepareation and good hygienic water prevnt the worm infestation. Amebiasis is spreading through contaminated food items so maintaining hygiene in the food prevent the amebic dysentery as well as bacillary dysentery.

We have enough protective power but removing this protection by surgery or collapsing immunity and in-flammation then we are unsafe to face any infection so need to recover this collapsed system first and education is need to the doctors to not to remove the immune organs for simple reasons (like no medicine so surgery).

- Allopthy doctors having no idea, why some time antibacterial works wonderful but few of them not so effectively recovered from the bacterial infections?
- Why some people only will have series infections all of a sudden which spread so rapidly.
- How the virus is staying inside the body without any struggle as if a guest? How the body and virus is compromise each other never fight with that.

Infections are divided as common and rare infections, but basically infections to human itself has to be rare because he is born with hyper protection in his body. Even though If the infection is happening to the particular person, it will be limited to particular site itself, may not allowed to spread all over the body and may not be allowed to multiply and produce severe infections, all is limited and controlled by inflammation and immunity. When the person is affected by an infection, he will recover on his own without any medicine. Most of the time doctors panicky when the person getting fever and he tries to prescribe something and especially he try to give antipyretic he believes that stopping fever, which solve all the infections [Indian doctors] he feels comfortable only he has to prescribe some anti-bacterial so the patient will be safe (irrespective of viral or bacterial no test in many cases) so he collapses patient and patient goes to ICU most of the time.

Antipyretic and anti allergic and antibiotic is the

classical prescription for most of the allopathic doctors in India. if a patient suffering with viral fever all these 3 drugs unnecessary and put the person in severe trouble.

Prescribing the above combination during an epidemic viral attack is something hyper foolishness makes lots of death in India. But doctors are not leaving this combination.The allopathi never accept their incabablities and ask others to do their works.

Doctors believing that tonsil or adenoid is the source of the infection , removing that will save the patient life [in India] tonsillectomy and adenoidectomy is the all-time duty of the surgeon. In the list appendix also carry the equal marks that lymph gland also removed almost maximum people.

They know,there is no effective medicine for the virus and to some bacteria's in allopathy. But feels happy only after prescribing something to the patient to collapse the inflammation they never allowed a self healing or curing power.Doctors are having highest faith, even the severe viral illness will be cleared by antibiotic and antipyretic in India.

NO QUESTION AND NO WARNINING TO DOCTORS from INDIAN MEDICAL ASSOCIATION.STOPPING SNEEZING, STOPPING RUNINING NOSE, STOPPING THE COUGH, STOPPING THE FEVER IS THE TOP MOST WORK OF MOST OF MBBS AND MD in India.

THERE IS NO REASERCH ABOUT THE DISEASE AND NO WORRY ABOUT THE PATIENT SUFFERING. THEY DO MORE REASEARCH HOW WE CAN CREAT MORE MONEY.

When you allow the fever to run germs will not multiply, when you not remove the tonsil germ will not go inside, when you don't prescribe anti allergic then running nose will try to wipe the virus to outside cough will try to expel the bacteria or virus along with sputum so all immune and inflammation will carry out their function. patient will be recovering normally. MAKING THE BETTER WAY FOR GERMS MULTIPLYING.DOCTORS ARE EDUCATING THE PATIENT TO TAKE ANTY PYRETIC AND ANTI ALLERGIC AS PREVENTIVE FOR VIRAL FEVER ? AND FLU ?

many people in india is carry paracetamol or cetrizen as preventive medicine for viral illness or acute febril attack this is what allopathy doctors teached to the public. PREVENTIVE MEDICINE ? what kind of prevention is this.

NON-OF THE DOCTORS IN INDIA OR IN THE WORLD IS REQUESTED OR ASKED TO HANDLE THE CRITICAL CASES BY AYUSH DOCTORS. (OF VIRAL ILLNESS OR OTHER ILLNESS WHERE ALLOPATHY NOT HAVING ANY MEDICINE FOR THE DISEASE).

Prescribing steroids, prescribing anti allergics and pray for the pneumonia [infection of the lung parenchyma] has to recovered without death. When you make so much confused inflammation this will prevent normal inflammation response, but will happen destructive inflammation response leads to death.

Say that HIV And AIDS is dangerous to the humans but make almost all children non HIV but AIDS Patient .Yes no tonsil, no adenoid, no appendix, removed many lymph node and remaining lymph node made hard and indurated all the lymph producing organs or failed child is bathing in steroid everyday and taking anti allergic as food for 3 times a day inhalers and nebulizers so a child made as ACQUIRED IMMUNE DEFICIANCY BY ALOPATHIC MEDICINE.so what is the surprice in the death of the children due to pneumonia,other lower respiratory tract infections and diarrheal disease or flue etc.

Every mild infection considered as mega life-threatening complication and make heavy drug exposure for the children.

Most of the Indian children are under chronic medication for some of the other complaints.2 episodes of acute bronchitis with sputum collection and if the child struggle for breath then they put on life long inhalers [bronco dialer and steroids]? or else regular nebulizer. why continues medication for acute bronchitis its all magic of Indian allopathic doctor.

(why I am using the word Indian allopathic doctors, I hope this may not happen in other country there is some genuine doctors at least they practice what system teached to them.But here everything for money only).

Allopathy consider that infections is possible by expose yourself to germs and need to clear by appropriate germicide, there is no idea if there is no medicine for some specific infections like viral.

If your body protective mechanism failed then the germs will multiply and give disease otherwise it is hard to enter inside the body and tough to survive and multiply inside the body and absolutely no possibility of germs living inside the body it will be cleared by inflammation and immunity. When the immune and inflammation system is in good condition there is no necessary for antibiotics and we should not worry about that.

- When the confused inflammation is rich it favors infections.
- When the lymph nodes are failed in the particular site then the possibility of the infection spread will be more.
- The body can able to produce

effective antibiotic [antibody] for each and every germ so it is unnecessary to worry about the germs. Our work is too making sure that the system is working properly or not.

•   DEFINE THE POST HOSPITAL STATUS LIKE PATIENT IMMUNE SYSTEM IS IN GOOD CONDITION THERE IS NO NEED OF ANY OTHER MEDICINE FOR FUTUER INFECTION OR mention patient needed massive antibiotic to recover and poor immunity so please consult a homeopath and improve your immune system.

•   When the immunity is poor patient never recover on his own his prognosis is very poor.

•   Deficiency of lymphoid organ makes the infection more and spread easily

•   Taking anti inflammatory, anti allergic makes easy spread and multiplication of the infection.

•   Steroid reduce the over all immunity so possibility of infection is more, so please consult homeopath and try to stop steroid.

All the chronic infections are fall under chronic confused inflammation

(exception is parasites and the pathogen really bigger size and need some medicinal support to expel like worm,unknown regular intake of contaminated food or water or other germ source.)

All the simple infections have been complicated much taking longer time to recover has to considered due to base of confused inflammation.

A virus staying inside the organ as reservoir [carrier] or host is indicating the failure of the inflammation system or the attempt to clearing by inflammation has been distracted by anti inflammatory drugs so once a foreign body, now made as guest to human by allopathic medicine.

Vaccinations Are Making Complications ?

Vaccinations are following pure natural laws to arouse a immune system against the specific viral infections.here dead or live germs given to a individual so now the immune cells will be formed to kill the germs.so this is the way the individuals are getting immunity against the germs. IN THIS WAY EVEN THE PERSON NATURAL EXPOSURE TO GERMS ARE GETTING IMMUNITY BUT WE GIVE THIS EARLIER AND WE WANT TO MAKE SURE WE HAVE PROTECTION AGAINST PARTICULAR NOXITIUSE VIRUS .THERE ARE SOME VIRUS IF ONCE ENTERES THIS WILL CAUSE LIFE LONG PROTECTION.

ONCE THE ARTIFICIALLY ENTERED GERMS ARE KILLED BY A IMMUNE SYSTEM THERE IS NO POSSIBLITY OF DEVELOPPING COMPLICATIONS. BECAUSE THE INFLAMMATION AND IMMUNITY HERE STARTED AS USUAL NATURAL VIRAL ENTRY AND THEN INFLAMMATION AND IMUNITY WILL KILL THE VIRUS THEN THE PROCESS END NATURALLY.so possibility of developing confused inflammation or immunity is nill.so no worry and suspecian about the vaccinations it is safe.Fever or diarrhea or other minor infections like syndrome immediately after the vaccinations are says that your vaccine is working well again this is not a fearing factor.

The impurity,expired vaccines complication I connot give guaranty.

Autisam is a confused inflammation disease never related with vaccination.

14.GENETICS

Genetics are more and most interesting and devolping field. When we doesnot know anything about even common, simple, minor ailments. why doctors are beliving and showing intrest in genetics ? because the whole world of doctors does not know the cause for the disease but unfortunately the allopathic text book is trying to explain the cause by a chromosome defect hence the genetic is getting more popular.

Sure there are diseases are caused by genetics but most of the allopatgic text try to explain every disease through genetics , this explanation is absolutely fake because the cause is allopathic medicine not the gene.But after reading my text book about cause of the disease, doctors will belive what I said.Then they will ignore genetics since they know they are giving medicine that will also cause disease (side effects).

When explainabale cause is here , then what is the necessary and demand to read and expect more from genetics ? .

Allopathic doctors at present beliving someone will find the cause for disease,and that cause will be the genetics.

The human are having exceedingly good gene but allopathi docotors are creating disease.Genetic study is highly welcome, but read my book and you will comprehend how many more diseases are going to be pending to genetic research its highly less number since all the diseases explainable by varias day to day medicinal preascription and its main and side effects.

15.VITAMIN / MINARAL DEFICIANCY DISORDERS

V itamin deficiency may not produce inflammation or confused inflammation. So, except a few signs and symptoms remaining a major part of the current vitamin deficiency disorders all are fall under confused inflammation alone. Since doctors do not know the confused inflammation, they started trying to find cause for the disease, they try to fit with something that they think as a cause. But vitamin deficiency may not produce confused inflammation. vitamin deficiency produces minor discomfort or functional disability.but what we read as vitamin deficiency are really a inflammation symptoms. A VITAMIN OR MINERAL IS A NUTRIENT NOT A GERM OR POISONOUS PRODUCT, so it's impossible to develop inflammation especially deficiency of the particular vitamin or mineral.

Or the deficiency or excess of particular vitamin triggers the confused inflammation to develop the disease in the vitamin dominant zone (particular part of the body like VITAMIN A DEFICIENCY INVITE THE CONFUSED INFLAM-MATION TO THE EYE, VITAMIN C DEFICIENCY INVITE THE CONFUSED INFLAMMATION TO THE GUMS).

Mineral deficiency and excess produce the functional changes but it may not produce any chronic inflammation or the ulcers or tumors.

Both vitamin and mineral deficiency blamed as the cause of disease in many diseases due to unaware of the wide range of unimaginable diseases creating the power of confused inflammation. Again, when administrating vitamin or minerals gives better relief to the patient all this considered as VITAMIN AND MINERAL DEFICIENCY CAUSES chronic diseases.

A true inflammation never considers that vitamin or mineral deficiency as a foreign body or enemy. Because true inflammation comes and takes active participation if there is a true enemy. Because you are reading and treating a confused inflammation as vitamin and mineral deficiency.

THIS CHAPTER WRITTEN FOR THE PURPOSE OF UNDERSTANDING AND CLARIFY OURSELF FROM INFLAM-MATION CHERECTER FROM OUR MISCONCEPTION AND THIS EXPLANATION GIVES CLARITY.

Without our knowledge we use many shields to protect ourself from escaping the real facts . like the person is had that illness ? we reply since his sugar level is more . why had this illness he had poor vitamin .why this disease since he is having genetic abnormality ? we used all this shield to protect our self from say some excuse. We don't know the real cause so we belived who ever and what ever they said we belived and accepted blindly. this is not necessary anymore.

16. CLASSIFICATION OF DISEASE

Classification of disease

A. Adynamic disease : accidents , mechanical injury.

B. Dynamic disease : this is major disese category.
1.true inflammation and immunity (infection disease)
2.confused inflammation disease (non communicable disease)

C. Nutritional deficiency & disease due to food excess

All these three disease groups are a major classification of disease

Adynamic disease - Accident

Emergency management in all the system is same.

Accident is the one in which the disease occurs due to hit or fall so the disease not arising naturally but in dynamic disease diseases occurring naturally.It means by deranging the vital force in other simple medical word diseases in a dynamic category disease arises due to inflammation and immune system failure.

More or less the treatment approach in any school either allopathy or homeopathy a fracture has to be unite by either open or close reduction. A open wound is switchered. a cut muscles or nerves or sheets and tendons again kept in porper place repaired where ever need switchering all are no difference of opinion to save the life by homeopathy or allopathy.

A swither is switcher, there is no homeopathy or allopathy switchering of the wound. If a person completely dehydrated and going to collapse due to hypo tension need emergency iv fluid management there is no difference of opinion in allopathy.

Heavy maceration and laceration and fecal and mud soiling and contaminations everything will be there so antibiotic is need since wound is massive surface and the protective systems not enough to hold the open thread to infections so legal advice to consume antibiotic is ideally supported here.

All other life savings drugs what ever it may be invented to save the life without worrying about the future complications is fully recommended and supported only on the basis of do maximum to save the life.

Either homeopathy or allopathy rule for save the life is same.

Artificial respiration, blood transfusion, everything and everything to save the life in an emergency situation is common for both homeopathy and allopathy.

Allopathy system and surgery is supported massively in a mechanical injury and disease.

Dynamic disease

All the disease arises other then accidents fall in this category. It is further divided into two.

1.Communicable disease (infection disease).

2.Non communicable disease (other then infections excluding accidents).

3. nutritional deficiency disease and disease due to dietery excess.

1.COMMUNICABLE DISEASE

Communicable diseases are included all the infections caused by

1.Virus

2.Bacteria,baccillai,spirochetes etc

3.Paracytes

4. Fungus ,,,etc.

2.Non communicable disease

Caused by taking allopathic medicines for communicable disease. These diseases again managed by allopathic medicines and till the orgon failure or till death of patient. EXAMPLE – Diabetes, arthritis,heart attack,stroke, cirrhosis of liver, psoriyasis ,,,, etc

New Classification of the disease

1.confused inflammation, immune chemicals, cells predominant basis

2.Diseases due to other waste dead cells formed during inflammation

3.Disease due to irreversible feedback mechanism and irregular regulation orders.

4.Disease due to wound healing cells and chemicals based.

1.Confused Inflmmation And Immune Cells And Chemicals Predominent Basis.

a.Diseases due to inflammation stopped in the early stage.

Itching eruptions, allergy, all the pains and nuralgias, bleeding diseases, blood vessal congetions, spasm,constrictions. Altered sensations, etc.

b.diseases due to distracting wound healing in early stage.

b.Effusive Disease

c.Dissease due to immunoglobulin disorders

d.Auto immune disease

e.Disease due to immune complex

d.Disease due to excess destructive chemicals (ulceration,necrosis) e.Disease due to cellular and humoral immunity activation.

g.diseases due to abnormal deposites

h.disease due to imbalance in feedback mechanisam.

4.Disease Due To Wound Healing Cells And Chemical Basis Late Stage.

a.Tumor

b.Indurations

c.Sclerosis

d.Cancers

disease classification also used based on prominent clinical signs and symptoms.

classification based on duration

- ACUTE INFLAMMATION
- SUB ACUTE DISEASEs
- CHRONIC DISORDER AND DISEASE
- ACUTE ON CHRONIC DISORDER
- ACUTE ON CHRONIC DISORDER [NOT KNOWN TO MEDICAL FIELD NEWLY ADDED]. running acute mild to severe course but with destruction more or less possibility of recovery due to confused inflammation.

Basically, we have to consider **acute true inflammation** is a not disease we have to name this protective mechanisam as acute inflammation rather then calling this as a disease. if we name this is as disease then there is possibility of prescription. Here the inflammation denotes (fighting with enemy,Regeneration and complete recovery all include). So, we can call this disease with denominations of end with IT IS like Rhinitis, Tonsillitis, arthritis,,,,,,,etc.

But don't call any chronic inflammation disease of present disease as it is like chronic hepatitis chronic, nephritis this will misunderstand this is as inflammation, they are not inflammation they confused inflammation disorders.

Acute disease means disease with short duration. chronic disease means disease with long duration.this is what the classification of present disease.

But the acute disease is self limiting it has a purpose to kill germs so all the process is over then the body will recover the damage and patient is completely alright now.

When we interrupt the acute disease, this self curing and self recovering power lost so the disease runining unusually longer period called chronic disease

SO CHORNIC DISEASE IS KIND OF FAILURE OF THE CURING OR SELF RECOVERING SYSTEM SO THE DISEASE IS RUNING LONG DURATION. So, if your chronic disease here after doctor will think that there are some obstacles is there to recover the acute disease so the doctors will try to remove the obstacles and achive the cure. But at present doctors are accepting and thinking that chronic disease means the disease which is there for long duration. He will just announce the disease.

Inflammation and immune system failure are preceds many years before the heart failure,kidney failure, lung failure and liver and bone marrow failure and importandly allopathy doctors does not the inflammation and immune system failed that is the basic reason for all this orgon failure and he does not understand this. So indirectly we can prevent all this failure by recovering failed inflammation and immunity in the very early stage.

The distracted confused inflammation is really not curing power so the disease created by this inflammation mimic like inflammation and do destruction but never cure so run a long course (chronic disease)

CHRONIC DISEASE :

There is no chronic disease and specially there is no chronic inflammation at all what we believed as chronic inflammation diseases are actually misunderstood. This is produced by existing confused inflammation cells which is formed for previous acute true inflammation but we distracted it ,so still it is roaming and producing the disease.so using the name again as inflammation makes lot many confusion for doctors, if we name like that then doctor will try to do the treatment by anti inflammatory or something arrest inflammation like what he did already. This is what happening now. Like doctors naming it wrongly and trying to heal wrongly so they failing. All this confusion raised because we do not know what we treat, we do not know the cause of the disease.

It is not inflammation, it will not going to do the functions of the inflammation, it will not support the human, it will not heal on its own, it will produce only destruction, the destruction may be mild or severe so why we have to name this is as chronic inflammation ? it's a wrong nomenclature's a appropriate name otherwise general name like confused inflammation disorder of the liver. Confused inflammation disorder of the brain ,,,,,,, etc.

KEEP THAT IN YOUR MIND WE ARE GOING TO REMOVE THE NAME ALL THE ITIS OTHER THEN THIS.BECAUSE ALL OTHER SUB ACUTE,CHRONIC ACUTE ON CHRONIC ALL IS NOT A INFLAMMATION AT ALL.SO CALL THAT CHRONIC LIVER DISEASE DON'T SAY HEPATITIS (INCLUDING VIRAL HEPATITIS SINCE THERE IS NO CHRONIC INFLAMMATION, A VIRUS RESIDE IN THE LIVER WITH OR WITHOUT ACTIVE HEPATIC DAMEGE, THE SYMPTOMATIC LIVER DAMAGE IS NOT BECAUSE OF VIRUS IF AT ALL IT WAS HAPPENED LIKE ACUTE ON CHRONIC CONFUSED INFLAMMATION BASE THAT IS ALSO NOT A INFLAMMATION ,A INFLAMMATION MUST SAVE THE HUMAN AND WITHOUT GIVING ANY RESIDUAL DAMAGE. SO CHRONIC LIVER DISEASE.)

CHRONIC LIVER DISEASE – WITH CONFUSED INFLAMMATION [PRESENT AUTO IMMUNE DISEASE].

CHRONIC LIVER DISEASE WITH HEPATIC VIRUS. ,,,,, ETC.

DON'T USE THE DENOMINATIONS ITIS WHICH INDICATES INFLAMMATION.

Chronic disease ? how the disease gets chronic or acute as a duration indicator's confused inflammation disease is not a acute or not a chronic once if it is formed we can remove it acutely at the same time if it is not removed from the body it will stay within our body life long.so the duration what we mean it is not indicates realism.

Acute disease is not an acute disease it is protective action taken by body going to end within short duration so inflammation of the throat or tonsil or something so it is not a disease it is good protective function of the body.

The current concept of General systemic and local disease classification by an allopathy doctor is not a usefull classifications.

Classification of the disease by Hahnemann.he classified disease in 3 main broad categories like

- Psora (similar to histamine excess disease of confused inflammation)
- syphilis (similar to diseases due to excess destruction stage of inflammation)
- sycosis (similar to disease due excess cell proliferation (distracted wound healing cells).

And other disease calculated based on mixture of the same like psoriyasis is mixture of all 3 miasm and there is some disease like comibination predominant 2 miasm psoro syphilitic or psoro sycotic like that.This classification we are following already in homeopathy.

Hahnemann classified diseases into 2 major categories like dynamic and mechanical disease. The all 3 miasms fall under dynamic diseases.

Allopathic Disease Classification

General disease

Systemic disease

Other pathological based classifications based on systems and symptoms identity in the disease like diseases which has excess exfoliation and excess congestion and tumors like that, there is no proper analytical and value-based classifications.

❖ ❖ ❖

Part -1 – physiology

1.VITAL FORCE (HEALTH,DISEASE,RECOVERY, DEATH)

2.NATURAL IMMUNE PROTECTION

3.GOOD INFLAMMATION,GOOD IMMUNITY

1. VITAL FORCE (HEALTH,DISEASE, DEATH)

VITAL FORCE

I t is importand subject has to be kept in the first chapter discussed here since it is new subject so I am giving importance to what we know already let us discuss new subjects now.

The concept and significance of vital force is explained for the purpose of understanding the man is not a single body part he is comprised of all, man as a whole. Structure and tissues and orgon is considered but given importance to functions of the humans.

Vital force first introduced in the medical field by

dr Hahnemann in 1810 in his orgonon of medicine. But till date allopathy doctors not reading life force or soul or aliveness in the medical books in general.

Until that time we are discussed about only anatomy and physiology of the humans. Anatomy is study of human body parts and tissues. Physiology is studying functions of the human body parts and its tissues. Brain is having master power brain is controling the body parts. If the brain is at fault then the disease will arise. This idea was dominated in the world sometime Then gained knowledge about the heart and blood vessals then the doctors divert their concept towards heart so they now belived heart is having superiar power heart is controlling everything if the heart is in disease then everything else will be in collapse ,, etc.

During that time the treatment aspect is focusing towards specialization and body parts and tissues. Either health or disease explained on the basis of anatomy and structural components (concept of meteriayalisam).

How will you explain the brain and heart functions and protective superior power in the living ovum during the development ? who is governing who is protecting the life of ovum before the brain development ?

Now Hahnemann said vital force is the governing superior power body brain and body parts is kept under the superior power of the vital force ? OK Then answere following question.

- What is vital force ?
  life force aliveness.

- how we can see that ?
  over all functions and sensation of the whole man he/ she breath, walk, run sleep and eating everything and everything represent

and understanding about the presence of his vital force.

- where it is located in the human or living being ?

The vital force is there inside every living creature in the world. But opposite to our popular opinion which is not present as a air or breath. its is just expressed and understood as functions of all the body parts. (a life force is not a good soul (representing godliness) or bad soul (Ghost). This is just united function and expression of all the human body parts that's all.

(why I am saying good athma and bad athma ? even though medical field is not included what is vital force or life force entire world is discussiong about vital force as their own many years before even many years before fully developed medical field. Mostly their understanding is life force is like spirit sitting inside the human body and it escapes from the human body after his death if the man is good person then it will go to the heven if it is bad person and then his spirit will go to the hell like that) as a doctor we have to break this mythical concept need to explain what is vital force, so that doctors have an idea about what is spiritual force or vital force. (this idea of ghost and godliness is developing indirectly pople thinking human mind is the life force or athma (soul). So, what is mind. Mind is nothing but functions of brain (thinking,memory, intellect, will ,,,,etc) so olden concept of life force is related only with brain and its function. So, this is partially true life is functions of heart and lungs and kidney everything included.

So man is not only protected by or supported by a brain it includes heart and at the same time heart is not the only orgon which is protect ,support the whole body it is also supported by lungs it is not only by lungs also by kidney so over all the whole human is supported and protected by varies body parts and interlinked with each other for doing service to the mega single orgon (human body) so all the body parts collectively united for the purpose of total human living and enjoying this birth. A vital force is nothing but collective and total functions of the and body parts of the this mega orgon is vital force. Vital force is not a single body part or not single body part function it is collectively comprises of every body parts and its functions togetharness. It is not living in any one particular body part.

So, don't try to explain the disease more and more towards body particular part and tissues try to explain and treat on the basice concept of man as a whole. Each boady parts depend upon each other fo their basic functions.

Anyone can say simple yes that man is alive, and we can understand easily if someone dead. But what makes the person alive ? medically we have many parameters to understand a man is alive or dead. But even medically no one has an idea that how the man is alive where exactly this soul or aura or life is present in the human body. Hahnemann is the first physician he is trying to give explanation about the human vital force or life force.

in the aphorism 9 of ORGANON OF MEDICINE.

In the healthy condition of the man the spiritual vital force, the dynamis that animates the material body.

Rules with onbounded sway and retains the all the parts of the organisam in admirable hormoniyas, vital operations as regards both sensations and functions. So, that our indwelling reason gifeted mind can freely employ this living healthy instrument for the higher purpose of our existence.

This example which will give what is life force. Now we will see the life of the bird and how that is getting aliveness from non alive egg or seed.

Egg is does not alive it is a on object now. When the egg is getting enough warmth, then the liquid part of the egg started solid, growing part. That is the time actually the starting point of aliveness [vital force is apearing] of the bird, new bird was created with vital force. Now the cells started growing and dividing and further dividing to form a tissues and body parts of the bird. The decision to grow how to grow, which part of the body has to turn into heart, which one has to form brain, how to get the food all decided by this vital force [at this point gene and its coding cell growth, division of cells altogether explain the aliveness].

At any point if the cell division is stopped and no further growth means that point is called death it means no vital force. The parameter of the life and dead here [at this level not formed matured bird or not as simple egg] is not decided by heart beat or brain death or respiration since these parts are not yet developped, So, when a ovum stops its growht saying death. If it is start growing then alive.

Here our concept of understanding death is because no heart beat. death is because no breathing is not true understanding (this medically ok allopathy doctors record death cessation of functions of heart,brain,respiration as death but what did you understand about the life force ?) but vital force is not only here it is representing the whole-body parts and its functions for single person living their life. If the heart beat is recovered by shock then the person starte live because the vital force still ther in other part also,when a person stop breathing can be given srtificial respiration can get the live then he lives,it does not mean that the person giving artificial respiration passing his soul to another person and waking him up.

What a common man or research people and even medical profession is expecting something more then that. It means they believe some extra force then what I described is there so they want to discover it and they have an idea that someone will discover that. But actually, speaking nothing like that.

A common man thinking about the vital force is only related with death and live like that but Hahnemann explanation of the same related with all level like healthy status and his functions and living and enjoying self protecting and etc and etc.

A birth of life force to a seed is starts, when dried seed is getting enough wet and warmth then it will start swell due to attracted water the dried molecule or tissues get bulge then they start suck water actively and start grow and start produce leaf and get preparing the food from the sun like that so the life beginning at the time of dried seed getting slight bulging and getting warmth started growing. SO, THIS IS HOW VITAL FORCE IS BEGIN THEIR JOURNEY.

Now let's discuss what is the role of vital force in the human after birth. Where is vital force how we can comprehend vital force? Vital force is not a one single solid tissue or body part, more then searching for new body part as a vital force, we could understand that, its nothing but collective integrated functions of all the body parts and tissues which includes genetic information's within the cells of human being.

Vital force is including breathing, heartbeat, digestion, neural functions excreation, thinking, protecting, healing „„„„„ etc and etc functions, collective data of all. We have to understand this. A heart controlled by brain, a brain dependent to heart and lungs for its need of food and oxygen. A lung functions carried successfully by blood and blood is purified by kidney, the kidney functions shared by skin all this organs nourished by Gastro intestinal tract again this Gastro intestinal tract is controlled by brain, oxygen supplied by blood and lungs so like wise each and every organ is almost dependent for all other organs for its routine functions so to say a man is alive is include all this. A vital force is denoting and comprise and include of all the functions of the human body parts for doing and living and enjoying this birth.

So when we treating we must understand this a complex city of functions and dependency of the organs each other and like wise.so we have to keep in mind that vital force is a mega dynamic organ which represent individuality of the person instead of treating or considering just single organ or body parts we have to consider man as whole [he is a mixture of complex of all organ or vital force].

❖　Health is good functioning vital force expressed as by normal functions and normal sensations.

❖　If there is enemy attack Recovery or repair done by our vital force alone so self cure or self recovery done by this vital force.

❖　When functions are deranged, we consider this as a disease [diseased vital force],expressed abnormal functions and sensations.

❖　when functions of all organs totally cased then we consider death [cessation of vital force]. No functions and sensation.

So, disease is not in a tissues or body part. but a vital force deranged so disease.when we fail to recover this diseased vital force then the disease progressed to a damage in the body parts.

Yes of course the inflammation and immunity are the process which is allowed to repair the body parts if this forcibly stopped then the inflammation will collapse start producing the disease. It lacks of power to recover. So here a vital force is sick. This sickness can spread across the whole body it makes the sickness and express by unpleasant sensation and functions. It is not stomach is diseased the system collapsed so expressed in the stomach it is not lung is producing disease the confused inflammation created disease to lungs if we use appropriate medicine then confused inflammation will be cleared from the human body and lung will be normal in future.

Always we have a concept that diseased eye part producing the disease no a confused inflammation moves towards eye and make sickness but we search cause within the eye searching the cause inside the eye. We think reading the each and every tissue of the eye will help in finding the cause, but not true. Technically if a person born with anomalies or trauma misshape the person body parts then that will attract the confused inflammation and produce the disease otherwise a good healthy tissue never produce disease on its own.

dynamic force which is keeping the body in healthy condition, which is starts its own at the time of conception itself. It keeps all the body parts in a harmoniyas healthy states.

We are awar this vital force yes when the vital

force or life force is not there then we say he/she is dead. We know some extend the person is alive. But DR.HAHNEMANN says the vital force is doing great many works in the human body part.Which we may not awar.

He says vital force is a automatic force it has created on its own during conception.This vital force is keep all organs healthy and this will regulate the human body and sense the defect and heal along with brain and recover the functions like wise it do lots of functions.he says it's a dynamic force we connot see that but when man alive we can perceive/ understand that vital force is there.

When the vital force is altered then it is disease if it is good condition then we consider a human is healthy if the vital force is nil then the condition called death.

Life is the whole movement and total function that takes place within man

When a person dies all the organs in his body are still intact but none of them are functioning so he is considered as dead. Even if any of the organs of the body are functioning (Dynamis) we make sure that he is still alive.

The organs just not simply exist and they must function. Life refers to movement, movement does not simply mean moving and walking, but the function of the organs,

Life of a plant is beginning when the lifeless seed attracts water.the water moves from external world to inside the seed impress us the seed is living.the water moves all over the plant so that plant is functioning and it is considered as life. When the plant stop absorbing the water and stop helping the nurturing the plant is considered as dead. A dead plant is still having the branch and to some days dried leafs also but they are lifeless since they stoped their functions.The seed grows with the absorbed water and then the root then the leaf then the branch then the flower, then the fruit continues as the fruit .The tree continues to grow. There is tremendous root. However, the root does not absorb water and the leaves do not produce greenery in sunlight and it does not grow. Its movement stops This stage is dead.

Although there are whole organs, they are all functioning. Life takes care of the body. Life only created the body. There is no brain when the conception was happened (the time of life beginning). The life decides the necessity of brain and designed and created brain. Life created the heart and used it in a time, if the embryo stops growing then before the brain and the heart deveolops then that is called death hear, the embryo did not do its job it stopped working so it is dead .The moment the work stops, the embryo is dead.

So, if the vital energy or life force is normal then that is called healthy state of the human. That is expressed as healthy functions and sensations. If this vital force is deranged then that condition is called disease.if the vital force or life force is ceased then the person consider as a dead.

So, disease is not primarily due to damage of tissues or cells of the orgon. That is primarily by deranged functions and dynamis (altered functions of the inflammaiotn) this is secondarily creates the orgon damage and tissue damage.

What we need to know about individuals based on two different philosophies here is that one group is based on substances (meterialisam) (which discuss much about the damage to organs and tissues - anatomy, pathology) .-- Allopathy.

Another group is the process, the mode of action,

the movement (functions-physiology-dynamis) (the group based on its motion regardless of the object) The group based on its movement regardless of the body. -- Homeopathy.

That is why the group based on materials and body parts has the greatest basic treatment of the principle of removal of the affected organ is allopathic medicine. Here too anatomy is read only plain reading.

Homeopathic medicine thinks that medicines should also be dynamic force when giving medicines to a patient. The living state cannot be restored by inanimate object (material substance). Homeopathy Medicine is dynamised so it will meet the diseased life force. Drugs are equivalent to the body and it is meterial, this material never meat vital force, difficult to recover the life, the drug (substance) must be prepared to be dynamised.

Gene and life force

Do you understand now that life is a gene ? or genetic based. No life is not at all genetic. A gene is a criterion or definition that determines how a body and organism should grow and function. This gene is present in the non-living seed as well as within living plant.

Am I human / animal / tree? It's deiced by genetic. to have accurate estimates of my hair's color, my height, and how far my brain should grow etc and etc.

Gene is coding or script of the human body parts not a life force. Functions and movements of the human is a life force.

◆ ◆ ◆

PART - 4 - DISEASE PROPER.

(Preventive medicine, speciality medicine, General medicine).

ENT,Respiratory   system,OPTHALOMOL-
OGY,DERMATOLOGY, CARDIOLOGY , THYROID,GASTRO IN-
TESTINAL SYSEM, ORTHO, GYNECOLOGY, CENTRAL NER-
VOUS SYSTEM ETC

Most of the disease in each system described based
on new research and discovery, few supportive documenta-
tions were taken from other authers work (like disease statistics and clinical futures).this work is mainly focused on

prevention so not much medicinal management is focused)

1. ENT DISORDERS

Nearly half of the Indian population (60 crors) suffering with ENT disorders and there is no single curative remedy in allopathy and the medicine what they prescribe for this ailment will creates lots of new disease and that will cause severe disability and lots of non communicable disease.

ENT disease is very common disease nearly 1/3 of the world population suffering with ent disorders .more are less they meet allopathy doctors to take treatment. Allopathy doctors prescribe anti pyeretics and anti biotics and anti allergics for this disease and produce non communicable disease from now. Nearly 45-65 % of the noncommunicable disease arises only from allopathy treatment given ENT and upper respiratory tract disease. That mild simple non communicable disease is asthma,pneumonia, brain disease including tumors (except infections) , deafness , blindness and vision disorders other then infections ,,,, etc.

Now dear doctors and world health organization, I have discovered cause for non communicable disease and I have given the reponsiblity to you decide how you are going to prevent the non communicable disease and you are going to save the patient.

Option A – continuing the same treatment spreading and creating more disease, earning money and good name by doing same treatment.

Option B – Banning the anti inflammatory and anti allergics and refereeing the cases to homeopathy.

Option C – Bannig the anti inflammatory and anti allergics and using homeopathy medicine for handling ENT and upper respiratory disease.

When a person exposes to dust or virus , inflammation system gets activated so fever, running nose, and sneezing will come [rhinitis], In this condition if that person takes anti-histamine then histamine will be blocked, so that affected person feel relived now he will not have any sneezing or rhinitis. but the blocked histamine will circulate entire nasal mucosa now, repeated intake of antihistamine makes huge collection of histamine, this histamine will make the nasal mucosa sensitive to dust and smell temperature changes ,,,, etc.so now patient will develop *allergic rhinitis.*

Allergic rhinitis

Its very common disease now a days , most of the persons suffering with this disease.Cause for the disease was not discovered this many diseases it is now identified, the cause of the allergic rhinitis is anti allergics and anti-inflammatory drugs.

Allergic rhinitis starts with continues sneezing especially in the morning as soon as getting up from the bed or sneezing in the change of weather and climate like summer to winter or winter to summer or sudden exposure to ac room in summer. Exposure to dust ,,,,.

In the initial days patient felt symptom free periods at least in summer, he feels sneezing and itching in the nose is tolerable , But as the year progress, patient felt the number of sneezes will become more and he becomes increasingly sensitive to several new house hold items like using perfumes, soap, sent, drinking cold water, even sitting under the fan,,,, etc.

He started experiencing huge collection symptoms like nose block, watering from the eyes, red and congested eyes, persistent irritation in the throat which makes the dry irritating cough, difficulty in breathing, head ache,,,,,, and recurrent out burst of severe attack also common.

usually allergic rhinitis will not respond to antibiotic . but anti-allergic gives the relief. If the symptoms more persistent and not responding to the anti-allergic then the doctor will keep the patient under steroid.

Prescribing anti allergic causes more histamine and more sensitive nasal mucosa so causes severe the symptoms but this can be observed after the medicine effect is over.so this is the reason why many patient is having worst allergic rhinitis despite the medicines since the medicine (anti allergic tablets cetrizen , cold act, nasivion otrivin) is the cause for allergy but this medicine will gives the relief so patient will keep taking the medicine disease will grow like anything so patient will have many complications like sinusitis, nasal polyp , allergic asthma .

Allopathic doctors keep prescribing allopathy medicine without knowing the medicine is the cause for the disease . so the cycle repeates and disease worst very severe.

But we name this dust allergy, pollen allergy, some patient says I have eosinophil so I am allergic to dust. all this is fake terminology. Your not allergic to anything you are made to allergic to many things due to anti allergic medicines it is not anti allergic they are allergic medicines they are causing the allergy.

Esonophil count is raised. Serum IgE elevated in some patient. all this test reports reveal the elevated blood count is due to sudden stopping of the inflammation in the mid. So, this cell is creating allergy but this is absolutely not because person exposing dust causing this ,this is because you have excess allergic cells that's created by prescribing anti allergics.

weather the patient under anti allergic or steroid or nasal drops or the nasal spray the complications of the allergic rhinitis keep on progressing in majority of the cases so the patient need to hospitalized often for allergic asthma or for the surgery for the nasal complications like polyp and sinusitis. operation here is may not give the solution for the polyp or the sinus ,it will grow again and the turbinate will be swollen again and produce the new polyp.

Since doctors again prescribe the anti allergic even after the surgery to controle the symptoms .I Hope the doctors may not do this unscientific prescription.

Homeopathic medicines remove the allergic tendency and the hyper sensitivity. so the patient become normo sensitive ,he is free from all the allergic symptoms. he will become completely recover by allergic rhinitis and its complications.

homeopathic medicines cure the allergic rhinitis completely.

when the patient is having multiple polyps with enlarged turbinates. He should kept under observation with homeopathic medicine if the patient is getting improvement with symptoms of the allergic rhinitis, then he should continue the treatment if the symptoms not reducing and the patient is worse then it is ideal to refer the case towards surgeon especially advanced polyp and its compulsory to continue the homeopathic medicine after surgery to eradicate the allergic rhinitis and remove the confused inflammation for prevention of further polyp.

Treatment is necessary till the patient is completely cured.

> • nasal mucosa will be act as a negative magnetism for attracting confused inflammation all over the body, so the confused inflammation reach all over the body to nose and make the strong confused inflammation disorders here then from here it sprayed over the face [due to sun heat attraction or hormonal attraction] causes acne, pimples [teen], facial discolorations and tumors and other eruption [others like elders and children's].

NOSE IS THE COMMONEST ORGAN WHICH IS EXPOSE FREQUENT INFECTIONS AND DUST EXPOSURE SO THIS THIS REPEATED EXCESS ACTIVITY WILL ATTRACT THE CONFUSED INFLAMMATION CHEMICALS / CELLS ALL OVER THE BODY TO TOWARDS THE NOSE.

It is not simply nose complaints end with nose itself. lets discuss how many organs slowly damaged by a confused inflammation spread from nose to other parts.

•   The confused inflammation from nose spread to **adenoid** and slowly damage adenoid so that recurrent adenoid infection. These inflammations try to spoil the function of the glands by depositing unnecessary cells and fibrous tissue so that the gland is become hard and swollen so that the protecting adenoid gland is become source of infection causes recurrent throat infection and adenoid infection or does not protect any more. RECOVERING ADENOID FUNCTION AND CLEARING THIS ABNORMAL DEPOSIT AND CURING ADENOID WILL HELP THE INDIVIDUAL PROTECT THEMSELF.THEN THE GOOD FUNCTIONING ADENOID CONTROL AND ARREST THE GERMS ENTRY FROM EXTERNAL POLLUTED ENVIRONMENT TO THROAT ITSELF SO NO SPREAD OF INFECTION.

Function of the adenoid is similar to tonsil; it helps in fighting against the bacteria's and protect the respiratory tract . This small lymphoid tissue located in the upper pharynx in the posterior wall of the mouth.

simple adenoid infection makes minimal discomfort and cold attack but in majority of the cases the adenoid is become permanently swollen and weak hence its the source of recurrent infection in children's.

adenoid starts develop at the age of 1 year and attain peak at 3-5 years and atrophied after 6-7 year.

Complication of the adenoid hypertrophy:

1.it produces the recurrent tonsil infection and tonsil hypertrophy.

2.persistent nasal infection and cold and sinusitis.

3.snoring and mouth breathing, nasal voice, protruded tongue, reduced cheek (due to chronic enlargement the maxillary sinus is poorly developed so the cheeks is not prominent)-ADENOID FACE.

4.dullness and difficulty in concentrating

5.persistent dry cough.

Diagnosis is very simple by the clinical symptoms alone but x ray cervical spine-lateral view clearly helpful find the enlarged adenoid.

if homeopathic medicines prescribed at right time then there is no formation of the adenoid enlargement if the adenoid is already enlarged and its giving complications, in that situation homeopathic medicines greatly helps in reducing the size of the swelling as well as gives the better result in complications also, so there is a excellent prognosis in adenoid enlargement and cures the disease permanently.

•   spread to **tonsil** and produce tonsil infections tonsil swelling . tonsil one of the most important immune organ but getting frequent infection so that surgeon remove the Orgon in the early childhood itself.

Don't fed up with recurrent infection , the recurrent infection of the tonsil indicates that the gland is having confused inflammation so that it lost its function so that infections not cleared and affected with infection and more ever entire nasal mucosa also equally affected act as bacterial and viral flor for multiplying the germs so that recurrent infection is possible.

There is good medicine in homeopathy to re-
cover the functions of nose , tonsil , adenoid . So removing
this organ is unnecessary.

Infection of the tonsils so frequent in the children's then adult. common infecting organism is like
streptococcus and staphylococcus. severe throat pain with
fever is common symptoms, dry painful cough, head ache
also present. difficulty in swelling and the pain is present
below the jaw in the neck (due to lymph node enlargement).tonsils are swollen and reddish.

occlussive tonsillitis : The tonsils very big .So the
whole mouth opening into throat is blocked by tonsil so its
tough to drink and swallow any foods. so the child will loss
the hunger. child is suffering to swallow the food. drooling of
the saliva will be there.

when the tonsillitis is treated with improper
medication like allopathic medicine then the tonsil fail to
recover themselves so that the accumulated cells within the
tonsil is become uncleared so the tonsil is swollen in the
similar way repeated tonsil infection and arresting infection with allopathy causes huge big tonsil swelling but children may not complain any pain no fever but simply tonsil
swollen.

sometimes adenoid makes the child become recurrent tonsillitis.

Adenoid -----> Tonsillitis -----> Otitis
media

Adenoid -----> Sinusitis ------> Tonsillitis

Homeopathic medicines most helpful in curing the tonsillitis and keeps the function of the tonsil is become normal and prevent the recurrences.

Sinusitis

sinusitis is very common disease.

Basically, sinuses are healthy hallow places in the skull bone. There are 4 pairs of sinuses (frontal, maxillary, ethmoidal and sphenoidal) in and around the nose and all this sinus has a small pore which open into nose. suppose if water or pus or mucus collects inside the sinuses it drains into the nose. because of this connection people get sinus attack when they have common cold (nasal allergy or inflammation).

The function of the sinus is giving normal good-looking alignment for the face and helps minimally for producing tone of voice. sinusitis is an inflammation of the mucus membrane of the sinus cavity. cold we commonly mean that nasal congestion sinus is nothing but it extends from nose to sinus.

nasal infection or allergy can spread to sinuses, not all the time the sinus gets involved. but if the sinuses got affected frequently then every nasal cold settle in the sinuses. Since we terminate the inflammation before it is completing, the nasal turbinates swelling and mucosal thickening , narrowing of the sinus pores and the development of sino nasal polyposis and loss of protective mechanism in the nose.

signs and symptoms of the allergic and infective sinusitis :

.   sinus usually makes the sufferer to be sick , feels sleepy, dull, heaviness in the face and head worse when lean forward , cannot able to concentrate.

.   **Nose block** on majority of the patient it will be in the night time, alternate sides will be blocked, if the climate is too cold or the congestion is heavy then both nose will be blocked so the affected individual cannot able to breath in this situation new born baby and children get up from sleep and struggle for breathing will cry over night avoids feeding. Elder children's and adults may sleep with open mouth or sleep with heavy snoring.

An anxious patient will get severe panic if both nose blocked in the sleep, their heart beat will go up and they think they are going to dye now. Even though they get nose block they describe that they had breathlessness and had heart attack or they say respiratory arrest. They un ware their nose is completely blocked so that this fear is happen.

HEAVY SNORING WILL BE THERE WHEN THE PA-TIENT IS HAVING NASAL POLYP OR TURBINATE SWELL-ING.

nose block will make the head ache worse. If the sinus and allergy is very longer duration nose block will be permanent. well pronounced by others due to nasal voice.

On targeting nose block many commercial pharma products sold in the medical markets. nasal in-halers nasal drops many nose block reliving allopathic medicine and many Ayurveda and siddha medicine. non of the external applications of any system is not in-dicated even if it is homeopathy.

Acute nose block indicates absolute nasal functions we must not attempt to prescribe the medicines. since turbinate's close if we expose dusty or unhealthy atmosphere to protect us so don't take medicine for that.

Prescribe medicine to eradicate the confused inflammation from the nose so that recurrent nose block will be relieved by medicines.

•   Head ache worse when you enter into the ac room , or sun especially in the morning better in the evening (frontal sinusitis).
•   severe deep pain in the eye ball and upper molar tooth when clearing the nose (heavy infection /or active confused inflammation in the maxillary sinus).

There are many people will have discharge like water from the nose and they wipe and wipe in the whole day with using lots of tissue paper.

Thick tough nasal discharge , yellowish or yellow green in color, sometimes blood mixed mucus discharge in severe bacterial infection.

Often complain of blood tinched sputum hawked up from the throat in the early morning on first time but further spitting may be clear sputum without blood.

•   Deep pain in the occipital region (back part of the head) worse in the night indicates (sphenoidal and ethmoidal sinus involvement).
Most of the time this head ache in the occipital region, especially in the middle-aged man will often

raises the suspicions about elevated bp or some deep brain damage or cervical spine pathology.

• Sphenoid sinus infection less common in compare with frontal and maxillary, the sphenoid infection produces dull vague head ache and there is lacking of classical symptoms of sinus like running nose and fever so misdiagnosed as migraine or stress head ache is common. pain felt in various location like occipital , eye ball or in the fore head.

• bad breath especially pronounced in chronic purulent sinusitis or active acute or sub acute sinusitis.

• Loss of smelling sense - in chronic sinusitis.(smell sense recoverable by medicine).

• dry cough and post nasal drip.

• Most interesting part but distressing problem in allergic rhinitis patient complaints of itching inside the nose and eyes and deep inside. children will squeeze and rub their eyelids often so that eye will become reddish. itching and tickling inside the roof of the palate is making severe uncomfortable, itching inside the ears so child will try to scratch but unable to reach the itch spots so getting anger and cry on pointing the ear and same when they have ear pain.

This itching directly start producing atopic dermatitis, first upon the eye lids then slowly within neck and behind the ears we can see extensive spreading nature of allergy every and dominating entire respiratory tract with different name and almost all parts of skin as dermatitis or allergy. itching and itching everywhere itching is the only sign of presence

of excessive histamine in the circulation due to anti histamine use.

> •   **Pan sinusitis** severe simultaneous infec-
> tion in all four sinuses. produce moderate to severe
> fever , with severe body pain along with heaviness
> in the head.

Cause For Sinuses :

> •   CONFUSED INFLAMMATION IS
> THE CAUSE FOR SINUSITIS BUT SINUS INFECTION
> CAUSED BY MANY VIRUS OR BACTERIYAS after the
> sinus mucus membarane is weakned and lost its
> protective power by confused inflammation.

>   When the sinus does not have protect-
> ive power to eliminate the germs effectively then this
> will cause a chronic infection within the sinus it could
> be anything like virus or bacteria or even a fungus cre-
> ate a chronic infection.THE MAIN OBSERVATION HERE
> IS THE INFECTION WITHIN THE SINUS IS CLEARED
> BY ON ITS OWN, IT INDICATES NO CONFUSED IN-
> FLAMMATION HERE.but when confused inflammation
> is there then the sinus cavity will become source of for
> the germs it will stay here and multiply and produce
> life long infections without any ressistance from the
> body.So remember confused inflammation is the indir-
> ect cause for even a chronic infection.

Complication Of Sinuses

(we read this is as a complication of the sinus but this is not sinus complication it indirectly mean that bacteria or virus causing this that is not true this complications are due to confused inflammation):

- symptomatic tonsillitis and tonsil enlargement, adenoid and adenoid swelling children (common) asymptomatic or minimal discomfort tonsil enlargement is observed in adults.
- meningitis (especially heavily infected complicated sinuses in children may complicate the meningitis)
- cellulitis (especially diabetics and immune deficient people)
- osteomyelitis (children are more prone to osteomyelitis)
- abscess (chronic heavily loaded bacterial sinusitis is the source of recurrent boils and abscess in the body).

Diagnosis

sinus symptoms alone is enough to make the diagnosis and there is pain when pressing involved sinus region. this can be done by gentle pressure over the cheeks (for maxillary sinus),pressing over the root of the nose (frontal sinus).

x ray para nasal sinus is helpful to diagnose the sinus clear sinus cavity in the x rays may not rule out the sinus. when stuffy and sputum loaded sinus gives clear cut sinus infection when you take x ray after the acute attack subsided no much sign of sinusitis in the x ray.

nasal endoscopy helpful in some cases.

ct scan will help in diagnosing the accurate pathological changes within the nose and sinus cavity and simultaneous changes in the surrounding structure of the sinus.

(like DNS (Deviated nasal septum), polyp , nasal turbinate swelling. Adenoid , tumor).

when the x ray or ct scan cannot able do detect the sinus involvement in majority of these sinus headaches are misdiagnosed as stress headache or cervical spondylosis or migraine or visual error or psychological illness.sinus involvement will be marked only during acute or sub acute sinusitis. If sinus opening is closed and loaded with mucus means the x ray is very clearly define the sinus-itis. or else x ray looks normal or insignificant signs of sinus-itis so here ct or MRI paranasal sinus is the best choice or doctor has to consider the clinical symptoms for diagnosis.

sinusitis is curable by homeopathic medicine;the success rate is very good.

Some common medicine used to treat sinusitis in homeopathy is kali bich ,silicia,nat mur,,,,,etc.

Consult the doctor and get completely cured. Dont take some temprory medication.

Larynx

When normal course of infection is spreads to the larynx then laryngitis will starts . Hoarseness of voice or loss of voice is the prominent symptoms and cough will be louder then usual indicates involvement of voice box . sufferer need to clear the throat often.

A acute loss of voice associated with cold will often get normal within 2-3days. Usually this will be heal on its own but when you prescribe to stop the inflammation then confused inflammation will start running as a chronic laryngitis frequent cold with loss of voice. Laryngeal tumor is formed over use of voice this will invite the tumor pro-ducing cells like fibroblast and hyaline material towards the vocal cord and produce the vocal cord nodule (laryngeal nodule).

A chronic confused inflammation turn into cancer easily by repeated acid entry (reflux esophagitis) .

• Confused inflammation spread to **Lungs** produce recurrent bronchitis , asthma , chronic bronchitis, prone to lung infections,,,,, e t c . [will discuss later].

• Spread to **Mouth** produce the mouth ulcers, gum diseases ,caries, oral tumors, etc.

• Confused inflammation Move to **Eye** and produce all kinds ophthalmic disorders.

• Confused inflammation Moves to **Ears** produce all type of ear complaints. All most all the ear disease secondary to nose involvement more or less the ear is not fall recurrent disorder un-less the nose is chronically affected .

THE EAR IS HAVING LOW POWER TO ATTRACT CONFUSED INFLAMMATION NATURALLY , SINCE IT IS NOT GOING TO GET PRIMARY INFECTION AND ALSO NOT GETTING RECURENT

DIRECT INFECTIONS OR INFLAMMATIONS.SO THAT EAR IS PRO-TECTED WELL DUE TO ITS ANATOMICAL LOCATION.

THE SAME ANATOMICAL LOCATION IS GIVING CHANCE TO SPREAD THE DISEASE FROM NOSE AND MOUTH TO EAR VIA EUSTACHIAN TUBE. BUT THE EAR IS PROTECTED WITH TUBEL TONSIL.BUT DUE TO CONFUSED INFLAMMATION THIS TUBEL TONSIL IS BECOME INEFFECTIVE TO PROTECT THE EAR SO THAT INFECTIONS CROSS THIS TUBEL TONSIL AND ATTACK THE EAR.

Both *acute and chronic suppurative otitis media* is favored by confused inflammation and super added with infection [the germ entry is secondary to confused inflammation]. The healthy ear is does not allow the infection to cross the infection from nose and mouth to ear.

TYMPANIC MEMBRANE RUPTURE in an acute otitis media is a normal phenomenon. The discharge within the ear is not having any outlet other then rupturing the tympanic membrane so that the ear discharge will come through ruptured tympanic membrane. But after this rupture possibility of direct spread of infections is high. for few individuals the tympanic membrane closes after some time but for many people tympanic membrane remains open for many years but without / with infections. Tympanic membrane rupture may not produce any hearing loss until the bone attachment is not affected.

Gradually the **Inner Ear** is getting affected with confused inflammation so that patient experiencing noise in the ear, giddiness now and then, slow deterioration of the hearing.

THE INNER EAR DISEASES VERY MARKED ONLY AFTER TREATING THE EAR DISCHARGE WITH EXTERNAL EAR DROPS.WHEN THE INFECTIONS IF IT

IS ALLOWED TO DRAIN EXTERNALLY THEN THE PER-SON INNER EAR WILL NOT GET AFFECTED SO EASILY AND SO QUICKLY. EVERY INCH MIGRATION OF THE CONFUSED INFLAMMATION HIGHLY SUPPORTED BY ALOPATHIC MEDICINES AND SURGERIES.

Ear pain is the one of the common complaints especially in children most of the very simple sharp pain indicates infection or inflammation crossing and entering into the eustachian tube along with stuffy ear, this stuffiness is temporary's before and during middle ear infection causes pain and it will be relieved by perforation of eustachian tube.

Frequent ear stuffiness and echoing of his own voice but there are no actual infection symptoms in the ear and nose but the history of nasal allergy and sinus infection indicates the confused inflammation cross the **Eustachian tube**. This stuffiness patient experience when expose to cold air and in ac room.

The tumor and other severe pathological changes unavoidable after application of the external ear drops and it helps in more confused inflammation to the ear. Even though the enough confused inflammation cells are available in the body that will be attracted in the mouth and nose so it will mostly stuck in oral cavity and nose and sinus will produce tumors or other deep pathological changes over there itself.so it does not come to the ears so easily there is no great attractive power in the ear to attract confused inflammation.so developing tumors is later than usual but using ear drops makes the confused inflammation which is enough to make severe pathological changes.

- Move to **brain** and produces psychological disease and brain disease. Most simple entry of the confused inflammation is via sinus to base of the frontal lobe, and to the base of the

325

brain by eye. And to base of the temple lobe from middle ear. Brain over activity and loss of sleep stress and strain will attract the confused inflammation toward brain from nose, eye and ear.

A medicine used for treating many bodily ailments directly increases the confused pro inflammation chemicals which will generate confused inflammation in future.

Example ; anti-histamine block the histamine so heavy histamine in the circulation as well as in the brain. This excess histamine will produce abnormality in the brain activity in the early then it will produce brain disease by inducing semi inflammation process. And the same histamine will attract the remaining confused inflammation to the brain.

Ear drops, eye drops, nasal drops highly support the confused inflammation entry into the brain from ear, nose and eye.

•   Confused inflammation move to the scalp and causes varies disease to **scalp**. Scalp is the one among the attractive force for the confused inflammation. The heavy heat or cold exposure attract the confused inflammation to the scalp and produce varies scalp skin disease.

Dandruff indicates easy notification of the confused inflammation to both patient and doctors.so the presence of the dandruff is the first step of the confused inflation treating the dandruff with with external application or other skin diseases like psoriasis and eczema will help to spread the confused inflammation to the remaining skin in the entire body.

Confused inflammation allows the scalp to

get infection especially fungus but the fungus spread to the chest and back by falling and producing disease by direct fungus not with the help of confused inflammation. A tiny recurrent boil is another indication that the confused inflammation has surfacing to the scalp, source is probably from sinus infection or caries tooth.

Alopecia areata is caused by confused inflammation, the recurrence and rapidity of spread is indicating strong supporting active confused inflammation in the nose or in the sinuses or caries tooth or the confused inflammation in these areas repeatedly tried to push towards face and scalp by strong medications. Treating with local steroid injections just temporarily relive the spots will appear in the same area or it may shift to other parts. THE NUMBER ALOPECIA AREATA CASES INCREASING IN NUMBER DUE TO INCREASING HEAVY ALOPATHIC DRUG USAGE FOR ENT DISORDERS MAKE HUGE CONFUSED CONFUSED INFLAMMATION.

Prematurely early graying is another indication of confused inflammation presence in the scalp. Gray hair may be associated with food and hormone deficiency minimally but confused inflammation makes early gray even to the children.

• Parotid and other **salivary gland** disease again caused by confused inflammation sprayed from nose to cheeks.

• Confused inflammation Spread from breast , hands and arms to axilla produce the generalized signs and symptoms of confused inflammation in axilla like atopic dermatitis and produce recurrent suppurative adenitis especially if the confused inflammation has the fibrous cell type which is destroys the basic protective mechanism and allows the infections so that abscess and indurations and keloid formations.

Recurrent adenitis , usage of deodorants ,frequent shaving, using some chemical for removing the hair, all invites the confused inflammation to the axilla. Treatment for fresh inflammation especially dermatitis or other boils by external application gives abundant confused inflammation so it helps deep and permanent pathological changes here.

NOSE IS ACT AS A MASSIVE SOURCE OF CONFUSED INFLAMMATION IN THE BODY THEN ANY OTHER BODY PART.ALMOST 90 PERCENT OF THE HUMANS HAVING SOME OF THE OTHER CHRONIC CONFUSED INFLAMMATION IN THE BODY OUT OF WHICH ALMOST ALL THE DISEASES [ORIGINATES FROM ABOVE THE DIAPHRAGM] IS COMING FROM NASAL MUCOSA.

SO, THE NOSE GIVES THE DISEASE FOR EVERY HUMAN EITHER IT IS A CARIES OR BALDNESS OR EYE DISEORDER OR LUNG DISEASE,BRAIN DISEASE ALL IS SOURCED BY NOSE ONLY.

NOSE IS ACT AS A MASSIVE SOURCE OF CONFUSED INFLAMMATION IN THE BODY THEN ANY OTHER BODY PART.ALMOST 90 PERCENT OF THE HUMANS HAVING SOME OF THE OTHER CHRONIC CONFUSED INFLAMMATION IN THE BODY OUT OF WHICH ALMOST ALL THE DISEASES [ORIGINATES FROM ABOVE THE DIAPHRAGM] IS COMING FROM NASAL MUCOSA.

SO, THE NOSE GIVES THE DISEASE FOR EVERY HUMAN EITHER IT IS A CARIES OR BALDNESS OR EYE DISEORDER OR LUNG DISEASE,BRAIN DISEASE ALL IS SOURCED BY NOSE ONLY.

2.RESPIRATORY DISEASE

Asthma

The cause of the disease has not identified till date. Due to the doctors consider this is again an inflammation, but not know how the inflammation has occurred. so, kept us unknown etiology.

Asthma is a common disease of the respiratory system. difficulty in breathing due to spasm [constriction] of the bronchus. Asthma is caused by confused inflammation excess histamine and subsequent confused inflammation together makes asthma.

The basic understanding of the asthma till date is some external or internal factors induce the spasm of the bronchus—pollution, exercise, germs, diet error. Allergy ,,,,etc. all slowly induce the real inflammation so that now the bronchus is sensitive and produce constriction and produces asthma.

But the reality is reverse. Improperly treated nasal congestions, interrupted true inflammations is spread from nasal and upper respiratory tract reach to the lungs and produce asthma or sub acute or chronic bronchitis.

Pathophysiology Of Asthma

Since the true inflammation is blocked by anti histamines but still the pathogen present in the circulation trigger more histamine liberation so patient try to take again anti histamine **so this excess histamine**, this excess accumulated histamine directly spread to bronchus and to the lungs and produce the entire bronchus is confused inflammatory chemicals. This chemical is hypersensitive to environmental changes. If bronchus exposed to minor or major pollution makes the hyper response so there by spasm of the bronchus.

Asthma is purely allopathic doctors induced disorder. Especially anti-histamine makes this diease.UNFORTUNATELY MOST OF THE DOCTORS AGAIN PRESCRIBBING ANTI HISTAMINE ALONG WITH BRONHCO DIALTER AND STEROIDS.

[what we think the dust invite the histamine but the true is inflamed bronchus (histamine rich bronchus) is abnormally sensitive to the pollution , a normal bronchus will hyper act to remove this dust but an abnormal bronchus initiate hyper abnormal constriction of the bronchus].

A GOOD FUNCTIONING HEALTHY LUNGS SLOWLY OCCUPIED BY CONFUSED INFLAMMATION BY TWO MEDICINE ONE IS ANTI INFLAMMATORY AND OTHER ONE IS ANTI HISTAMINE.

BRONCHITITS

A normal physiological inflammation [*acute bronchitis*] within the lung will have purpose it means a fever will control germ multiplications, an inflammation kills the germs and excess mucus wash away the dust and germs in the bronchus and it will end within a week time. Here there is congestive phase [with fever and tiny blood tinged sputum],a swelling phase marked with white clear mucus with cough, so then resolution phase the patient cured without any medicinal support.

If we use anti histamine and anti-allergic then slowly, we used to get recurrent cold attack due presence of confused inflammation. A real inflammation saves us from infection but confused inflammation favors inflammation. A constant inflamed bronchus and lung tissues undergoes gradual reversible pathology and then over period of time irreversible pathology.

The patient started experiencing difficulty unbreathing when ascending stairs and cannot able to breath in closed room and difficulty in breathing during winter season before diagnose the person as asthmatic or COPD.

some times the inflammatory signs will precede asthma but the inflammation is used as a trigger for the asthma it does not come to help to clear the germs or dust. Since it is single cell or chemical dominant [eosinophilic / histamine] partial or confused inflammation.so it makes only the constriction of the bronchus.

severe irritation within the bronchus so dry teasing cough. Spasm and cough, spasm and cough this episode last for weeks to months. But the confused inflammation temporally stops due to over antihistamine or Broncho dilator or steroid use.by using this drugs helps in form more histamine and confused inflammation cells so even non episodic silent symptom free period this confused inflammation remain inside the bronchus will slowly destroy the bronchus will lead to irreversible bronchus damage over a period of time patient deteriorate towards chronic obstructive pulmonary disease [**COPD**].

Other lung diseases also similarly induced by anti histamines and anti-inflammatory drugs which will produce histamine rich lung disease and more confused inflammation. but anti-inflammatory drugs will prevent this inflammation temporarily . if the person exposed to dust and minor or major germ infections then this accumulated confused inflammation chemicals dumped into the lungs will produce severe painful sub acute inflammations [bronchitis , pneumonia,,,,etc.] recurrent bronchitis over a period of time will produce **COPD.**

So non of the respiratory diseases arises as we study in the text all the diseases arise because we sprayed the confused inflammation chemicals either histamine alone or in total inflammation chemicals this is occupy in the lungs and produce mild to severe lung diseases for many years.

Pneumonia and other lung infections

A lung is protected with multi level guards so it is not that easy to produce the infection within lung. Then how the infection and how the death.

Instead of how to prevent pneumonia and infection related death better we study how to make death so that it will be easy for Indian doctors to understand.

• Prescribe anti inflammatory and anti allergic drugs if there is any running nose and sneezing and fevers and train the public to take on their own.so this will collapse the basic protective mechanism and patient become Hypersensitive.

• Once the patient is hypersensitive, they definitely come with hyper response to dust and climatic changes so they often fall upper respiratory tract infection and then end with lower respiratory tract infection so its easy and legal to prescribe anti allergic and anti inflammatory along with we can prescribe what ever may be the anti biotic available in the market.

Use all nasal drops, nasal sprays and paracetamol syrup must they must carry this paracetamol syrup in hand all the time because it will cure viral infections, bacterial infections and all other gram-negative bacteria's and lot more,,,,,,etc. When the congestion in the nose put anti-allergic syrup otherwise nasal drops or nasal spray so stop running nose sneezing. This will cure all the allergy and infections.

Use steroids if the fever and running nose and cough is not arrested within 2 days.We have to bath the children with all of the above drugs.

• Mean while remove the tonsil,adenoid,lymph nodes around the neck one by one.

• Prescribe antibiotic for all upper respiratory and lower respiratory tract infection either it is allergy or viral or bacterial or any other germs so our duty is prescribing some antibiotics.

• When the child cross about 2-3 years now anti inflammatory and anti allergic and anti biotic may not be effective in controlling the infections and hypersensitiveness so **ask the patient to use nebulizer and bronchodilator and Steroids**.

• When the child is become 3-4 year now you make one apartment in the hospital to stay along with their family in the hospital itself it will be easy for them to reside and take the treatment then visiting weekly once or twice.
Child will loss total immunity and addicted to allopathic drugs.
Allopathic drugs also loss its effectivity.

• Now we can say patient perfectly fit for death. We are attained our goal.
No immunity, drug addiction, drug resistance,hypersensitivity,high tendency to get infection, easy spread of the infection from nose to across the

respiratory tract and all over the body,

We can certify that person definitely fall in ICU and attain quick death.

•   We have to prescribe all the available medicine for simple cold and viral fever is the basic standard.one anti allergic, one antipyretic, one cough syrup mucolytic and steroid all is needed if the cough is persist more then 3-4 days keep that in mind we have to prescribe this drugs otherwise patient fall in collapse from acute cold.

A HOSPITALISATION IN INDIA AND MEDICATION IN INDIA NOT TO CURE THE SICKNESS IT IS FOR GETTING THE SICKNESS.YOU ARE GOING TO HOSPITAL TO GET THE FOUNDATION FOR SICKNESS NOT TO CURE YOUR SELF.

YOU ARE ADMITED IN THE HOSPITAL NOW A DAYS FOR STOP FEVER,RUNINING NOSE, COUGH,VOMITING,DIARRHEA .ALL ARE BASIC BODY PRTECTIVE MECHANISAM TO HELP YOU TO COME OUT FROM SICKNESS THEY SUPPORT FOR YOU TO KILL THE GERMS.BUT HOSPITAL DOING MAGIC TO THE PATIENT FEEL PROUD TO THE PATIENT BY STOPPING THIS.

SO, THIS IS THE FANDAMENTAL CAUSE FOR YOUR FUTURE ADMISSION FOR HOSPITAL.A HEALTHY MAN FORCIBLY FIGHTING TO THE GERMS IS NOW ALLOW THE INFECTION TILL THE LUNGS HE WILL NOT RESSIST IT.

YOU WILL BECOME HYPERSENSITIVE; HYPERSENSITIVITY IS THE DOCTORS MADE DISORDER BUT THEY WILL SAY YOUR BODY IS HAVING SOME SPECIFIC GENE AND YOUR FATHER OR GARAND FATHER IS HAVING ASTHMA AND SO YOU ARE HAV-

ING THIS.

PASSING STOOL AND URINE IS ALSO A GEN-ITIC DISORDER SINCE YOUR RELATIVES ARE PASSING IT SO YOU ARE ALSO PASSING IT.

1.Infection reach to the lungs only by breaking the protective functions of the upper respiratory tracts.

2. Confused inflammation is the top most reason for germ entry and its multiplication and death.

3.Steroid prescription to children's especially for respiratory infection is too high,this will again reduce the immunity over all fighting capacity to infections so germs entry and multiplication so easy.

We have to read and understand death rate is more in case of respiratory illness but we have to score and create all top most reason for respiratory tract infections and allergy asthma and COPD.

A child affected with viral pneumoniya then there is no medicine in allopathy but they never send this case to homeopath.this patient again will recive antibiotic ? more the doctor is sure about the disease is fatel then more the doctor will prescribe antibiotic and steroid this will kill the child sure.

Presvention of death rate in case of pneumonia and other respiratory illness is simple .

1.Avoid stopping fever and runining nose.

2.Take homeopathic medicine

3.Take homeopathy and remove confused inflammation from your body.

A INFECTION NEVER KILL THE PATIENT BUT THE

CONFUSED INFLAMMATION CREATED BY DOCTORS WILL KILL THE PATIENT ,SO THAT RECOVERY OR DEATH IS NOT RELATED WITH WHO IS HANDLING THIS CASE OR WHAT VIRUS OR BACTERIA IS GONE IN BUT HOW MUCH CONFUSED INFLAMMATION IS PRESENT ,WHAT IS THAT IS MAKING A CHOICE DEATH OR RECOVERY.

More then sufficient time is there to save your childrens take homeopathy in advance save the child life.Since all the childrens under allopathic medicine sure they will have confused inflammation in the body.

Tumors in the lungs

There is another group of inflammation cell will reach to the lungs this will produce excess infiltration of fibrous and gelatin matrix tissues inside the lungs and produce tumors. This is caused by treatment of the skin diseases/ulcers by external applications like strong ointments so the material used for wound healing [fibrous, gelatin material] and skin diseases sprayed all over the body is attracted into the lungs by repeated infections or dust and pollution exposure [hyper functions or irritation in the lungs].

So now this chemicals and cells will infiltrate inside the lung tissues and impair the total lung functions bronchial secretions will impaired and protective mechanism is impaired and the normal respiration functions is impaired [purifications] prone to infection to varies virus and bacteria's lead to severe pneumonia or abscess and total pathological changes of the entire lung.

A lung is become lost its sponge nature it become solid [hepatization] unable to carry out simple inflammation due to collapse of circulation ,inflammation ,immune system collapse so that long run of the inflammations and abnormal entry of more powerful inflammation cells into the lungs which will again makes the healing as well as damage so the disease produce severe necrosis or produces severe chronic lung disease like **tb** or **chronic lung abscess**.

The abscess formation and healing are not a normal response of the lungs. an abscess formation is actually indicating failed inflammation due to excess accumulation of confused inflammation with excess germs allowed.

" *We study and treat and search the lung disorders in the way that asthma is inflammation, bronchitis is the inflammation, pneumonia is the inflammation ,lung abscess is the inflammation, tuberculosis is the infections. But the true all are secondary not the primary all are not a inflammation it's a pathological inflammation it means confused inflammation. It gives all the disease in the lungs*

So, the way we are looking into the disease is persist again then non of the disease is curable by any drugs it may give temporary relief but long-standing chronic disease.

We drain the lung abscess we can heal the lung abscess but we have to think why abscess ? . How this pathology is happened, how all the multi level protection is failed ? how the infection reached to the most protected organ so easily .

Who broken this many barrier layer? what measures we taken to rebuild every layers broken by germ or medicines ? before the fibrosis or abscess formed ? why we read simple congestion and abscess and fibrosis is same degree ? how we can think fibrosis of the lung is a normal inflammation mechanism ? how we can think an abscess inside body is normal inflammation ? when we study in this manner patient will not get proper treatment from the doctors.

A lung is dumped excess fibrous gelatin tissues before the active inflammation begin so that it does not allow the inflammation to carry out normally, we cannot expect the resolution or recovery phase.patient will die sooner or later by recurrent lung infections.

A staphylococci or streptococci or tuberculosis or pseudomonas makes the lung abscess. this bacterium killed and digested when the lung is in good condition that we name it acute bronchitis up to this level is considered inflammation is physiological. But when the lung is full of confused inflammation chemicals and cells like excess infiltrations of fibrous tissues and other cells inside the lungs will prevent to carry out normal immune , inflammation functions now if the entered organism is even a influenza virus can kill the person and staphylococcus will make the huge abscess similarly streptococcus and pseudomonas and TB All will stay inside the body and makes the huge long standing severe diseases.

A tuberculine baccillai is inactive to produce a tuberculosis in the healthy human. A full-blown tuberculosis is highly possible even if the person is having otherwise healthy but within the lungs there is a collection of fibrous and inflammatory material.it means A tuberculosis is almost always secondry to heavy chronic inflammation cells within the body.

Draining the abscess, recovering from acute illness recovering from tb is not a cure, eliminating the confused inflammation from the lungs is a right way of cure otherwise patient will suffer again and again with the lung ailments.A Tuberculine baccillai removel helps to stop the confused inflammation cells entry into the lungs,this is like we gave some artificial enemy to the lungs so all the cells are reached here now we are eliminating that so the patient is recovering.

So, don't panicky about the germs all are second-ary treat the primary cause and don't support anymore confused inflammation chemical formation.repaire the in-flammation and immune system to act normally, cure the hard and indurated non functioning lymph node to func-tioning .repair the indurated non functioning tonsil to work normally. cure and repair the nasal congestions and al-lergy ,cure and repair the adenoid and recover the function of the adenoid so now all protectors act well will not allow the virus or bacteria's entering so easily inside the body.

If you don't interrupt in the true physiological inflammation no confused inflammation inside the lung .so if the lungs are healthy can handle any inflammation and germs easily and kill them without great disturbance to the patient and heal without an abscess cure without any fibro-sis. Fibrosis and abscess inside the lung are multi level sys-tem failure not just an inflammation aware this it means you are given many years for reaching this worst stage so treat and cure before reaching this stage and if you don't have medicine send someone who is having this medicine.

Identifying and removing the tumor early is ne-cessary but need a question mark why the tumor here. you are so hasty and prescribed many medicated creams for the ulcer which is going to heal normally.So, the wandering con-fused inflammation settled in the lung makes the tumor. We make the trouble in the name of treatment and we act like we are giving treatment .

Why are you going in depth and too long to search cause from genetic ? when the cause is readily visible ? and recently you collapsed system ? are you forgot that ?

I am listing out so many illegal treatments, If that medicines is following rule of biology, then all this diseases may not come to the public. ofcourse I understand genetic but read the whole book and go to your practice come to conclusion who is right who is wrong.genetics having extremely minor role in disease producing you are blaming all the disease as genetics.

Always doctors have to keep in mind that recovering the failed system is an important aspect along with or after the treatment of the main disease for which patient came.

Failure of liver, failure of the kidney and heart is given great importance to the doctors but they are not aware that before kidney failure there are many system failures happening we are least bothered about it, before the liver and heart failures there are many minor to major system failures happenings we are least bothered about it, before the lung failure and heart failure many system failures happening we are least bothered about it that's why the organ failures unavoidable.

Failure of inflammation is a key factor for major diseases, failure of lymph node function is important you have to cure that and make that alright,but you are ignored and not felt guilty that you are not having medicine to recover that,more ever you felt happy when removing diseased lymph node (failed physiology teaching) failure of tonsil function you are ignored it and felt happy that when you removing tonsil as if you did something great to patient (failed physiology teaching). So, now the inflammation is the only disease you are handling everywhere inflammation cells or immune cells but no idea why this disease ? this cell here ?

Copd and cor pulmonale is indicates that India is not having any one single doctor or a copd patient never met doctor in his life time. both or not true in fact the cause for COPD is allopathic treatment. ignorance and negligence are not only neglecting the treatment but making the disease by knowingly is a crime and negligence. Allowing the disease to spread fully and mature its full course and the doctor is giving many prescriptions which gives the relief but the disease will progress to worse what kind of observation is this.

Hypersensitivity pneumonitis and occupational lung disease

A true inflammation is functioning against the humans has to be accepted in these 2 categories. A Noxious agent's entry is continuing so that the inflammation has to be maintained for never ending so that if the inflammation is not closed within a period of time then the particular body parts will suffer due to inflammation. This excuse is not acceptable anywhere else in the body since. There is no continues voluntary and knowingly allowing the organism to enter inside if we did without resting phase for inflammation to repaired and regenerate the inflammation area sure it reaches worst damage like fibrosis and lung failure.

We can say the only one ideal example of the inflammation and immunity may produce danger.

Every time when we worried and feared about inflammation or immunity is danger we have to ask our self why the inflammation is worked good to us, now it is the enemy [we should not simple think auto immunity all time] the above example is make the doubt very clear .yes the person will go heavy industrial dust which is more micron size then the ordinary dust every day without rest so the inflammation has to work continuously will damage the lungs .here the inflammation has the aim and target but the mistake is the target is never ending ,it keep coming so it has to work ,work need to send more powerful cells.

Yes, it does not able to digest is so granuloma ,yes of course we have accepted it. but I am not accepting the tuberculous granuloma that is made by confused inflammation .Our body immunity has highest power to digest this tb bacilli but since the inflammation has been confused the granuloma is formed but in occupational and hypersensitivity pneumonia the situation is some thing wrong and acceptable.

A continues exhausting war will sure collapse the entire country.

But doctors always keep the difference between power of solider in protecting the border in the peaceful country , here there are few fights now and then, and the real war between two country for many years.

Don't try to prevent death rate don't focus on major life-threatening disease, focus on minor ailments and minor mistake, since this minor mistakes over a period of time growing like mega death producing agent. A minor ailment we treat illogically in the nose and skin is causing life threatening cancer or heart attack or tumors in future.

3.VASCULAR DISEASE AND HEART

- STROKE / MYOCARDIAL INFARCTION
- CORONARY ARTERY DISEASE / ATHEROSCLEROSIS.

Cardio vascular disease is number 1 in cause for death.Nearly 17 (1.7 crore) million people died due to CVD in 2016.

Doctors beliving that reducing risk factors will reduce the possibility of the cvd like stop smokking, reducing unhealthy diet and maintaining ideal body weight,stopping harmfull use of alcohol, doing regular exercise will reduce the cvd risk and again keeping blood sugar ,blood pressure and cholesterol under control will prevent the CVD risk.

Myocardial infarct (heart) and stroke within cerebral blood vassals are preventable.so easily and simply, since these 2 diseases reserve their dominance in middle age and elderly, we have so much enough time to give 100 % safe coronary artery (heart) and cerebral artery (brain).

SO, THE TOP MOST KILLER DISEASE IN THE WORLD AND IN INDIA IS TRACED AND GOING TO BE ELIMINATED FROM THE UNIVERSE, BE HAPPY YOU ARE SAFE NOW.

In a single day, a life in the middle-aged or the elderly aged person suddenly changed due to these attacks the whole family is in suffering the individual will become have lots of disability. Bear the sufferings to some extent in the young age then you will not suffer in the middle age or elderly period.

Meet the homeopath and take treatment with them to recover from minor acute attacks. Keep in touch with them to trace and eliminate the confused inflammation.So, no possibility of chronic disease. It means the root cause of the vascular disease is confused inflammation. So, prevent vascular disease by avoiding allopathy or take homeopathy to existing confused inflammation disease.

We don't want speedy recovery, allopathy is not giving speedy relief, dear they stopping the natural healing process so that we feel the temperature is stopped, the pain is gone, the sick feeling is relived, we surprised and believed those who are doing magic in the human body. For doing magic and forgetting science and natural healing power, why we have to study 6 years basic medical science I don't know ? . So, honey we don't want any magic to happen to our body bear the suffering or else meet the homeopath take the treatment.

And remember that heart attack may not happen on the next day when you suppress the fever or suppress the skin disease with ointments it happens many years after the treatment, I hope you may forget that event in total. Even a doctor will be forgot that event. so that you and along with your doctor considered this disease is happened today and there is no relation with your

old treatment and searching the cause for today ailment. search-
ing, searching and searching, till date they have not detected the
cause.

I appreciate the humbleness of allopathy doctors they
accept at least many diseases are coming immediately after the
acute illness. But beyond that, the confused inflammation dis-
order may take unusually longer time to resurface so that doc-
tors forgot to correlate this disease with past occurrence. But
even though they are not accepting that it was happened due to
their medicine. but the disease having clue and evidence to say
that doctors created this disease by wrong treatment,and its not a
fresh natural disease.

All the Confused inflammation diseases are not the
complications they are the primary first work of the medicine.It
means the single dose of paracetamol will produce confused in-
flammation before the stomach burning happen, the fever is
stopped (then confused inflammation ready) the pain is stopped
(then confused inflammation ready).

Honey you won't believe along with you, your doctors
are also hearing this mal the function of the medicine, I hope
he will not do this anymore for just making satisfaction to the
patient.

Why the doctor prescribing the anti-inflammatory
and anti-histamine because he does not aware deepest main
effect of medicine, like you, so he is doing this. You are admit-
ted in the hospital with suffering but now you are going to home
without any suffering so you and your doctor believing that we
are safe and we did something good to the patient, but honey keep
in your mind you are admitted for getting life long-suffering not
to cure.

1. There is no possibility of coagulation within
the blood vessels in a healthy person and there is no inflam-

mation within the artery is maintained as normal functions. But this normal protective function is disrupted due to inappropriate usage of medicines especially external applications and anti-inflammatory anti-allergic etc.

The blood coagulation happens immediately near to the injured site to arrest the bleeding, but when we use anti-inflammatory or any other chemical or ointments in the wound then the coagulation chemicals reenter into the circulation. The chemical which is there inside the blood which helps in preventing intravascular coagulation may not work upon this reentered coagulation factor leads to intravascular coagulation and thrombus formation where ever it sticks and attracted.This intravascular coagulation is highly minute and subtle except if it is affect importand vital organ we may not aware this. THE STROKE OF CEREBROVASCULAR DISEASE IS HIGHLY MINUTE MICRO BLEEDING AND SUBSEQUENT INFARCT AND THE MYO-CARDIAL INFARCT AND PRECEDING ATHEROSCLEROSIS ALL VERY MINUTE AND MICRO LEVEL but it is not normal it may not happen as the age progress or due to wear and tear malfunction. This microbleeding,micro thrombus and following micro infarct all happen due to confused inflammation and inward receded clotting factors . AGING OR GENETIC IS NOT HAVING ANY ROLE HERE EATING CONSTRUCTING food ELEMENT IS NOT A CAUSE (it means cholestrole is not a cause for atherosclerosis). nothing is there to do further research. it is crystal clear what is the cause for the ailment.

The intravascular coagulation / emboli formation is an emergency condition. This will create lots of diseases within the blood vessels. Along with confused inflammation chemicals, this intravascular coagulation chemicals will induce inflammatory changes within the blood vessels.

2 . Vaso constriction one of the earliest process of the injury so by using an external application this vasospasm inducing chemicals will re enter into the circulation and will cause vasospasm in many unnecessary

places (frankly speaking there is no allopathic medicine to stop vasospasm, bleeding and many more sequences of the wound healing and inflammation than how I am saying the vasospasm chemical allowed to re-entering ? using or applying any chemical to an injured site other then water is not allowed all the chemical used for the purpose of dressing the wound will distract the accuracy of the wound healing and promotes wandering confused wound healing cells and chemicals). Simple vasospasm will induce angina pain and produce signs and symptoms similar to a heart attack but CAG (coronary angiogram) will disprove vascular disorder in the brain it produces TIA transient ischemic attack with faintness and giddiness.

3.When we disturb the wound healing then the fibrous tissues gelatin matrix and fatty materials all will be allowed to roam within the circulation. If we not disturb it might close the wound and make the wounded parts equal surface without any barrows or deep pitting. The superficial fatty layer of the skin is constructed with this gelatin matrix as well as this fatty tissus the broken skin tied with fibrous tissues since we use heavy medicated or chemical ointments this process disturbed so that thw wound may be closed but the fatty tissues,gelatin matrics,fibrous tissues all will allowed to roam within the circulation.

So this 3 material is almost enough material to make mini tumor or micro or even macro indurations to many sites. This 3 material along with any epithelial cells or any other regenerating cells will produce mini to gaigantic tumor within the body.in the same way this material produce the vascular deposites and athrosclerosis. (now read the character of the confused inflammation).

The circulating confused inflammatory chemicals why chooses the blood vessals to deposit and more ever why it chooses middle layer of the blood vessals ? the construction is attracted by either another fresh wound or it may be attracted towards a hyper working site (all the confused inflammatory cells and chemicals will be attracted by slightly more then hyper functions of any body parts is the character of the confused inflammation cells. So, it reaches the muscular coating of the blood vessals rather then despositing within the lumen of blood vessals. It penetrates and reaches the tunica media and produce atherosclerosis. A fat and matrix and fibroblast start wound healing where it is not necessary and the intravascular coagulation happen any time to this site. It is not that paerson food (cholestrole either good of bad cholestrole is depositing here.It is actually distracted confused construction fatty material depositing here keep this information in mind.

(it is unnessary to think that atherosclerosis is peeling of and produce wound so that the macrophage or the platelets coming and producing the thrombi formation all are not happening here)

A slight even normal turbulence within the artery is highly enogh to attract the confused inflammation to invite wound healing in an absolutely normal region.it is the standard of every tumour ,yes every tumour is a wound healing but in an unwanted parts. All this collapse is happening after inappropriate and illogical treatment.

But even though we take anti-inflammatory from childhood, we never had a heart attack or stroke in the early life, the reason behind it the inflammatory chemicals pushed away from original inflammation site is choosing the skin or joint or microvasculature and veno arterial junctions or mucocutaneous junctions' similar sites of the periphery.

(But endocardia are fall in damage in early childhood (rheumatic heart disease) one of the confused immune disorder) but the trend is changing now there are so many childrens now a days fall in chronic diseses.

It gradually gives the disease in skin or extremities again we try to push away by strong medications kind of we do not allow to surface the disease in the skin mucous membrane so after many folds strong allopathic drugs then the confused inflammatory cells are finally choosing the sites of deeper organs like heart , brain, kidney, etc. here also it does not make the symptoms immediately it takes a longer time to develop angina or myocardial infarct.

In comparing to normal blood vessels, the confused inflammation attacked blood vessels (artiritis or atherosclerosis) are vulnerable to break and bleed because it is losing basic elastic property and more ever due to inflammation within the blood vessals.

The atherosclerosis is formed by confused inflammation in many cases atherosclerosis itself make some vascular insufficiency (angina-chest pain if you run or climb stairs or heavy work, exertional giddiness or blockouts). Mostly the anastomosis will help in promoting the proper vascular supply of the heart. atherosed vessel is the more vulnerable site for thrombus formation due to losing its basic protection against the internal clot's mechanism due to internal receding of the clotting factor during the allopathic treatment favors the thrombus formation within the artery STROKE IN THE BRAIN, HEART ATTACK IN THE HEART (MAYOCARDIAL INFARCT). So, leading to death or recovery with disability or without disability.

The blood vessels which are supplying to the brain are blocked due to emboli or atherosclerosed artery gets blocked.So, thereby no blood supply to the brain cells and stroke comes / or leaking of the micro bleeding to the brain causes a stroke. The bleeding again not related to any blood disorders it is happening due to breaking of the vessel wall like in congestive phase of inflammation actively.

Prescribing medicine for preventing intravascular coagulation is absolutely unnecessary.again this intravascular coagulation prevention [blood thinner] may not work effectively , because of the intravascular coagulation is happening due to confused inflammation chemical this may not respond for blood thinner. If enough intravascular clotting chemical is there then sure the patient will have intravascular clots despite current allopathic preventive medicine ,we can describe this in olden terms swallowing iron rod and then drinking zinger water to digest that iron rod.its similar to that.so prevention is don't allow the confused inflammation to happen that is right prevention if at all it is happen use homeopathy to remove that confused inflammation from the body is a right step.

Whenever the bleeding is happen whenever the clotting has happened inside the body we always search in bleeding and clotting factor may be at fault, so we wright a test immediate bleeding time and clotting time and vitamin K and INR platelet and Prothrombin time like that bleeding and clotting inside the body [intravascular coagulation] happen only because of confused inflammatory chemicals. Which was created by taking anti-inflammatory tablets or external applications to the wound especially applying any chemical in the fresh bleeding wound cause inward receding of the bleeding, clotting factors and chemicals cause this.

Early detection and clearing the confused inflammation within the circulation helps in preventing atherosclerosis so that stroke and myocardial infarction is preventable.

Atherosclerosis is looks like inflammation within artery here more than early stage of confused inflammatory changes It looks like the late constructive stage of inflammation, the available microscopic future of the *ath-*

351

erosclerosis is mimic like a mini tumor [ATHROMA] inside the blood vessels deposits of

- fat
- fibroblasts
- smooth muscle cells
- inter cellular matrix.
- Some inflammatory cells like macrophage.

do you still thinking some germs or some genetical malformation or excess cholesterol induce all this issue then medicine induced confused inflammation?.

So smoking or hyper cholesterol or eating rich diet or no exercise blood disorders all are just a triggering factor. THE TRUE CAUSE FOR THE DISEASE IS CONFUSED INFLAMMATION WHICH IS REMOVABLE FROM THE BODY AND WE CAN ASSURE AND ISSUE A CERTIFICATE TO THE PERSON THAT HE WILL NOT SUFFER HEART DISEASE IN FUTURE.

WE CAN PREVENT CARDIO VASCULAR DISEASES MORE THEN 10-20 YEARS BEFORE NOT AT THE ICU OR AFTER ESTABLISHED PARTIAL STENOSIS IN THE CLINIC THIS IS GOING TO BE THE FUTURE.

Symptoms Of Heart Attack (Mayocardial Infarct)

- Pain or discomfort in the center of the chest.
- Pain or discomfort in the left shoulder arm, jaws, elbows and back.
- Difficulty in breathing

- Shortness of breath
- Feeling sick or vomiting
- FEELING LIGHT HEAD OR FAINT
- BREAKING INTO A COLD SWAET AND BE-COMING PALE

Common Symptoms Of Stroke

- Numbness of the face arm leg especially one side of the body
- Confusion ,difficulty speaking or understanding speech
- Difficulty in seeing one or both eye
- Severe head ache with no known cause
- Fainting or unconsciousness

Summery

Distracting confused inflammation causes vascular changes the distracted inflammation induces the chronic inflammation and atherosclerosis along with available chemicals and produce atherosclerosis. This atherosclerosis narrowd space become narrowed due to emboli formation this emboli formation again encouraged by distracted clotting chemicals.(see under scleroderma / vasculitis for further detail)

Prevent the vascular disease and save the public by not producing confused inflammation and eliminate the confused inflammation earlier by taking homeopathy medicine before it taking internal disease like heart and brain vascular disease.

If atherosclerosis is preventable then nearly millions of life in the world is saved. Sure, it is highly possible to prevent atheroscleroris.

Prevention progrome by WHO : for cerebro vascular disease :

The cerebro vascular disease is increase steadily from 594 million in 1975 to 1.13 billion in 2015.

Under the leadership of the WHO, all Member States (194 countries) agreed in 2013 on global mechanisms to reduce the avoidable NCD burden including a "Global action plan for the prevention and control of NCDs 2013-2020". This plan aims to reduce the number of premature deaths from NCDs by 25% by 2025 through nine voluntary global targets. Two of the global targets directly focus on preventing and controlling CVDs.

Homeopaths will help in achiving reducing non communicable disease burden for sure. This achievement will be more strengthened if allopathy ready to prescribe homeopathy.

HEART DISEASE

Many orgon in the body is fall in sickness often but the heart is not so easily fall in disease when comparing with other orgon. The cardiac diseases mostly trouble in old age that disease also due to blood vessal of the heart not directly by heart tissue damage by confused inflammation. Tumor within the heart and cancer withing the heart everything is too low when comparing with other orgon.

When you read over all in the whole text

book I use to fry allopathy doctors like anything but not with heart disease but all either respiratory disease or liver or kidney. But the chance developing confused inflammation is too high in heart why ? since the only massively shakking and vibrating orgon in the body, hyper mobile orgon in the body is heart by this action the bad inflammation sure will produce the disease but it is not happening since extremely poor possibility of bad inflammation catching or trapped within heart. (but this is not good since the recived blood forcibly pushed towards one chamber to other chamber with more turbulence and vigrouse shaking suppose if the confused inflammation present in the blood then that will get activated to develop disease by this violent procedure but not giving option to develop disease so this will cause disease immediate to the next possible site like within the blood vessals).

Since too frequent prescription of the antibiotics and anti inflammation then the blood is having heavy confused inflammation and antibodys for that almost half of the world childrens fall in rheumatic heart disease and valvular heart disease but the rheumatic heart disease incidence is less. Then what about this confused inflammation that is busy in making disease in ENT and skin and other orgons.

So there by very poor chance of direct heart disease be the confused inflammation. Comparing to other orgon heart is located deep that might be cause for less disease occurance ? no.

Then what ? eventhough the heart is deep and in safe location brain is located too safer than heart but brain is affected very worst and very often either pscychologically or brain tumors of epilepsy in that way more coomnoly affected then heart.

We can say all the blood including bad inflammation and immunity will come and pass through the heart only but still there is less possibility disease tendency then rest of the orgon. The reason is

The kidney is having many parenchymal tissues (neprons more then 1 crore neprons the bad inflammation chemical when passes through the minute structures and the bad inflammation produce confused inflammation disease.

Actually, speaking all the blood is recived by the heart with mega large blood vessals and pumped out in the same mega large blood vessals. So extremely less possibility of trapping or resting option of the confused inflammation.

A liver is damaged so there by secondarily blood flow stagnated then the disease occurring (right heart failure). Peripheral vaso constriction then more hypertension then left heart failure

The blood which is passing through extremely tiny alveolar blood circulation so here more intimate contact of the bad inflammation within the alveolai and bronchiyoles causes severe disease. For example, over all capillary strength of lungs is more then 100 times then the heart.

Each orgon in the body recieve the blood-through the aretery. Then artery blood passes through the arteriole then the blood passes minute blood vessal called capillery more then capillary further tiny structre is alveolai and nephrons.

But heart recive the blood through bigger vein then all the veins and pump the blood bigger artery then rest of the artery. A blood enters into the heart and leave the heart less then 1 second. Heart act as a bigger blood vessal nothing more then that just pumping. Kidney has to filter and completely seprate the waste product. lungs has to remove CO_2 saturate the oxygen so it takes some time. Liver has to collecte the all food mixed within the blood and it also has to send needed food within the blood so there is blood stayes within the liver bit more time then the heart.

What is disease fighting between two group enemy with soldger so where ever soldger is more the fight will be more and disease will be more

Appendix is fall sick due to presence of lymphatics so this will kill the bacteria and fail some time so disease.

Tonsil is having lympahtics so this will kill germs if it is failing then disease so either inflammation or infection or non communicable disease all are possible here. A liver is having immune cell kupfer cells a lung is having macrophage and so many other immune and inflammation fighting cells within.

A brain having astrocytes,microglia and so many macropahges all will kill the germs so possibility of infection and inflammation so there by non communicable disease if allopathy treat.

A lymph node is having such fighting chance so frequent disease possibility luckily our heart paranchyma is not having such great macrophage system and there is no great huge microcapillary circulation to expose the heavy infection or fighting mechanisam is the cause for less possibility of the confused inflammation disease then rest of the body orgons. The spleen is dead opposite to the heart it means having heavy macrophage system so the frequent killing functions of the germs and infections and recurrent disease then heart.

Still there are some disease like endocaridyal disease and some infections and some auto immune disease. But heart is nearly 90 % protected then rest of the body parts that's why the heart is safe until 50 + then also the heart attack is not happened due to disease of heart .the heart attack is caused by cardiac vascular system disease. There are childrens fall in cardiac disease mostly congenital and again. The heart disease is bit more those who have valvular disease then infections and non communicable disease possibility chances within the hear increases. Heart disease is more those who have liver disease and alcoholic and cirrhosis. Chronic lung disease will give stress cardiac disease (cor pulmonale).

Heart muscles dialted or hypertrophied due to hypertension that is again vascular disease followed by heart disease.

RHEUMATIC HEART DISEASE

Rheumatic fever occurs in about 3,25,000 children each year and about 33.4 million people currently have rheumatic heart disease.

Is causing damage to the heart valve and heart muscles from the inflammation. In 2015 it resulted in 3,19,400 deaths down from 374,000 deaths in 1990. Most deaths occur in the developing world where as many as 12.5% of people affected may die each year.

When a person infected with streptococcal sore throat then the infections treated with anti inflammatory and antibiotic then the immunoglobulin circulating within the vessals and heart is damaging the heart valves (auto immunity).

Symptoms Of Rheumatic Heart Disease Including Shortness Of Breath.

- Irregular heart beat
- Fatique
- Chest pain
- Fainting
- Symptoms of rheumatic fever includes fever, pain, swelling of the joints.
- Nausea, stomach cramps and vomiting
- Rheumatic fever is attack between ages of 5-15 years adult also will suffer with rheumatic fever.

The antibody developed during this condition attacks the myocardiyam and valves and slowly impaire the normal structure of the valves and so there by the fibsrosed and short valves does not close properly so that the regurgitation or due to extensive stricture of the valves leads to short openining so that heavy pressure and less cardiac output so that impaire the perfusion.

Major Criteria

1.Migrating inflammaiton of the large joints
2.Inflammation of the muslce of the heart
3.inflammation of the pericardium
4.subcutanes nodules

5.erethema marginatum
6.sydenhams chorea

Minor Criteria

1.fever
2.arthralgia
3.raised ESR
4.increased white blood cells,Elevated ESR, Elevated CRP.
5.ECG Abnormality

Prevention of rheumatic fever has to be encouraged by stopping anti-inflammatory drugs and stopping anti biotics.

The olden days development of the same disease without anti biotics anti inflammatory is due to poor immunity with drinking impure water makes the recurrent streptococcal throat infection causes unusually longer period of streptococcal infection leads to self destruction but the current auto immune destruction is due to ant inflammation and antibiotic administration.

> why the auto immune cells and chemicals attack the valves of the eandocardiyam most prominently ? The distracted active immune cells are hyper active and most ready to initiate their action when minimal stimulus given. Within the heart the opening and closure of the valves in the body is the highest turbulence mechanisam in the human body so this will attract and initiate the destruction in and around bicuspid and tricuspid valve of the heart.

Hypertension / Hypotension

Blood pressure is controlled by vasomotor center (BRAIN) and maintained normal by the sensors within the blood vassals called chemoreceptor's and baro receptors and aortic body and carotid sinus.

The cause for high blood pressure is unknown except high bp in case of kidney disease but almost 95 % of the high blood pressure cause is unknown. Again if we trace the cause for kidney disease that is again unknown etiology it means no idea why this disease.

When the cause is unknown for bp , but they are very sure that bp is the cause for many cardiac ,kidney and cerebral disorders ?

The cause for hypertension and hypotension is caused by confused inflammation.The circulating confused inflammation damages the blood vessals and alter the vaso-constriction and vaso dialatation capacity when this happen in the early days the high and low bp is unstable in the early days of the vessal attack but at the later time the blood vessal is losing this capacity permanently and permanent hypertensive. These changes are evident many years before the atherosclerosis development.

Atherosclerosis is contributing high bp in extreme old age with majority of the arteries is become atherosed it may contribute another 1 or 2 percent but high bp is so commonly present in many adults and young people even with healthy artery (spasm of the bloodvessal and artiritis like changes begins long before the true atherosclerosis)

The carotid sinus mal function is one of the causes for the high bp.[need research final support to this theory].

Since the confused inflammation cells which is originate in the nose spread in the face and induce lots of disease and spread to the thyroid and parotid, produce the disease over there similarly it affects the carotid sinus. This changes like micro fibrosis or thickening of the carotid sinuses so that it sends permanent wrong signal to the vasomotor center to elevate the bp.

It is not only that , even permanent or temporary low bp is again caused by involvement of these receptors , syncope caused by involvement of this receptors (already accepted).

A food & oxygen carrying artery, signal carrying nerve, vein together tied with explosive defense fighting zones [lymph node] in the neck.so when the lymph node is enlarged then the carotid sinus get pressure and long time inflammaed lymph node will give direct permamnt pressure upon the carotid sinus will lead to permanent elevation of the bp)

Pressure receptors will help in reduce the BP ; chemo receptors will help in increase the BP according to the situation it will act. There are very important blood controller and maintainer in the body Barro receptors and chemo receptors in the body but anyway the signals carried and reciprocated by nerves [vagus, herrings] The higher centers [Vasomotor Center] works based upon the signals given by this receptors and nerves.

Disturbance in these signal centers and the nerves causes disturbance in maintaining the Blood pressure. Unfortunately, there is no disease recorded with suspecting swellon lymph node create the pressure to the receptors and there by possibility of the disease.

Only the neck region is having high possibility of getting trouble .because the nerves and the neck pressure/chemo signal centers all together passes along with deep cervical lymph node. when this lymph nodes get inflamed or infected or swollen then these signal centers and nerves will get damaged temporarily or permanently.

When this signal centers are damaged the body will develop high BP. [IT HAS BEEN PROVED ALREADY ALOPATHS BY STOPPING TOTAL BLOOD SUPPLY TO THE SIGNAL CENTERS WILL INCREASE THE BP].

The bp elevation initially fluctuating then it will be permanent after both sides nerves or signals are damaged. There is no great surprise that how both sides will affect.it is so simple that lymph nodes will get infect very frequently.

In fact, both signal centers will be in trouble even around 5-10 years age of childhood life but a repeated inflammation possibility makes indurations [it need around 10 more years to develop indurations in the nerve and signal centers after initial inflammation].

These theories again give further more possibility of various gastric disease and heart arrhythmia, palpitations in the nerve disturbance without real cardiac disease without any pathology in the stomach but just irritating the vague nerve at this point.

Possibility of neck pain and spondylosis without real cervical spine involvement. Due to pressure in the nerve but without involvements of cervical spine.

2. Failure of feedback and reciprocating mechanism.

In any situation when body elevate the bp to maintain temporary critical situation by this time prescribing medicine to stop the functions will disturb the reciprocating mechanism so there by elevation of bp.

For example, when heavy blood loss or loose stool then to save the person brain produce peripheral vaso constriction and central vaso dialatation.when administering medicine for stopping the loose stool will reduce the possibility of recovering the elevated bp to normal again so there by possible high bp in this way.

High bp is another important disease. we can say another scary diagnosis when patient is troubled a lot and he was put on allopathic medicine for life long.

Doctors assuming hypertension is the cause for many severe life-threatening diseases like

- Myocardial infarct
- Cerebra vascular disorders
- Hypertensive retinopathy
- Kidney diseases-hypertensive nephropathy
- Cardiomegaly

• Hypertensive retinopathy

(unfortunately, both hypertension as well as the the diseases suspected is caused by this hyepertension, all are unknown etiology but doctors are very sure that bp is causing this (?!) so to prevent that you have to take bp medicine). so that patient kept under hypertensive medicines.

Cardiomegaly [both dilatation as well as hypertrophy is possible] may be caused by hypertension due to heavy work load for cardiac muscle and few kidney diseases causes bp.

But other disease like cerebra vascular disease and myocardial infarct as already discussed in the diabetes chapter all this caused by confused inflammation not because of hypertension. The role of hypertension act as a trigger for developing this complication due to hypertension but even if the hypertension is not there the disease will be formed. So reducing the hypertension is having negligible role. It means after many years of hypertensive medicine the inflammation remain inside the blood and blood vessal sure will develop this complication since we are not removed the confused inflammation.

Why I am stressing removing the confused inflammation will relive the hypertension as well as complication listed by allopathy also prevented, so need broad sens of knowledge to understand this. Do you think the vasculitis will be stopped if we prescribe atnelal and amlong?.

Hypertension is caused by again confused inflammation this might happen due to vaso constrictive confused inflammation chemical induce this. If confused inflammation causes the hypertension it always fluctuates. Since this vasoconstrictive element keep shift and migrate and according to the environment.Patient come with highly elevated bp when we prescribe anti hypertensive then the bp will drop and goes to hypotensive satate in the next visit. Patient often gives certain period or certain situation causes bp related symptoms.

If hypertension caused by infiltration of the abnormal inflammation cells and dead tissues within chemo receptors and baroreceptors then hypertension will be a permanent one. Again, in the same receptor if there is any abnormal stimulation due to adjacent lymph node swelling then the bp elevation or bp drop is transient one, the bp will be normal immediately after the inflammation is withdrawn and swellon lymh node is shrunk after the inflammation is over but induration and swellon lymphnode may cause pressure towards carotid sinus.

Hypertension again has to keep a parameter for curing confused inflammation. If it is alarmingly raising it may risk the bleeding and leaking possibility in the atherosclerotic blood vessals,already confused inflammation damages the blood vassals. hypertension is secondary , primary reason was not discovered this many day , But the primary reason for cardiac and cerebral disorders vascular disorders, found and kidney failures again caused by confused inflammation.so treat that. Automatically bp will come down.

Confused inflammation of the vital organs like kidney,brain,heart again alter the pressure within the artery when the person affected with confused inflammation the kidney will be usually affected in the early life. Comparing to the brain and cardiac.

Kidney is targeted by confused inflammation by many ways

1.All the confused inflammation chemical will reach to the kidney for sure for the purpose of filtrations so if there is any confused inflammation is there in the general circulation will stuck here and may produce the disease.

2. All the medicine we consume has to be excreted through the kidney this will attract the confused inflammation towards kidney.

3. Genito urinary tract infections and the treatment by allopathy gives excessive confused inflammation so that will be attracted by the kidney.

When compare to heart kidney is affected more by allopathic medicines directly and confused inflammation too .. So, BP precedes the Heart attack.

It is not necessary to create heavy kidney damage to doubt or suspect kidney disease. Mild kidney damage is almost always possible, if the confused inflammation within the body.

Then now tell me are you going to give treatment for hypertension or you are going to give treatment for the confused inflammation. Are you agree my point that hypertension is the parameter?

Either in diabetes and hypertension I am stressing to give the treatment for cause don't give the treatment for effect or one single symptom of the mega disease. Since treating the symptoms never prevent the same disease itself then how you will prevent the complication arising from that ?

Hyperemia / vasoconstriction

If the vasospasm or vasodilation during the inflammation or wound healing is not distracted then this kind of local vascular disorders will not happen. So that vaso spasm lead on to *gangrene* or poor blood supply to the periphery or particular affected part is reduced or stopped. In the early stage of the disease the affected part is become dark and blue. The disease is showing their worst face in cold country and too low weather in any place where the temperature is too low,ischemia of the major organ is a prominent series disease,mayocardial ischemia, cerebral, kidney ischemia causes slow deterioration of the function of the body part and signs and symptoms worse when demand need especially exercise and fever.this vasospasm will attract the roming confused inflammation cells to make disease over the site. The vasoconstriction is normally happening in injured site to prevent blood loss.

Local Vasodilatations causes hyperemia to that part like acne rosacea and erethema.telanjectasia is a condition in which only single or few vassals particularly dilated and it is visible and this change occur in extreme tiny part all this is produced by confused inflammation.This local vascular dilatation disease worst during summer or in sun exposure,drinking alcohol.

There are many diseases which is similarly gets worse in sun heat and summer and again many diseases worse in cold and winter is may be having similar pathophysiology under the other major disease (asthma worse in winter and cold air and climate exposure).

4 . DERMATOLOGY

D isease free world is possible ? or not ? possible because the diseases are created, not truly and naturally heppaned. All the diseases are doctors made disorders. if the doctors are regulated in their treatment then
Disease-free world is possible.

There are many diseases for the humans but no
idea how it was caused. But doctors are keep treating the
disease without knowing how it was caused, they never
stopped, so this in turn causes many diseases. They never
waiting to know the cause. So, the doctor must know that he
is the cause for all this disease. There are many disease doctors know the cause but misunderstood wrongly, will discuss few diseases.

We have not discovered any cause for many diseases in dermatology. Thinking most of the disease is caused
by germs, so the search is in that aspect or it is searched
in the genetic or hereditary base or the auto immunity. So,
we are distracted from reality (or) blaming the environment
sun is the cause or weather change is the cause. This are all
the stimulating factor but the true cause is confused inflam-

mation which is created by allopathy medicine.

All my research related with cause of the diseases is nothing but disruption in the original system, this disruption makes the disease. To comprehend this, we no need to do great research or no need even great depth of medical knowledge and in fact the medical course itself will reduce from 6 years to 3 years. Because we read a text which says no cause but explain multiple theory of guess work it could be this or that, but for this guess work occupy 2-3 pages and again many unnecessary theories which confuses and distracts and wasting the time of physician. Doctors are habituated to live with unknown medical world and accepted these confused, unknown medical facts and treating the patient. This inturn create the new disease.

When you clue less what caused it, just trace the disease characteristics and what is there in the tumor or inflammation, like what type cells or chemicals involved in it, just do research or observe the diseases or use the knowledge of physiology when this cells or tissues will come and do in normal pathology [like neutrophil will be called for phagocytosis, fibrinogen will called for wound healing like that] but there is no wound healing or there is no bacteria then why here that cells ? some cells or misbehaving like giving wrong signals to brain or nerves or something else ?

USE THE KNOWLEDGE OF CONFUSED INFLAMMATION AND ELOBORATE ENTAIRE MEDICAL SYSTEM FROM, BRAIN OPTHO, ENT, DENTAL, GIT, RESPIRATORY, ORTHO, DERMATOLOGY , IMMUNOLOGY,ETC ALL SYSTEMS. I AM GIVING FEW EXAMPLES HERE TO UNDERSTAND NOT GOING INDEPTH JUST SUPERFICIAL TOUCH OF FEW SYSTEMS AND MINIMAL EXPLANATIONS of the disease how it was caused.

Almost all the skin disease is secondary not the primary ailment except few skin infections, all are caused by confused inflammatory immune diseases, we can say on other words all or autoimmune / auto inflammatory disease but created by medical professionals [Iatrogenic].

It is not only secondary, tertiary and penta disease. It means the disease crossed to heal from first time then started another disease (secondary) then same inflammation caused another disease (tertiary). What is the significance of knowing this facts? The true inflammation, first time produce a disease if we allowed it, this disease complete their functions and removed from the body tottaly so there is no seond or third disease. Another significance single inflammation product causes many diseases we have no clue that all are same so that we have consider everything is different disease, and confused how this disease coming why this disease , no idea . since we don't know much about this disease, we kept unknown disease, the medical text book is full of unknown disease. 3rd significance since we don't know the cause for the disease (allopathy doctors making disease) so we are doing same mistake again and again and produce many diseases, the true disease is less then 10 % but doctors created disease is like more then 90 %. Since doctors are not creating disease accidentally or rarely most of the allopathy medicines are disease producer not a healer or curer).

Almost all skin disease is secondary nothing is primary disease except wounds / infections and their complications chemical accident.

Is not that simple we can move simply saying all skin disease secondary, why ? because the current medical concept of disease and their treatment everything is considered as primary disease.so dermatitis means they conclude it happen as an allergy or contact or some climate like that doctors are thinking. Pimples happen as excess oily secretion and due to closing of the sebum secreting glands like that.vitiligo,psoriyasis,pimples,pigment disorders everything is secondary.

Secondary ? a good functioning inflammation is

primary, collapsed by strong medication so this distracted inflammation is creating the disease in skin secondary.

Then how the secondary disease [skin disease] is treated they try to treat almost by external aplications again. what will happen this inflammation [confused inflammation] pushed inside the circulation now the same confused inflammation will occupy the joints or liver or heart or kidney and strated produce the disease [tertiary disease] like wise the professional doctors playing with disease.

But in most of the cases the disease will be most stubborn and produce again the skin disease in many situations a single patient is having almost Penta [5 time suppressed], hexa [6 time suppressed] disease will ideally goes to cancer since the true inflammation cells and chemicals constantly stressed so this cells will create cancers so quickly.

I AM GIVING EXPLANTION THAT HOW THE SKIN DISEASE CAUSED AND THEN TO COMPREHEND I AM GIVING POSSIBLE EXPLANATION [CHRACTERS OF THE CONFUSED INFLAMMATION DISCUSED ERLIER]. SO NOW YOU WILL BE CLEAR HOW THIS MANY SKIN DISEASES ARE PRODUCED SO MY DEAR PROFESSIONALS TREAT SKIN DISEASE ITS GOOD BUT UNDERSTAND THAT IT IS A INFLAMMATION BUT NOT TRUE INFLAMMATION IT'S A CONFUSED INFLAMMATION [SECONDRY] SO AIM IN CLEAR FROM WHOLE BODY DON'T HIDE JUST FROM SKIN.BECAUSE ALL THE PUBLIC IS GOING TO READ THIS SO THEY WILL TEACH US SO HANDLE THE DISEASE CAREFULLY WIPE THE CONFUSED INFLAMMATION FROM SECONDRY DON'T SEND THAT INTO INTERNAL ORGAN AS A TERTIARRY DISEASE.OR ELSE ALOW IT TO STAY THEY THERE.

Psoriasis :

Cause is not identified till date but the cause I found is prescribing anti inflammatory drugs.so that the inflammation stops and inflammatory chemicals sprayed all over the body and produce psoriyasis. AND IT IS NOT A INFLAMMATORY DISORDER IT IS A CONFUSED INFLAMMATORY DISORDER.

• Characteristics of psoriasis Redness, silvery scaling ,plaque formation in the skin and pitting in the nail.

• typically mimic the inflammation especially stage 1 congestive phase, but lacks many signs and symptoms of the real inflammations like no fever and no pain].

HERE PSORIYASIS HAVING 2 TYPES OF INFLAMMATORY PHASE IN SINGLE DISEASE LIKE CONGESTIVE PHASE AS WELL AS REGENARATIVE PAHASE. SO CONGESTIVE PHASE PRODUCE VASODIALATATION SO REDNESS AND REGENARATION PHASE SKIN IS NEWLY FORMING.

• few special types of psoriasis have the typical relation with strepto coccus [guttate psoriasis develops after the streptococcus infections it gives the clue to source could be related with streptococcus infection]

• commonly worse in the winter, stress after throat infection ,better in summer but this modality may alter in very few cases. [it de-

notes the sensitivity of the disease ,a cold air exposure bring the psoriasis open up third dimension like
no need of injury or infection just normal environmental changes bring the psoriasis [contradictory
to the real inflammation stimuli, usually it has to
come either germs or nudities agents entry].even
friction or injury or pressure causes the psoriasis].

Hyper sensitive skin [produced by confused in-
flammation] react to the cold environment and invite
all the confused inflammation chemicals and cells to
the skin and produce the psoriyasis.PRIMARY CAUSE IS
THE CONFUSED INFLAMMATION BY ALOPATHY MEDI-
CINE, secondary cause or inviting factor is cold environment.

Pressure or friction or micro injury micro
cracks in the palms and soles in winter all produce
the psoriyasis in a thick leathery sites we give more
pressure so soriyasis develops here (knee,elbow,scalp)
scalp ? when we lye down our scalp and back is toucing
in the bed so psoriyasis in the back and scalp and especially it starts in the occiput and then spread.

Almost a wound or nearly wound like heavy
pressure is need to develop a psoriyais but in dermatitis
it comes in the folds like neck befind the knee and front
of the elbow here just a minor pressure is enough to produce the eruptions and sweating react with histamine
enugh to produce the dermatitis. (in both psoriyasis
as well as dermatitis alopaths searching for bacteria
or virus or atleast some antibody but my dear just
scaratch or sweat or claimatic changes enough to cause
disease since this is not immune or inflammation disease this is confused inflammation disease.

So, this 2 factor is etiology here. We have to

understand that it is not a normal inflammation so we no need to expect any virus or germs or no need to expect a real injury is caused this so please close the file don't confuse doctors as if we are in search of cause for disease.

[read carefully the characters of confused inflammation].

•　　　　　　commonly present in the extensor as well as leathery thick skin areas and pressure site. But it can also appear abdomen and thin skin areas even flexural origin is not uncommon. [location is explainable like simple throughing out of psoriatic spots will choose any ware in the body either thin or thick but mostly not extensor usually trunk. but the characteristic distribution extensor is almost related with pressure (most pressure bearing sites recive the psoriyasis like soles and palms and back and front of knee.and then the spots appear [kind of binarization] the confused inflammation is attracted by friction in the hands (injury). The pressure and friction and cracks will attract the psoriyatis spots since the presence of wound healing cells will attracted to heal the wound (cracks) that is why kobnarisation is works well.

•　　　　　　itching is not a marked symptom but it will be there when the skin is dry almost mild itch ? why lacking histamaine .dermatitis and lichen planus and ringworm all will have heavy histamine so itch and itch and itch as you wish.

•　　　　　　Para psoriasis red spots less scaling ,or scaling with hypo pigmented spots etc. [similar pathology like psoriasis but lack of proper chemical or inflammation material to produce exact identical with psoriasis]

•   now psoriasis characteristics resemble inflammation [either infectious or wound healing or inflammation of any other reason] but does not progress with aim or does not completed ,keep recurring with/without infection in fact for minimal environmental changes like winter ,pressures .T cell infiltration again confirm the inflammation [immunity] origin, but without any much reason why T cell ?.But this confusions and question marks will be cleared that it is not a inflammation but scattered, interrupted, confused inflammation .it is not a real inflammation It is not a real immunity it is confused or collapsed, incomplete confused inflammation or immunity with respective chemical or cells.

A confused inflammation reaches to the pressure and friction sites and stayes over there so the inflammation trigger immunity (no need of any explanation since always inflammation preceds and initiate the immunity) so T lymphocytes activated and produce skin disease.

A skin is choosen by this ailment not to attack but for attraction so they does not come here to destroy so body is not produced any antibody cells against the skin. Infact skin here is growing excess not having any ulcers or destruction of the skin so absolutely no damage to the skin we see this when psoriyatic spotes leaves the skin is turns normal within a month as if a completely normal skin.

If at all you are seeing destruction and antibody don't name this auto immune it is altered immune or confused immune disease because of alopaths medicine.

•   So, the chemical involved in inflammation sprayed all over the skin produce the vasodilatation and congestions since it is not a real inflammation of the system proper it could not progress and complete as an inflammation. Since true inflammation has the target so the target is killed then the inflammation is withdrawn but here the inflammation is attracted by pressure and cold exposure suppose if the cold is not there or the fricthion and pressure is not there then the sotes will disapear

•   important reason is collapsed inflammation system itself when we interrupt inflammation in the mid then the signals will not be received by a brain weather the inflammation purpose is complete or not no feedback so that the chemical keep coming to the inflammation site and also all over the skin surface from the point where it is interrupted [same chemical or cells].so every pressure and winter exposure body will send only that particular chemicals. This is the reason why some patient not getting severe spots and even complete symptom free period for many years. but few patients are having severe outbreaks of psoriatic spots.

•   So, psoriasis as medical profession already thinking it's an inflammatory disorder but why it does not fit with real inflammatory signs and symptoms is it caused by just distracted few chemical or cells of inflammations from original site of inflammation .so inflammatory disorder but not a real complete inflammation itself IT IS CONFUSED INFLAMMATION DIS ORDER.

Dermatitis : ATOPIC DERMATITIS

CAUSE WAS UNKNOWN - BUT DISCOVERED THE CAUSE, the cause is distracted inflammation chemicals pre-scribbing ANTI HISTMINE MEDICATIONS – Excess hista-mine and other pro inflammatory chemicals induce pruritic inflammation . to solve the discomfort itching and burnin-ing inflammation patient takes heavy anti histamine so the the disease getting accentuated. The disease will get worse like anything, but giving comfort in itching temproriliy. So, the cycle will continue and disease get worse. The cause of the disease is anti histamine, but it give the result and relive the complaints so patient keep taking that medicine to re-live but really the disease getting worse.

Preventive medicine ? a preventive medicine prevents the disease not to create the disease. How to prevent skin disease stop prescribing medicine against the inflammation and immunity. Learn how to remove the in-flammatory remenents from the body is the right way of prevents. Anti histamine and anti inflammatory is dir-ectly anti human medicines and making sickness so it is against the medical profession. Yes there is negative impact also happening due to inflammation process by creating some distracted inflammation chemicals but don't use that option for creating further trpuble all the anti inflamma-tory drugs are not removing troublesome inflammation chemicals instead it increases the more and more dis-tracted inflammation so it creates so many disease directly and by triggering stimulating the immunity directly. Anti inflammatory and anti allergics dumping the unnessory in-flammation chemicals is the only cause for lot many dis-eases. Understand and act, take necessary steps. I don't want just 6 hours satisfaction. Remove the bad inflammation (confused inflammation) chemicals from my body. Is that possible then speak, don't sale the medicine in the name of anti inflammation. The antinflammation act 6 hours, this drug prevents the action of inflammation and collect the inflammation not to act so we will not have the pain and fever but this collected inflammation is the cause for the 100 of disease in the body. The function of the anti inflammatory is converting good functioning inflammation into self destructing inflammation why doctors using this since it relives fever for 6 hours. This medicine is creating poison from our body to destroy our body by blocking the good and right function into the wrong and self destructing function. So this is not a side effect of the drug. The main aim itself to stop the inflammation for 6 hours by just preventing inflammation formation only 6 hours but during this 6 hours the inflammation chemicals dumped inside the body will create the inflammatory disease so we prescribe again inflammaition preventing medicine.

A future medicine will allow the good inflammation and support the inflammation and never produce the distracted or bas inflammation chemical. A future medicine will remove the confused inflammation from the body – at present we have that future medicine that is called homeopathy. Homeopathy medicine is there in present but people are not consuming popularly so that when public using it then only it is present medicine. The current dominant medical system is allopathy. Which is creating many diseases to the humans.

Inappropriate usage of medicine for nasal inflammation will lead to allergic rhinitis [secondary disease], allergic rhinitis makes severe running nose and itching in the nose so patient rush to the doctor and take repeated anti-allergic by using this medicine slowly the mild allergic rhinitis will slowly spray the confused inflammatory cells /

chemicals histamine this will produce itching in the throat, ear, face, neck, eye ,,,. Patient started experiencing dry cough which will not ease as easily it may stay more then a month [usually after a mild cold] with tickling and itchy feel in the throat. Patient by this time slowly experience dry cough with lung involvement with slow wheezing episode [asthma].over a period of time patient develops dry skin and itching in the skin especially when expose to cold air. **ESON-OPHILIC OR HISTMAINE CONSTITUTION or ATOPY.**

[Dr.Hahnemann explain this is psoric miasm and itching will be predominant, he says psora makes the platform for the diseases, without psora there may not be any disease psora is a mother for all disease, we have to understand the histaminosis produce severe disease].

Atopic dermatitis is choosing the skin fold as the site of attack earlier but more widespread involvement with severe itching is possible.

The child is sleepless and annoyed cranky and itch and itch continuously all are happening just antihistamine usage. We study and understand that a allergic rhinitis patient will also have atopic skin but how and why we never asked any one day. Excess accumulation of the histamine in the circulation spread across the skin and start producing itching in the flexor surface due to accentuation by folding the joints this temporary stagnation of the histamine in the folds produce itching due to considering there is enemy this signals invite the IgE to the affected site and initiate the dermatitis.

(excess histamine in the circulation alone is the cause. Histamine is more hypersensitive then rest of the hypersensitive a simple example is angioneurotic edema and airborne conduct dermatitis PSORIYASIS NEED STRONG PRESSURE OR AT LEAST SCARATCH TO CREATE ERUPTION BUT HERE MINIMAL CONTACT AND FOLDING MAKES THE DISEASE).

Type 1 hypersensitivity is the rapid quick hypersensitivity since the chemicals involved here act directly to produce symtoms and disease.Type 2, 3,4 everything all are more or less slow and delayed hypersensitivity because they develop disease slow due to inflammation has to trigger this immune system and then it has to produce the disease.Histamin,bradykinin all are act quickly and respond directly to the environment but immune system activation always after the inflammation. There are many time the immune system may not triggered by inflammation so some times immune system may not be activated.

Every scratch will invite more histamine activation (dermographism). Scaratching is keep the dermatitis active child or adult scratch until it bleeds or the skin become lichenified.

Patient now will have severe irritating disease. The sprayed histamine will not only produce the itchy eye actually it collapses basic protective mechanism so that red eye, with mucus formation in the eye, slow micro deposits within the eye, (the infection is favored by this confused inflammation, the infection alone connot make the heavy infection disease, the recurrent heavy infection is supported by confused inflammation, a fully protected good inflammation never allows the viral or bacterial multiplications). we started using anti histamines again this will inturn create more confused histamine it will goes deeper into the eye due to [topical eye drops] a oral anti histamines just allow the histamine into eye and produce external ophthalmic disease like dermatitis, conjunctivitis, styes in the lids, lachrymation, ,,,etc, but the usage of eye drops will push and hide the confused inflammation cells within deeper tissues of the eye so the patient sure will suffer many ophthalmic disease in the childhood and teen itself this diseases again met with foolish handling like selling some glasses and prescribing some medicine if there is inflammatory or infectious sign or call for surgery but never aimed to clear the confused inflammation but the worst factor keep increasing the confused inflammation by prescribing same anti-inflammatory and anti-histamine. The confused inflammation cells will collapse the internal barriers and allow the minor infections to go deeper internal eye parts will produce severe ophthalmic disease. ALMOST ALL OPTHALMIC DISEASE ARE TERTIARRY AND DETRA,PENTA DISEASE [IT MEANS THE DISEASE REPTEDLY ALLOWED TO TAKE REATTACK , MAXIMUM PRIMARY DISEASE SOURCE IS FROM NOSE].

The A to Z psychological complaints and brain diseases are comes just because of this spraying of inflammatory product into the brain. A GERM WILL NOT ALLOWED TO ENTER INTO THE BLOOD BRAIN BARRIER [BBB] BUT THE INFLAMMATION CHEMICALS AND CELLS IS ALWAYS CROSS THE BBB easily.

A EYE DROPS FOR CONFUSED INFLAMMATION DISEASE A EAR DROPS TO DISEASE,A NASAL SPRAY,NASAL DROPS WILL EASILY THORUGH THE CONFUSED INFLAMMATION INTO THE BRAIN.A oral medication and injection of anti allergic anti inflammatory produce more or less superficial or minimally invasive disease but the external solutions,sprays,drops will take the disease to the deeper organs like eye, ear and brain.

But the diseases not necessarily have to produce only histamine related disease it can be anything and what available chemical or cells present in the body now and which organ affected will decide the pathology and decide the signs and symptoms.

But all the time doctors will say that cause is allergy or infection or auto immunity they do not have insight that their medicine is creating all , they keep produce disease.

ANDROGENTIC ALOPECIA

Hair follicles closed earlier so no hair groeth so lead to baldness. This is hapen due to premature degeneration created by confused inflammation. This androgen induced alopecia is gradually increasing in too early age due to more confused inflammation due to widespread allopathic drug usage.

Rightly named as androgen induced hair loss ok.how many of them is affected few of them severely affected few of them affected mild rest of them escaped. The escaped person is not having any androgen ? those who have baldness is healthy others are unhealthy ?

I am not making fun on this observation androgen inducing the alopecia. But the name will induce the doctors to prescribe unnecessary medications.

Actually, the confused inflammation cells are attracted by androgens and sun heat. So this confused inflammation produce androgenetic alopecia and many more scalp disease, based on the confused inflammation cells availability.

A shampoo wash will retain the confused inflammation within the scalp, hair oils help in conditioning the hair. Onian paste, herbal applications helps confused inflammation remain within the scalp and produce hair loss instead of hair growth. More vaso dilatation by minoxidil and mintop will invite more the confused inflammation cells reach to the scalp may be the excess blood supply help hair growth but more confused inflammation cells to the scalp make speedy baldness after stopping the minoxidil and mintop.

Urticaria

if a person eating some food which is not suitable so the urticaria develops, urticaria (allergic to some medicine) for some medicine, urticaria when applying hair coloring all this says another truth. Even though the allergic substance is there somewhere else but the allergic reaction appears in the in the skin. This is a small understanding of events for explaining how seriously the inflammation system is collapsed.

Vomiting is a right step if the food is dis agree (its happen in most of the case) ,if hair coloring has some bad chemical then rashes must appear within scalp not in the legs and abdomen and arms. This is what happening every time when bacteria or virus enter inside the body instead of attacking the germs and virus the histamine [chemotaxis happen all over the body]. This is the true nature and character of the confused inflammation. Simultaneuse accentuation of confused inflammation present all over the body. some times it spreades all over the body that is accepted.but anyway no target for enemy.

In simple we can say excess histamine or itching producing chemicals rich so for many food and external factors like hair dye ,soap,metals in the cloths for all it produces reaction and itching will come.it means actually we will accept this thing but we have now enough confused inflammation which makes the sensitivity.

Redness and itching in the pressure sites [pressure urticaria] indicates confused inflammation spread across the body and in the pressure sites.

The Dermographism indicates generalized histamine pooling in the skin. MAY GIVES VARIETY OF modality like sun exposed urticarea,rash when exposed to cold climate .

Emotion or anxiety makes urticarial rash indicates histamine within the brain within the scalp.

Similar to eosinophilic esophagitis makes the urticaria in the skin. A stress or anxiety makes the urticarial rash indicates hyper eosinophilic deposits in the brain.

A true inflammation due to infection is targeted and completed without any interruption. but in many other cases every time the infections flared up it gives the urticarial rash.

The dermographism or the urticaria is act as systemic or generalized disease spreader by spraying all inflammatory chemical or cells which is produced by every allopathic medication.

Say for example a person having dermographism is now had pustular infections somewhere so that it was treated with external creams now massive fibroblast cells are slowly allowed to the circulation actually this fibroblast and gelatin is coming for healing purpose of the pustules. This fibroblast easily attracted to the demographic skin person easily so the fibroblast easily taken to allover the skin surface so now when you scratch, we can find itching similar to dermographism but within 2 days he will see thick leathery eruption in the skin.

Mast cell and esonophil releases histamine that will attract the circulating T cells the accumulated t cells along with protease enzyme the keratine leyar destroyed is the some of pathology underneath lichen planus, severe itchy, polygonal flat-topped eruption in the skin (lichen planus).

The histamine in the skin (dermograph) stimulate the macrophage and there by inflammation starts and produce variety of skin disease.

A histamine is a chemotactic factor will invite all confused inflammation cells which is produced now and in future to all over the skin surface and mucus membrane. Kind of dermographism is the base and in which all further skin disease is going to form.

Demographic skin highly vulnerable to infections. But gives the hyper inflammation response then normal regular inflammation response.

Contact dermatitis

immune and inflammation system is collapsed so the person slowly experiences uncomfortable to many things, this is because a heat or cold or pressure created by the ornaments invite the confused inflammation cells to the site so there by dermatitis is formed. Using many shampoos ,body spray, lipstick, hair coloring previous to collapsed inflammation is normal humans enjoyed that, no allergy but now the confused inflammation is triggered by this chemical agent and produce mild to severe allergic reactions. A confused inflammation is hypersensitive (due to presence of excess quantity of histamine and readymade instead of liberation of histamine after identifying germs and then releasing) and again it is contact directly to an object then since abundant in the skin.

It is not all over the periphery is rich in histamine once the germ enters then eosinophil and must cells migrate from somewhere and reach here and then release histamine and other chemotactic chemicals and then this will help in dilate and breaks the blood vassals to invite the other inflammatory cells so everything will come one by one with order and with necessary if it need more then more cells will come if the condition under control then cell migration will be stopped.

But here everything is there on the spot more or less within the capillary bed and tissues [so hyper respon-sive, quick and speed inflammation for extremely tiny irri-tation] more the pressure and more the histamine and other confused inflammatory cells present in the site how much confused inflammation cells present in the body all will come here and start produce the inflammation there is no measurement how much is need and when it is going to stop this confused inflammation has no control over anything. It stays longer time, sometime clear early, it may be due to there is no continues stimuli to this particular part.

A food allergy, drug allergy , contact dermatitis, dust allergy all will says the inflammatory systems is collapsed so we have to identify that and we have to repaired the collapsed in-flammation and cure the disease permanently either prescribing anti-allergic or just avoiding the food or things which causes al-lergy may not be the medical profession work.

If the food or chemical or some other contact not triggered the dermatitis, we may not aware this confused in-flammation at all.

So urticaria or contact dermatitis is not a dis-ease to treat instead treat the confused inflammation to set right the repaired confused system into normal. After the troublesome suffering is calmed our aim is to bring back the normal mechanism of inflammatory system.disapearing ur-ticarial rash or disappearance of the contact dermatitis is not an aim of treatment.

Acne vulgaris / pimples

The acne and the pimples appear in different types of eruption papules , comadones , pustules, keloid in face . There are individual will have either papules or cluster of all.

Why acne ? there is no clear-cut cause yet identified but believed that excess activation of sweat and oily glands in the face and also think that there is closed pores in the oily glands causes this, corynibacteriyam in the face also linked in pustular acne.

Usually starts in the teen age so that believing hormonal influence with the acne.

Patient is worried about the scars, dark pigments repeated pimple attack so makes the person to seek varies medicine to cure this applying so many creams and ointments, herbal paste in the face, face wash (this treatment are having it has great marketing to the Doctors and other cosmetologist)

Explanation of the real facts :

The circulating Confused inflammatory cells/ chemicals (is the cause for the pimples) always choose the face as the one of the common places to settle.

This is because the face is one of the exposed part of the body so that heat and cold will invite the confused inflammation cells to the face, so there by not only the acne all type of so many skin disorders will appear in the face before the teen and before the pimples even all through life time.

The confused inflammation is readily available just beneath the face of the individual who is having allergic rhinitis and sinusitis or as caries tooth so that when the oily glands is become over active during the adolescent's time then automatically the confused inflammation cells present in the sinus and mouth attracted towards oily glands and started producing eruption.

The type of rash is due to presence of confused inflammation cell or chemical type like it is red based painful ,itchy papules in the face indicates [predominance of 1 set phase of inflammation chemical] if the pimples are more in pustules indicates that predominance of phagocyte cell predominance ,fibrous and keloid like hard pimples indicates that more of fibrous, gelatin cells in the confused inflammations.

Sycosis nuche

A thick rubbery papule in the nape of neck.

A long-standing confused inflammation together with fibrus and gelatin accumilation causes this sycosis nuche.its looks like a mollascum cantagiyosam in some individual ,rubbery in nature.present in the nape of neck.

There are many teenagers giving histry of pimples in the scalp and entire back this type of pimples usually associated with fungal infection in the scalp where ever the fungas fall they develop the pimples in the back.

Usually the confused cells in the face, they come to the face after improper medicinal usage. Blocked the regular protective functions any ware in the body or within the nose itself but usually the suppression again by usage of anti-inflammatory creams ,through away this cell to scalp or brain or to thyroid gland or sinus or to caries tooth ,to testes to ovary to the breast.

[I can trace some of the psychological patient give their disease arises during teen age I was misunderstood this is could be over study or due to stress is the cause for the psychological disease it may be a trigger but simple stress may not produce long time psychological illness the disease may be disappear after the disappearance of the stress but it continues even after surely a shifting confused inflammation from the body to mind]

Usually alternate with sinus and face for many years. Uncomplicated with confused inflammation may recover soon ,but those who have excess confused inflammation carry this for many years until shift either to brain or to other body parts.

In the medical history suppression of skin disease carry the highest number of internal disease but almost all the people having pimples and acne in the face and taking external application for curing the pimple again is common.WARNING SUPPRESSION IS NOT GOOD FOR HEALTH IS SOMETHING VAGUE TERM HAHNEMANN STRONGLY OBJECT THIS BUT AS A HOMEOPATH EVEN I AM NOT CONVINVED HIS WORD SINCE I AM A HOMEOPATH I AM ACCEPTING THIS BUT NOW I AM CONVINCED WHAT HAPPENING WHEN WE DO SUPPRESSING THE SKIN DISEASE.YES all the disease we discussed now is bad effects of suppression .supression ? it means not allowing the natural process to happen and again blocking the disease in an unscientific way all will lead to disease .i am giving examples and explanation throught the book what will happen when we do suppression.

This confused inflammation cells are easily move to other secondary sexual organs which is developing at the same time [breast,testis,ovary,uterus]

Hypo pigmented spots to vitiligo

what we try to understand when we start reading hypo and hyper pigment disorders we read lot about the melanin and melanocytes like that but the complaints comes somewhere else then the malonocyte,the confused inflammation underlying the skin makes hypopigmented spotes,but the confused inflammation just stays here stagnant that's all.so that discoloration of the skin.

Here we can see a complete lack of inflammatory sign but it's an inflammation. The spraying of confused inflammation in the skin will produce vitiligo.

[example in chronic sinus infections variety of hypo pigmented spots in the face but it fades away .in contrast to vitiligo a complete loss of functions of pigment cells with rapid spread of the vitiligo thorough the body. The confused inflammation present in the skin surface causes rapidly spreading vitiligo, in my observation the pressure , frictions ,heat ,cold , chemical exposure all invite the chemical of the confused inflammation to any pressure sites or injury site causes hypo pigments or depigmented spots.

The usual response to depigments is immediate depigmentation of the skin if its is superficial affection but in most of the cases the white spots spread slowly and make big patch and also many new spots here and there.

I have seen in many cases depigments also happen and close without any treatment especially if the spots is smaller in size and in early cases, here I have an another finding that the body can replace the damaged organs or tissues even without any real trauma or true inflammation it means the recovery or cure may happen even in confused inflammation but here it will happen only if the inflammation is leaving the spots or it is too weak or superficial, the similar findings I have observed in alopecia areata in this disease the spots created by alopecia will be replaced full hair again without any treatment, but this will not happen after repeated spots.

The same thing happens in psoriasis ,when the psoriatic spots disapered completely from the body then the spots slowly recover to completely normal skin.

THE REASON BEHIND THE RECOVERY OF THE

DISEASES IS,WHEN THE CONFUSED INFLAMMATION IS MI-GRATED TO THE PRESENT LOCATION OR EXPRESSING ITS PRESENCE IN THE PURELY HEALTHY TISSUES SO THAT IF THE CONFUSED INFLAMMATION IS LEAVING THIS SPOT OR LESSEN THEIR INTENSITY THEN AUTOMATICALLY THE CURRENT LOCATION START WOKRING THEIR FUNC-TION .SO IT IS NOT A RECOVERY OR REPAIR OF THE USUAL INFLAMMATION PROCESS,IT IS JUST STARTED WORKING AS USUAL AFTER THE INFLAMMATION CROSS AWAY IT WILL WORK IF THE DAMAGE IS LESS . IF IT IS SEVERE AND DEEP ENOUGH DESTRUCTION THEN THERE IS NO POS-SIBLITY OF FUNCTION SO NO REPIGMANTATION NO NEW HAIR GROWTH,ETC.THIS IS THE MECHANISAM HAPPEN HERE.

Example :

First few times the alopecia spots getting hair growth but over a period of time the alopecia is operantly bald this is because the hair follicles damaged permanently so that even though there is no confused inflammation there is no possibility of hair growth.

there are few good and complete recovery of the white patch in vitiligo but this is may not happen if the spots are repeated over there or if it is bigger spots like that.

The psoriatic spots all the time recover [start func-tion] completely as if nothing was happening to the patient. The skin looks smooth and function as usual, it does not mean the inflammation producing the spots and it repairing the damaged tissue so that the spots is become clear. The reality is just withdrawing the effect upon the skin causes the skin is start working as usual not over or not under func-tion of the skin.

The eczema spots in the skin are coming to the

normal stage after withdraw of confused inflammation [except infectious eczema the infectious eczema invite the true inflammation in super added with confused inflammation so that the skin repaired after the infection process]

WHEN TRY WITH GOOD HOMEOPATHIC MEDICINE POSSIBLITY OF THE RECOVERY AND REPAIR IS THERE IF IT IS RECOVERABLE DAMAGE.HOW ? WE HAVE TO SAY THE NERVES THAT THERE IS A DAMAGE IN THE PARTICULAR TISSUE BY THEIR LANGAGE [MAKING PSUDO INJURY-HOMEOPATHY MEDICINE SO THAT NOW BODY WILL START THE INFLAMMATION PROCESS AND COMPLETE THE INFLAMMATION PROCESS BY RECOVERING THE REPAIRED AND DAMAGED ORGAN TO NORMAL].*of*

But in the contrast depositing abnormal fibrous and gelatinase material in the scalp causes permanent closure with additional tissue deposits in the scalp so that permanent scared alopecia [lichen alopecia].so there is no possible normal function and limited scope even with medicine. But we have to administer medicine to clear the excess fibrous deposit in the circulation or we have to stop active fibrous cell sending signal of the inflammation process.so that possibility of wound healing by keloid or over growth will not be there.*the ivy died righie send by t, so no more white ne to recover t spots to block spots.*

But all school of physician aiming to recover the skin become block will always fail or succeeding to bring the normal skin is considered as wrong direction or illegal to the human body without clearing the confused inflammation.

The **hyper pigmentation** of the skin is happening due to again presence of confused inflammation ,this will react with sun rays and produce tanning causes over all darkening of the skin.

Sun tan is usually happen those who are affected with confused inflammation. Especially uncovered and exposed parts of the body, just dark color discoloration is the simple variety if there is variety of confused inflammation cells available then will get so many skin eruptions as sun allergic rash, we read this under photo sensitivity. A human is having friendly relation with his surrounding environment but having enmity relationship after the confused inflammation.

Most of the time sun tan is ignored by a man and we can see his face is too darker then rest of the body [to the Indian climate]. but females are sensitive about their colored so they hide their face and skin with cloths it gives the partial results and they use the sun screen lotions.

A doctor aim is not to sale the sunscreen lotion removes the confused inflammation from the body and give the cure to patient and avoid the medicine which is creating the confused inflammations.

But truly speaking allowing sun tan is good and it collects all confused inflammation remain inside the body to skin so that internal organs free from disease. Take the treatment without using sunscreen lotion observe the skin discoloration getting normal then the skin is now free from confused inflammation, HERE AGAIN AIM IS NOT TO BRING THE NORMAL COLOR GIVE THE TRETMENT FOR REMOVING CONFUSED INFLAMMTION FROM BODY.

THOSE WHO HAVE DEEP INTERNAL DISEASE BETTER TO TAKE SUN BATH.BUT WHEN YOU DEVELOP SEVERE SUN ALLERGY BETTER TO AVOID SUN BATH UNTILL RECOVERY.

THE CURRENT GENERATION IS FULLY INSIDE THE ROOM CAUSES ALL CONFUSED INFLAMMATION REMAIN INSIDE THE BODY DESTROYS THE INTERNAL ORGAN.FREQUENT USAGE OF THE EXTERNAL APPLICATION OF THE MEDICINES AGAIN SEND THE CONFUSED INFLAMMTION INSIDE THE DEEP ORGON.

Translocation of the destruction of the pigment cell destruction and pigment stimulation is another important aspect of the hyper and hypo pigmentations.

An injured site repaired by body it will begin like destroying the pigment cells which is partially damaged in the injury if this destruction distracted then where ever it goes then the white or depigmented spotes. Similarly when the regeneration of the pigments and stimulation of the pigment is happen somehere then we distract it then distracted pigment cells stimulation produce the hyperpigment where ever it is going.

ACANTHOSIS NIGRICANS

Dark, thick skin that develops in the neck, armpit and in the groine can be caused by an confused inflammation, exacess pigmentation on the skin, and increasing skin growth is the reason behind the development of this disease (the pigment formation and new skin development is distracted and producing the disease here). THE DISTRIBUTION OF THE ERUPTION IS SIMILAR TO ATOPIC DERMATITIS BUT EXCEPTION IN THE KNUKLE SPACE OF THE HANDS.

Skin Tag

Warts like skin growth on the neck is made up of similarly confused inflammatory cells, caused by chemicals that stimulate the growth of the skin.(skin growth distracted from wound healing or inflammation site to here)

Seborrheic warts

Another skin change, such as dark warts , is found around the neck and eyes Caused by confused inflammatory skin growth and pigmentation.Most people in their 30-40 begin to see this in and around the eye and cheeks and warts started appearing in around the neck and abdomen. Initially reddish and then dark brown

Unnessary usage of ointments and eye and ear drops stops the inflammatory process and shifts all chemicals and confused inflammation process from the real inflammatory sites to non inflammatory healthy sites causes warts and skin tags and seborrheic warts, lentigens, pitriyasis alba,,,,,etc.

5. SOLES AND PALMS

When bacterias or other germs is the cause for disease then we can consider route of entry or source of infection of the germs and their specific seat of locations. But after the discovery of the confused inflammation, the cause is could be anything of day to exposure. Anything related with food or our daily intake or physical contact. So, we are directing our disease discussion based on this.

Palms and soles having high contact with external world by touch, walk, exposed to different temperature when holding cold or hot in the hands walk in the cold room or warm floor all will bring the confused inflammation to the this parts and then produce the disease. So, we are discussing palms and soles here. From now, we are going to give equal impartance to parts which is act as route of infection and producing disease by excess stimulation.

Soles and palms is having high attractive power to confused inflammation, so that it produce diseases. This is because of expose to heat and cold and bearing whole body weight [soles] and using the hands for various day to day activities like gardening and cooking pressure and heat and cold exposure varies chemical exposure like detergents, etc [palms].

Soles are expose to varies germs when walking in unhealthy roads and possibility of getting wound by thorn, glass piece so that we are going to use sure external application for all sole ailments so it has its own confused inflammation and mostly retain their confused inflammation and make disease like corn, eczema , shoe bite , cracks in the soles, heal pain,,,,, etc.

A people working in damp weather or living in damp marshy weather possibility of fresh foot infection is more.(Soles scores top mark to attract and retain the confused inflammation then rest of the body similar to nose). In the same weather soles getting wounds in the web spaces of the toes allow the infections and germs to enter into the body. When the people living in unhealthy damp weather makes the possibility of germ entry so most of the lymphatics in the legs spoiled frequent inguinal lymph node enlargement will be there so that **filariasis** comes [filarial parasite infection is secondary to previous lymphatic damage]. We can say in better word, the full fledged filariayal attack is can be seen better those who stay in marshy damp living claimate then dry place. This weathere also better wether for masquito.

So, the lymphatics as well the veins are carry the confused inflammation from sole to thigh but it will roam again from pumped blood from heart. Varicose veins is formed when a persons standing long time along with confused inflammation present in the body will produce the vericose veins, this vericose vein development is more sever if the person is pregnant due to pressure upon the veins in the lower limbs then the vericose veins formed or it will becom worse.

Cracks in the soles or palms is formed due to the

presence of the confused inflammation present in the soles having direct contact with external environmental changes so it breaks easily then constrict. It will pain and bleed if you have some confused inflammation chemicals or else it will be simple cracks if the skin in the soles proliferate and new scales keep form (psoriyasis) if the enough inflammation chemicals or stimulation is there.

presence of confused inflammation within the mucus membran of the GIT makes the ulceration simply, but the same confused inflammation does not have power to produce ulceration here it can able to produce just cracks. A cracks is not simply indication of claimatic changes it means winter is not producing cracks,a confused inflammation produce cracks. So this is the reason not everyone is having cracks few of them having cracks not all of them so it is not simply indication of deficiency of some mineral or vitamin or skin is losing elasticity it is purely a confused inflammation presence.

Nail changes

like discoloration, dystrophy, thikening, breaking mostly reflect local pathology, it means presence of confused inflammation in the fingers & toes. But anemia, cyanosis, jaundice reflect systemic disorders.

Mosquito chooses legs and foot, hands, arms since it is uncovered part . mosquito bites invite the confused inflammation it is diagnosed **mosquito allergy** , mosquito bite uses the available confused inflammation and produce itching ,mild papules and heal with scar looks like severe skin disease especially in children's ,mosquito act as one of the confused inflammation attractor to skin but we use external applications so it will go to deeper tissues or change the location.

Frequent **Felon** and other infections of the palms and soles indicates presence of confused inflammation and most importandly loss of protective functions here, so that recurrent infection. The germs like staphylococcus and strepto coccus produce felon but the onfused inflammation gives the better field for develop the felon well. Since confused inflammation reduce the accurasi and killing power of the normal inflammation.

Corn or callosity

is caused by excess availability of wound healing and growth factors in the soles. And this corns and callosity is developed due to pressure of soles attracted this wound healing and growth factors.

So,the germs enter through NOSE, MOUTH, REPRODUCTIVE ORGANS so this gersm produce the disease. But palms and soles,skin,jonits ,,,etc also produce disease but by using confused inflammation.

Arthritis is beginning in the hands due to repeted touch to different parts so that pressure in the hands and expose handling warm or cold water objects attract the confused inflammation from all over the body and produce the **rheumatisam** in the hands. There are many other arthritis or pains or sufferings or disease in the hands and wrist all are caused by confused inflammation.

In most of the cases of Palms and soles act as a beginner for **vitiligo and psoriyasis**,what is there in the palms and soles to cause psoriyasis or vitiligo why it is choosing plams and soles ? what special chemicals or some germs is there in the hands and foot to cause this disease. A circulating confused inflammation stuck within the capillary of the palms and soles and due to pressure and frictions and varies other stimulus causes to retain this confused inflammation here and initiate the disese.

Peripheral neuritis is an importand disease which is arising in the palms and soles but having connection with diabetes and kidney failure and vitamin B12 deficiancy. But it is an individual disease of the palms and hands due to confused inflammation presence in the hands and palms.

So the nose , mouth ,genitals is having high possibility of the entry of the germs and there by disease produced in the same parts but hands and jonits and skin is having so many ailments this was not identified till date how the disease is produced in the hands and soles why some diseases will be there allover the body but started in the hands and soles ? since the confused inflammation will getting attracted and retain the confused inflammation and produce the disease over there.

6. CONNECTIVE TISSUE DISORDER

Lupus erythematoses [SLE] :

SLE is a most notorious disease ,affecting women of childbearing age. This disease causes severe morbidity and suffering and affects many vital organs like heart ,kidney,brain,nerves and blood vessals ,,etc . the active disease damage these organs, produce organ failures and many individuals affected with this disease died.

Urban women affected more then village women.the disease get accentuated or worse when expose to sun rays.affcted individual need to take heavy allopathic drugs to controle the disease and prevent the active attack.

So these disease produce many suffering and even to death so we have to plan thise disease to prevent. Nearly

10-400 women in 10000 women in America is suffering with this disease (prevalence).

How to prevent.at present we can protect by avoiding sun exposure and avoiding estrogen pills too some extend helps but this is may not be a true preventive measure. So better we will understand this disease fully first.

Why Sle ?

This disease is having full of inflammation and immunity but without any infections.the explanation is given by allopathy doctors is

The sensitive (susceptible) women when undergoing to un normal external environment but she is specifically reacting to some environment factors in an abnormal way so she is started producing abnormal immune response (auto immunity).

So that,

1.innate immunity develops (monocytes and macrophages formed)

2.T AND B Lymphocytes losts their tolerance so that early reaction to even mild environmental exposures.

3. apoptic cells and immune complexes clearance is delayed.

4.CD4 AND CD8 T lymphocytes controle is modified.

These basic factors are basic for development of auto immunity.

Why female since they have estorgen thse estrogen is causing long time activation T And B lymphocytes and they found women who consume the estrogen pills for avoiding pregnancy or other purpose having more possibility of developing SLE.

I am actually not contradicting these factors and observation but the reserchers are struggling to give explanation how this happen they use some strange terms like susceptibility (some individual person having abnormal tendency to react normal external environment as the enemy) but these evidence less guess work is not acceptable and again trying to fit observed evidence with their imagination or some other similar simultaneous occurring factors but not really proved this is related with that. The observed facts is SLE disease and its pathology with this true facts they trying to explain these could be genetic or some basic body nature or something of their own imaginations these factore are imaginary manipulative theory so it does not fit with research.

So then what happens ?

Now we have sle disease observations and pathology and luckily doctors observed the fact that the disease is run many year course without producing strong clinical evidence of SLE.

True Explanation

1. Stopping inflammation by any medicine then inflammation is stopped but the inflammation chemicals circulating within the body but without ability to produce strong disease.

2.These circulating chemicals have chance to meet the enemy and day to day external factors like sun rain cold food and other cosmetics and our medicines etc and etc.

3. As the reserchers thinking there is no specific tendency or susceptibility which is that particular person is having (belived this is gentic origin) really the control less chemicals of inflammation is started acting towards natural environment or our chemicals ingetions what ever it may be the reaction or induction of another inflammation or immunity is not because of particaulr person inherent special cherecter this is a simple mistake we did in the present or in the past medication is the answere.

4.a histamin and other pro inflammation chemicals (bradykinin,leucotriens,,,,) safely libareted from the monocytes and esonophil is blocked by anti histamines so these histamine libaretaion is keep formed by the monocytes again and again they keep prevented by our prescription so that excess pro inflammation chemicals circulated within body and now it is ready made.

5.These chemicals usually allowed in a negligible amount and cleared from the circulation after their function is over. So, there is no possibility of these chemicals intereact with our body daily exposures. So no SLE OR ANY OTHER INFLAMMATION OR AUTO INFLAMMATION. But unluckily we stuck with this disease and sigma .

6. the enemy is entered so there is a invitation of warriers to kill the enemy to the eney entrance site. For inviting the warriers we used pro inflammatory chemicals they have power to dialate the and break the blood vessals and invite the inflammation and there by immunity my deat now you see the inviters and destructers are living all over the body.

7.so any factors which is naturally dialting the blood vessals (sun heat) will first attract the pro inflammation chemicasl and there by these pro inflammation chemicals will gather in the skin exposed to sun massive gathering of these inflammation chemicals now invite the inflammation and immunity.

8.but before producing any inflammation and immunity it takes several such attempt or mild vague illness or just sun allergy or heat allergy ill defined ailments.since there is no strong good amount of proinflammation chemicals to produce the mega disease.

9.but any way we never allow the disease to surface we advise the patient not to expose to sun and prescripe many creams and externa applications to stop thise secondary confused inflammation.

10.so the indore living avoiding sun but taking many strong medication or hormones attract the chemicals and these chemicals invite the inflammation and immunity inside the body and destroy the internal organ.it will produce internal as well as external and manifestation in general now it has power to produce a genaralysed systemic disease SLE or any other disease.

11. SLE or other inflammation disease or immune disease is decided by what chemicals or what einvironmental factors or what medicine we consume.

12.So the sun exposure,estrogen tablets and female is a risk factor not a real cause for the disease. The real cause is purely distracting the inflammation and confused inflammation is the cause for the disease.

13.so avoiding sun exposure,avoiding hormonal pills and other chemicals may not stop the disease but help in minimize the disease but it is absolutely imposible any way may take some food some chmicals without our knowledge make the sickness.either SLE or if try to triggering factor of SLE in total other disease will come we name the disease differently could be rheumatoid arthritis or vasculitis etc.

14.when we stop the inflammation then all the process associated with this left in the same level including apoptosis and immune complex clearing so that this is the cause again there is no other reason for non clearing of the immune complex.dont manipulate your imaginations.

15.stop the original source eliminating the confused inflammation from the body is the first step.

16.avoiding furdher inflammation distraction is the Top most importand preventing factor for the SLE and other disease.

17.Recomended to consult homeopathy since before it is going to be a fully developed SLE can easily treat and cure the disease pre SLE.

Clinical Future Of The Sle.

Systemic:

Fatigue, malaise, fever, anorexia,weight loss

Musculoskeletal:

- Arthralgias/myalgias
- Nonerosive polyarthritis
- Hand deformities
- Myopathy/myositis
- Ischemic necrosis of bone

Cutaneous :

- Photosensitivity
- Malar rash
- Oral ulcers
- Alopecia
- Discoid rash
- Vasculitis rash Other (e.g., urticaria, cuta-

neous lupus)

Hematologic

- Anemia (chronic disease)
- Leukopenia
- Lymphopenia
- Thrombocytopenia
- Lymphadenopathy
- Splenomegaly
- Hemolytic anemia

Neurologic :

- Cognitive disorder
- Mood disorder
- Headache
- Seizures
- Mono , polyneuropathy
- Stroke, TIA
- Acute confusional state or movement disorder
- Aseptic meningitis, myelopathy

Cardiopulmonary

- Pleurisy, pericarditis, effusions
- Myocarditis, endocarditis
- Lupus pneumonitis
- Coronary artery disease
- Interstitial fibrosis
- Pulmonary hypertension, ARDS, hemorrhage

Renal

- Proteinuria,cellular casts
- Nephrotic syndrome
- End-stage renal disease

Gastrointestinal

- Nonspecific (nausea, mild pain, diarrhea)
- Abnormal liver enzymes
- Vasculitis

Thrombosis :

- venous,
- arterial.

Ocular :

- Sicca syndrome,
- Conjunctivitis,
- episcleritis,
- Vasculitis.

Rheumatoid arthritis

The common present symptoms of the rheumatoid arthritis is

- Chronic inflammatory disease but the cause of the disease unknown. (cause dicovred discussed below)
- Common disease affecting joints and also heart [pericarditis], lungs, anemia, peripheral neuropathy, etc.
- The cardiac affection of the rheumatoid arthiritits makes high possibility of

coronary artery disease and increase the death.

• 　　　　　　Early morning stiffness and pain, affecting smaller joints,etc. This disease affects many joints not necessarily smaller joints or symmetrical distribution but sure the damage to the joint is several patients are suffering with severe pain and stiffness joints severely deformed swollen and tender joints, nodules near the joints is another hall mark of this disease. Joints deformity due to severe long-standing chronic inflammation of the joint.

• 　　　　　　Rheumatoid factor positive.

• 　　　　　**Allopathy doctors identify that in the joints and synovial fluid- T CELLS, B CELLS, FIBROBLASTS, MAST CELLS AND GRANULOCYTES PRESENT IN THE SYNOVIAL FLUID OF THE AF-FECTED JOINTS? But no idea why this cells here, so they concluded that body is producing this cells to destroy the our own body cells.**

Concluding again it could be genetic in origin ,related with estrogen pills and other environmental factors.

Discussion proper

No need to worry (read the confused inflammation charecters under Risk factor or triggering factor of confused inflammation or the cause of the disease)

we are seeing the inflammation cells and immune cells in the joints without any infections or injury, so the doctors guess this disease may be due to self originating inflammation / immune system , and they found the body tissues are damaged more so they decide inflammation targeting the own body tissues   so they classified as auto immune disease. But this is not true.

I will explain in detail, Rheumatic arthritis (RA) is is not inflammatory disease, it is again confused inflammatory & immune disease . The confused inflammation created by allopathic medicine. This confused inflammation produces group of signs and symptoms in connection with joint involvement.

Next to nose and mouth the extremities especially hands are more prone to attract the confused inflammation towards the hands and fingers. This is due to holding / handling many thinks in day to day works, which is attracting the confused inflammation (B cells,T cells, Mast cells and granulocytes,etc).

In a family female more prone to handle household activity and expose to handling cold and hot objects while cooking, washing and many more works by hands bring the confused inflammation to hands so there by rheumatism is more common in female then male. Mostly the women resides indore and so that no possibility of sun exposure ,if the person is do regular sun exposure then inflammation choose the site of disease In the skin not joint and cardiac and internal organs.so in future may change since indore residence is more and male cook and all other factors change the incidence towards equal sex ration in future.estrogen tablets is a risk factor it will attract the confused inflammation towards the female reproductive organ or bone and estrogen dominant zone but there is no much female reproductive organ affection then joints and connective tissues.estrogen and other hormone excess including different hormone during pregnancy and lactations (natural hormones secreting for pregnancy and lactation has the role in attracting the confused inflammation these harmones in general is lacking to men it means no great new hormones after puberty to andropause but there are heavy natural exposure to multi hormones all these hormones attract the confused inflammation to initiate the disease either in female genitalia or extra genitals since the pregnancy and lactation hormones reduce within 1-2 years then these accentuated confused inflammation produce disease all over the body.

A women is having confused inflammation is not fit for carrying pregnancy due to all the good hormone will induce disease to female and again consuming any other hormonal pills and any allopathic medicines will induce many disease not only RA.

now a days modernized cooking utensils and cooking machineries made the household activities is become less so there is less likely to get rheumatism to female but house maids still have the possibility of the rheumatism. but it is not happy news since the confused inflammation started troubling internal organ like lungs, heart and blood, those who leading a sedentary life. But the workaholic and heavy manual labor works gardeners, sweepers etc. people will have joint manifestations sedentary life style people will get more internal organ manifestations.SO WHAT SHALL I DO NOW SHALL I START WORK VIGOROUSLY TO BRING THE CONFUSED INFLAMMATION TO SKIN AND JOINTS ? NO THAT'S NOT A RIGHT STEP.DONT ALLOW TO CREATE CONFUSED INFLAMMATION.DONT ALLOW UNSCIENTIFIC PRESCRIPTION DON'T ALLOW THE BODILY NATURAL FUNCTIONS DISTURBED.WE SHOULD NOT AFRAID TO HEART OR JOINT. WHY JOINT OR WHY HEART? I WANT ALL MY BODY PARTS SAFE AND IN GOOD HEALTHY CONDITION.

Sun exposure relive the pain due to skin attract the confused inflammation to skin wheather it is producing skin disease or not.

Stiffness of the joints and muscles and tendons usuall response of the muscles and tendons to inflammation is stiffness since we take whole night rest then the stiffness is more accentuated so when we try to initiate the first few movement is tough then gradual working or work out causes the relaxation of the muscleas and tendons so that the stiffness and related pain obliterated by movements and still more this stiffness is exaggerated in winter and cold claimate then summer and hot days. The stiffness remein more hours in winter and few minutes to few steps walk in summer. Cold increasing the stiffness of the muscle as well as increase the inflammation itself. It is not only early morinining stiffnes , precisely we can say rest stiffness mostly the arthritis gives the rest stiffness when we sit long time then when we try to walk, we have pain so this pain can be elicited better when tryin to get up from sitting.

Rheumatism has better future to develop disease to all over the world since we generally use the ac . So, no much sun exposure, women, working more fine hand works or physical activities, staying in cold claimate or using ac, using allopathic medications all are risk factor for rheumatisam.

Symmetrical distribution? having extremely tiny importance not great surprise it happens due to we use both hands simultaneously for majority of the works. If it is not then definitely disease will choose single side also.

Inflammation ? Or Something Else ? :

WHAT HAPPEN TO JOINTS ? SWELLON,ITS RED ,THEN WHAT ? I CONNOT DO ANY WORK AND IT IS STIFF AND I have FEVER.

SO, ITS LOOK LIKE A NORMAL INFLAMMATION ALMOST COVER ALL PARTS OF INFLAMMATION. [RUBAR, DOLAR, CALOR AND LOSS OF FUNCTIONS.

But it is not an inflammation ? How ? How do you say this is not inflammation and how sure you are saying this is came only by allopathic medicine?

yes, almost cover all classical symptoms of inflammation, but it has come without any natural invitation. Inflammation must start when any germs or any injury nothing is happened here, But it has come to the joints due to pressure in the hands and cold climate means this inflammation show hypersensitive to environment and pressure of the hands.

Chronic Inflammation ? :

Then this inflammation is chronic it means it is continuing for many months / to years. A true inflammation will run acute or sub acute course not as chronic.chornic means it is not body generated inflammation ,a body generated inflammation will have target (kill the enemy) and after completion of the target the inflammation will complete, it may not run for a life long course. end to end the inflammation process is governed and run till its completion. Since we forcibly stopping the inflammation the inflammation distracted. Now the inflammation is created as passive inflammation not having any governance not having any target it will run their course till the trigger is present or sometime the inflammation may be present in the site for even life long. The chornic inflammation or chronic disease is because there is no goal or target or aim and no one is runining this inflammation or process it has started on its own due to some triggers if the trigger is present long time then the disease also presents. The confused inflammation from the day one it is chronic disease. If the True inflammation is interrupted then the inflammation chemicals and cells remain inside the body unable to remove by anyone it stays in our body till the end of our life will prduce different disease it could be RA or SLE or any other disease.

A True inflammation will not give damage and destruction, this rheumatoid arthritis is damaging the joints and deform it. The readily available inflammation (C Inflammation) has begun here and do their action.

There are many wound healing cells here (fibrus and gelatin cells) of wound healing within joints who called this cells here then where is the wounds ? since we started using many external applications eventhough the wound will heal automatically we will never happy if we not apply anything to the wound so this will distract the wound healing cells so they come here and produce the joint become permanently immobile over a year.what happening here wound healing is happanining without any wound.germ killing is happenining without any germ.inflammation is happenining without any targed enemy to the body.

Yes, ofcourse all this process is a auto inflammation and auto immunity and auto wound healing is happening due to unnessory and non scientific allopathic medicines. Not the body is producing some cells to destroy the body. All this immune and inflame cells if we allow it abnormally longer period in an normal surface it will destroy that since they are asked to work in the needed damaged site so this special cells are not similar to the cells which is remain in the blood vessals they will be ready to work so they are working you are killed bacteria so they are not having target. But they are not going to remove from the circulation and not going to withdraw so they will destroy your body cells.WHO IS REMOVED THE TARGET (BACTERIA).Who is having medicine for remove the target.who is using antibacterial.

chornic disease it means failure of healing power and failure of the protective system .tell me now who is prescribing against the healing power of the human inflammation and immune and wound healing process.why are you blaming the body.who is prescribing medicine before completing the acute disease.who is stopping the fever and terminate the inflammation in the mid.you are doing more then enough service then the violent germs in the world.

Joints and fibrous rheumatic nodule but it has trying to heal without any injury and without any precision causes deformity and loss of functions.Excess collection of confused inflammation chemical and cells to do a near normal classical inflammation. Highest possibility of allopathic treatment for fever and external application for skin disease or wound healing produced this cells.NO ONE IN THE MEDICAL FIELD INVENTED MEDICINE FOR STOP THE NATURAL PROCESS OF HEALING OTHER THEN ALOPATHY.

We do head to foot wrong treatment everything against the nature and against the biological process so allopathy doing wrong treatment so cells stuck somewhere and really unite with some available chemical and cells start doing damage so we find it and name it but interpreted wrongly. Now that also we discovered.

SO, WHAT IS THE POINT IN DISCOVERY? WE HAVE TO PREVENT DISEASE BY NOT USING THE MEDICINE AGAINST BIOLOGICAL NATURAL HEALING POWER OF THE HUMANS.WE SHOULD NOT MAKE CONFUSED INFLAMMA-TION.PREVENTION IS BETTER THAN CURE.

Many fold suppression of disease

Chronic Inflammatory joint disease, unknown etiology . when we prescribe anti-inflammatory at the age of 10 and the rheumatoid arthritis develops slowly around 25 to 30 years then how we can suspect that rheumatism is caused by a shifted inflammation from selected location to all over the body. **It does not mean all this 15 -20 years inflammation is been silent for many years it keep gives the trouble we give the different diagnosis name but**

we ignore it or we may diverted these disease are some deficiency or some skin disease again we prescribe same anti-inflammatory and steroids so the disease matured as rheumatism .rheumatism usually tetra or Penta disease [the primary disease repeatedly suppressed so the rheumatism developed as 4 th or 5 th time suppression]

Doctors are getting benefit by collapsing the system but the patient are suffering, we have all evidence of what we done in the patient, but we close our eyes we search the cause for the disease as a genetic or something else no reason so auto immune disease. There is inflammation in the joints but no bacteria or germs or no wound then why inflammation? so we are name this as auto immunity. We found some immune cells which is against the joint space so we have evidence now to say this is auto immune disease.

We should not conclude that the present lymphocyte or immune globulin's are appointed for this purpose to do damage to the human body.actually speaking most of the cases the presence of inflammation and blood cells are self-appointed it means either they stuck or it is attracted due to creation of confused inflammation in joints or thyroid or in the skin. Why auto immune disease since readymade available immune cells attracted towards confused inflammation site or stressful sites and create the destruction.

But my dear doctors this is not appointed for destroying any organ from order by brain it has joining to the existing inflammation or this cells alone damage where ever they attracted. [don't say we found immunoglobulin say confused immunoglobulin, don't say lymphocytes say confused lymphocytes)

We collapsed the system many years before and we forgot that now we this is different disease.We forgot that we are violated by prescribing medicine.People with rheumatoid arthritis don't get that much in the near term. But this is not good news.

Arthritis can occur in the hands or feet but if the affected cells do not hit the hands and feet we cannot be happy because now it can go into the body and start attacking the body's organs, heart attack or kidney failure causing liver damage.blood cells are at targets now so thaw omens will suffer with many blood cells failure.

rheumatisam is a deadly disease, and it is the worst disease to affect the internal organs so its better to remove the confused inflammation from the body.

Consult best homeopaths to do this. Rheumatisam is one of the disease which will demand to take many pain killers and heavy stroids which is not necessary. The first aims is we have to prevent the disease.

If the disease is start giving trouble like vague joint pain and arthritits then consult homeopathy they will clear it before it is formed as RA. If the ra is developed better consult homeopathy don't complicate the disease by strong allopathic steroids and pain killers and external applications.

Using data from the Global Burden of Diseases, Injuries, and Risk Factors (GBD) 2017 study, researchers examined the trends in global, regional, and national prevalence, incidence, and associated disability-adjusted life years (DALYs) in patients with RA. No such global study has been published since 2010.

The GBD 2017 study included 195 countries, 7 super regions, and 21 regions across the globe, from 1990 to 2017; data on 354 diseases and injuries, 282 causes of death, and 84 risk factors were systematically analyzed.

Results of the analysis indicated that there were 19,965,115 globally prevalent cases of RA in 2017 (95% uncertainty interval [UI], 17,990,489-21,995,673 cases).

Osteo arthritis (OA)

OA is caused by confused inflammation disorder, every human can bear his weight, there may not be any chance of erosion of the bone due to unable his own body weight.So don't have misconception that we are having erosion of bone due to excess body weight. **The normal bones strength Is reduced due to administration of steroids and other drugs is one of the important causes for osteoporosis and related OA.**

Mild to moderate confused inflammation in the joints produce the weakening of the soft tissue of the joints as well as bone of the joints will lead to osteo arthritis.

Osteo arthritis pain worse when walking or doing work. Can be explained the inflammation is near the bones so when more the walk more the complaints worse.

Prescribing calcium tablets not necessary.It helps minimally in some osteoporosis cases . Correction of mal aligned joints due to trauma or birth anomaly is necessary otherwise this will attract the confused inflammation somewhere in the body to joints and increase destructions of the joint.

Obesity gives the over strain to the joints but it is bearable to healthy person but if they have confused inflammation then that will come to joints and increase the oa. So obesity is a risk factor only those who have confused inflammation.

Osteo arthritis is makes the disability and reduce the working capacity so it is better we have to prevent the oa before it takes place. We have to rectify the mal aligned joints.

Osteo arthritis related with confused inflammation can be well cured by homiyopathy medicine and recover the patient and prevent falling in disability.

Calc flour , rhus tox , calc phos ,benz acid is some

remedy but better to consult a doctor and remove the disease from the core.

Scleroderma

A man was cursed by some evil, then the person is become wood or stone , I was saw in many movies. In the same way in sclerodemra most of the soft parts of the body is lost their elasticity and become thick & hard . it is not like stone or wood but the affected part is losing their elasticity and free movement it become hard. Scleroderma is a mega induration of the skin and soft tissues with deposites Excess collagen and fibroblasts.

Why this disease ? explanation by allopathy :

The explanation for scleroderma is same old story like genetics and environmental and immune dysregulation by allopathy doctors.

When explaining pathological process of this disease by allopathy they keep using many chemical and cells name which is involved in inflammation and immunity and complete their explantion but they never use the word this is similar to wound healing or almost all futures of wound helaing is happen. And they fail to understand almost there are many different type of vasculitis each has different pathology outcome. but all is inflammation and immunity alone which is targetes the blood vessal everytime doctor is giving explanation by using some chemicals and process, without understanding why the same trigger, has to produce different disease and different out come in the endotheliyam (this is because availability of confused inflammation chemicals).

There is a vascular changes in scleroderma patient what happen there are many triggers (like virus toxin,im-

mune complex , any chemical or other environment exposure) so that the endotheliyam damaged so now vaso constriction and vasodialatation process is abnormal and then
the vascular permiblity is increased and luecocytes are lib-
erated and internal cloting is happening then the muscular
layer is proliferates and then excess fibroblast and gelatin
has formed but due to chronic long standing nature of this
disease the vessal lumen is completely obliterated over all
excess fibroblast is the prominent futre in this process.

Now if you see what will happening when you have
wound first vaso constriction and then clotting and inflammation process like vasodialation and increased vascular
permeablity, white blood cells entry and then germ killing
then fibroblast and gelatin entry then regeneration of the
damaged cells and that's all the wound healing process this
is what happen here. But without any real injury (we assume
that viral antigen or other environmental we are not having
sufficient proof of this viral antigen) but all this whole process happening like starting from vaso constriction to final
regeneration. But without any proper sequence and order
and some process happen excess some process is happen too
less but not correct level. If the ednotheliyam is damaged by
any trigger it has to heal or repair. but why the repair is not
happening here eventhough there is a minimal attempt to
fibrinolysis of removing the clots within the blood vessals
it is not succesfull and fail ? why fail ? it is subnormal not
sufficient to obliterate the blood vessals. But excess fibroblast cells occumilation which is not necessary here why this
unnessary accumulation .vaso constriction and vaso dilatation process has to be adjusted according to the need but it is
altered why this altered. Without explaining all you are trying to explaining abnormal pathology as equal with normal
pathology.

Vascular injury and then injured part will be repaired here the pathophysiology is normal pathology. Vascular injury but keep destruction partial recovery ,partial destruction excess regeneration abnormal proliferation all happening but you are completed pathophysiological explanation without explaingin why thise happening. a reader can easily / hardly understand something is wrong you need to explain what is wrong why it is ?. All the abnormal pathology is happening is due to confused inflammation. A warier is fighting in the war is something different from zombiya warier war. But you are explaining zombiya war as if normal war. You need to add one importand one line that is all this process is almost happen in wound healing here it is mixed and confused and happen in incomplete way not having any purpose not doing any repair because this is not a normal pathology this is abnormal pathology. The available confused inflammation run the process so it will be like this, there is no surprice in this.

What Will Happen By Scleroderma ?

classified into one of two major subsets based on the pattern of skin involvement Moreover , while systemic sclerosis is associated with prominent and early internal organ involvement.

Local scleroderma presents with long-standing Raynaud's phenomenon, indolent skin, limited internal organ involvement, and a better prognosis.

Morphea presents as solitary or multiple circular patches of thickened skin and, less commonly, widespread induration (generalized or pansclerotic morphea); the fingers are spared.Linear scleroderma—streaks of thickened skin, typically in one or both lower extremities—may affect the subcutaneous tissues with fibrosis and atrophy of supporting structures, muscle, and bone. In children, the growth of affected long bones can be retarded. When linear scleroderma lesions cross joints, significant contractures can develop.

Initial Clinical Presentation

The initial presentation is quite different in the diffuse and the limited cutaneous forms of the disease. In patients with dcSSc, the interval between Raynaud's phenomenon and appearance of other manifestations is generally brief (weeks to months).

Soft tissue swelling and
intense pruritus are signs of the early inflammatory "edematous" phase of dcSSc.
The fingers, hands, distal limbs, and face are usually affected first. Diffuse hyperpigmentation and
carpal tunnel syndrome can occur.
Arthralgias,
muscle weakness and
decreased joint mobility are common.

During the ensuing weeks to months, the inflammatory edematous phase evolves into the "fibrotic" phase,
with skin induration that is
associated with loss of body hair,
reduced production of skin oils, and
a decline in sweating capacity.

The subcutaneous tissue becomes affected,
with fat atrophy and fibrosis of underlying fascia, muscle, and other soft tissue structures.

Progressive flexion contractures of the fingers ensue.
The wrists, elbows, shoulders, hip girdles, knees, and ankles

become stiff due to fibrosis of the supporting joint structures.

While advancing skin involvement is the most visible manifestation

of early dcSSc, important internal organ involvement develops during

this stage. The initial 4 years from disease onset is the period of

rapidly evolving systemic involvement and greatest risk for pulmonary

and renal damage. If organ failure does not occur during this

period, the systemic process may stabilize.

ischemia,ulcerations, and auto amputation of the fingers.

Organ Involvement _ Raynaud's Phenomenon

Raynaud's phenomenon is an episodic vasoconstriction in the

fingers and toes that occurs in virtually every patient with SSc.

Vasoconstriction may also affect the tip of the nose and earlobes. Attacks are triggered by exposure to cold, a decrease in temperature,emotional stress, and vibration. Typical attacks start with pallor,followed by cyanosis of variable duration. Eventually erythema develops spontaneously or with rewarming of the digit. The progression of the three color phases reflects the underlying pathogenic mechanisms of vasoconstriction, ischemia, and reperfusion.

Raynaud's phenomenon, is more frequent in women.

Breakdown of atrophic skin leads to chronic
ulcerations at the extensor surfaces of the proximal interphalangeal
joints, the volar pads of the fingertips, and bony
prominences such
as the elbows and malleoli.

Healing of ischemic fingertip ulcerations leaves characteristic fixed digital "pits." Loss of soft tissue at the fingertips due to ischemia is frequent and may be associ-ated with striking resorption of the terminal phalanges (ac-roosteolysis)

Calcium deposits occur in the skin and soft tissues. Calcinosis
cutis is most common in patients with lcSSc who are positive for
anticentromere antibodies.

Pulmonary Feautures

Pulmonary involvement can be documented in most patients with
Scleroderma and is now the leading cause of death.

- aspiration pneumonitis complicating gastroesophageal reflux,
- pulmonary hemorrhage due to endobron-chial telangiectasia,
- obliterative bronchiolitis,
- pleural reactions,
- restrictive ventilatory defect due to chest wall fibrosis,
- spontaneous pneumothorax,
- lung cancer, particularly bronchioloal-veolar carcinoma, may be increased.

Interstitial Lung Disease (Ild)

ILD and pulmonary fibrosis cause restrictive pulmonary function defect with impaired gas exchange The most common pattern in SSc, nonspecific interstitial pneumonia.

Pulmonary Arterial Hypertension (Pah)

Approximately 15% of SSc patients have PAH that can occur in association with ILD or as an isolated pulmonary abnormality. The natural history of Systemic scleroderma-associated PAH is variable, but in many patients it follows a downhill course with development of right heart failure and significant mortality.

Gastrointestinal Involvement

The gastrointestinal tract is affected in up to 90% of Systemic scleroderma patients with both limited and diffuse cutaneous forms of the disease. The pathologic features of atrophy of smooth muscle, intact mucosa,
and obliterative small-vessel vasculopathy are similar throughout
the length of the gastrointestinal tract.

Upper Gastrointestinal Tract Involvement

reduced oral aperture,
resorption of the mandibular condyles are fre-

quent.

Symptoms of gastroesophageal reflux disease (GERD) develop early .

diminished motility in the distal two-thirds of the esophagus,

delayed gastric emptying accounts for GERD.
Severe erosive esophagitis
Esophageal strictures and
Barrett's esophagus may complicate chronic GERD.

Gastroparesis with early satiety,
abdominal distention, and
aggravated reflux symptoms is common.

Lower Gastrointestinal Tract Involvement

Impaired intestinal motility may result in malab-sorption and chronic diarrhea secondary to bacterial over-growth. Fat and protein malabsorption and B12 and vitamin D deficiency ensue. Colonic involvement may cause severe constipation,fecal incontinence, gastrointestinal bleeding from telangiectasia and rectal prolapse.

In late-stage systemic scleroderma, wide-mouth sacculations or diverticula occur in the colon, occasionally causing perforation and bleeding.

Renal Involvement : Scleroderma Renal Crisis

Scleroderma renal crisis, the most dreaded com-plication of Scleroderma
Patients characteristically present with acceler-ated hypertension

and progressive renal insufficiency.

Normotensive renal crisis is generally associated with a poor outcome. Headache, blurred vision,and chest pain may accompany elevation of blood pressure. Urinalysis typically shows mild proteinuria, granular casts, and microscopic hematuria; thrombocytopenia and microangiopathic hemolysis with fragmented red blood cells can be seen. Progressive oliguric renal

failure over several days generally follows. Oliguria or

a creatinine >3 mg/dL at presentation predicts poor outcome, with

permanent hemodialysis and high mortality.

Cardiac Involvement

The endocardium, myocardium, and

pericardium may be affected separately or together in scleroderma.

- pericardial effusions,
- atrial and ventricular tachycardias,
- conduction abnormalities,
- valvular regurgitation,
- hypertrophy,
- heart failure.
- Systemic and pulmonary hypertension

MUSCULOSKELETAL COMPLICATIONS

Carpal tunnel syndrome
Generalized arthralgia and stiffness are prominent in early disease.

Joint mobility is progressively impaired (prominently hands) Contractures develop at the proximal inter-phalangeal joints and wrists.

Movement at the elbows, shoulders, and knees is frequently reduced. True joint inflammation is uncommon; however, occasional patients develop
erosive polyarthritis in the hands.

Muscle weakness is common and may indicate de-conditioning, disuse atrophy, and malnutrition.

Other Disease Manifestations

Dry eyes and dry mouth (sicca complex).

Hypothyroidism is common and generally due to fibrosis of the thyroid gland.

sensory trigeminal neuropathy due to fibrosis or vasculopathy can occur, presenting with gradual onset of pain and numbness.

Erectile dysfunction is frequent in men with systemic scleroderma and may be the initial disease manifestation.

malignancies is increased in systemic sclerosis. Some studies have indicated that cancers of the lung, tongue, and breast occur more frequently in
patients with Scleroderma. Barrett's metaplasia is associated with increased
risk for adenocarcinoma of the esophagus.

Diagnosis :

The presence of skin induration, with a characteristic symmetricdistribution pattern associated with typical visceral organ manifestations,

establishes the diagnosis with a high degree of certainty.

Occasionally, full-thickness biopsy of the skin is required for establishing the diagnosis of scleredema, scleromyxedema, or nephrogenic systemic fibrosis.

Vasculitis

Inflammation within blood vessals is vasculitis. Till now the inflammation is observed and found many inflammation and immune cells and chemicals and mediaters participating in this vasculitis but the cause is unknown. So, suspected as auto immune disease.

There are many classifications like wegeners granulomatosis, churg ,giant cell poly arthritis ,serum sickness and cutanues vasculitis syndrome,poly arteritis nodosa ,,.henoch shonlein pupura,,,,,etc.

Allopathic doctors concluded that it caused by genetic predisposition and environment and the immune cells acts in a different way to antigens in this particular individual.

Generally, most of the vasculitic syndromes are assumed to be mediated at least in part by immunopathogenic mechanisms that occur in response to certain antigenic stimuli **(Table 326-2)**.

However, evidence supporting this hypothesis is for the most part indirect and may reflect epiphenomena as opposed to true

causality. Furthermore, it is unknown why some individuals might develop vasculitis in response to certain antigenic stimuli,

whereas others do not. It is likely that a number of factors are involved in the ultimate expression of a vasculitic syndrome.

These include the genetic predisposition, environmental exposures,

and the regulatory mechanisms associated with immune response to certain antigens.

- HORRISON TEX BOOK OF GENERAL MEDICINE -18 TH EDITION.

Discussion :

What changes is happening within the blood vessals.there is some trigger initiate the inflammation so that the blood vessals attacked during this inflammation and immune process the blood vessals damaged and blocked so there is no blood supply to the particular part is stopped. This is process is not due to any germs but belived that it could be some viral or bacterial chemicals (enemies' chemical - antigen) may induce this process. But this is happening to very specific individual not all that's why they say it could be genetic or environment.

They named auto immune because they destroy us instead of protecting us it is destroying. So allopathic doctors belivingthat inflammation and immunity will do good to humans so there is a normal protecting immunity and there is a destructing immunity . We see lot of malfunction of immunity so that we have prepared many numbers of medicine good we have medicine to stop bad inflammation and immunity that is anti inflammatory and steroids good . I have one question do you have any single medicine which you commonly use to support the immunity & inflammation. Ok now I am saying stopping inflammation will cause auto immunity and will cause many diseases so repaire immune system rather then stopping repair the term included what is needed in that particular part to recover its normal function rather then hiding the disease is the right choice.

As I am saying frequqntly the vasculitis is partial inflammation and distracted confused inflammation and it is not a inflammation at all. So how I can say this a inflammation is having target that target is not our body a inflammation is regenerate the blood vessals damaged, this is we observed in every inflammation cases but here we saw the vessals damaged and it is not recovered and regenerated more then that the blood vessals allowed to close completely so we named this is self destruction forgot about name but see clearly only the destructive part of inflammation is happening which is usually normal but neo vascularization after apoptosis is usual process of any inflammation which is not happening here this is because this is partial process and see first leaucotrience and other chemicals damaged blood vessals and nutrophilic chemicals further damage the blood vessals and again what ever may be the blood and immune cells or other chemical intermediaters targeting the blood vessals it damages further but this process happen only once in normal inflammation process after liberation cehmicals from must cells once for natural fighting cells has to come out of the blood vessals to targeted site. So observing everything vomiting in the text book saying this is reserch or using this throry to the upcoming medical proffesion will spoil future of medical profession. Observe and interprate and then announce.

Right Interpretation Is :

1.The chemicals which is used for inviting warrier by minimal destruction of blood vessals is allowed to roam within the circulation. There are enough anti-inflammatory medicines will do these functions so there is no need to blame genetics or environment or immune modification on its own.

2. These chemicals are triggered by any natural bodily excess or hyper functions or even normal functions this is not related with inborn predisposition. This is related with their chemical functional analague like vaso constriction (exposur to cold) or vaso dialatation (sun exposure) ,pressure upon the particular vessals like any trigger. Why this hyper response this is because we spill the acid in toilet and nutralise that with water and flush enough

water and then we sit in the toilet imagine what will happen when we spill acid in the whole house and then we walk in the floor. This is not something genetically our foot is predisposed to wound because of acid this is so normal we poured acid we are not cleaned or removed it. Similar way blood vessal destroying chemicals are allowed only to the negligible amount in the inflammation site like tonsil or nose or the boil or abcess site but when we stop this now then this blood vessal destroying chemicals allowed to roam all over the blood vessals they are not removed it. But they will not do damages immediately it will take many months to years to develop vasculitis since need enough chemicals to do proper disease but mean while it will try to produce minor changes here and there but allopathy doctors fail to identify that.

3.even though blood vessals destroyed not sequentially all steps will happen again what ever it may be the confused roaming blood cells available only will help in run the process here neutrophils and monocytes and macrophages come and form granules. If you read carefully the cheracters of confused inflammation that will say this what exactly happening. Destruction is happening but no repair by body .

When the same person falls in the ground there is minor injury or abrasion in the legs immidiatly there are many recovery systems and regenerating system so the blood vessals stopped bleeding then closing the wounds regenerating the blood vessals everything happens. But still its happening but why destruction is happen in the vital part and here also the blood vessal is damaged but no recovery ? since this is body design, the damage is induced by our own body chemicals and that is appointed to destroy the blood vessals, they are doing their function so body may not interfere their functions. Since this is not enemy. Like we create tumor in an unnessory part we create ulcer or destruction in unwanted part by getting aprovel from the body in the name of some infection in the nose and infection in the tonsil but we stop that infection and inflammation and we take them to do damage within the blood vessals here (all over the body in general). So this is not a auto immunity, this is distracted immunity or confused immunity.

4.After repeated stopping of inflammation we never allow the inflammation or rash or skin disease in the skin and mouth or repeated medications then the confused inflammation chemicals allowed to stay within blood vessal will do this function naturally we not allow the superficial inflammations we keep suppress that by ointments and medications inturn started destroying blood vessals more.

5.so now it is very clear that distracted inflammation alone produceing this disease so it is highly in our hand like patient and doctor they can decide wheather they need vasculitis or not . the prevention is largely depend upon stopping the inflammation . you stop demanding the doctors to prescribe medicine and doctors must say what is the consequncess of stopping inflammation and infections then sure vasculitis will be preventable. Vasculitis and many other auto immune disease is preventable so we can live without any kidney failure or storoke or heart attack or asthma attack induced by vasculitis and auto immunity.

" I have designed to protect the people health,during fight with enemy I might damage the body parts, I will regenerate my damage but I don't have access to regenerate when the damage is purposeless or without my controle even if the damage is happen by my body tissues " – DEFENSE MECHANISAM.

"INFLAMMATION DAMAGES WILL BE REGENARATED & REPAIRED BY BODY"

BUT CONFUSED INFLAMMATION DAMAGES WILL NEVER RECOVER.SINCE ITS OUT OF BODY CONTROLE.SO THE DAMAGES HAPPEN WITHOUT BODY

WILLINGNESS SO BODY MAY NOT RECOVER THAT ,till the end of life in most of the cases.

BACK AND SPINAL CORD

Back ache / neck pain is the one of the common complaints for many people but leading many tests I am surprising that many of the poor people also demanded to take MRI spine they have MRI spine in their hand when coming to my clinic. MRI report says some finding or no finding, but not much relief of their pain.

Often the diagnosis in India is comes like disc bulge , disc prolapse, disc erosion and osteo arthritis [for young teen/middle age stout person sitting in office] neck bone erosion ? everyone is having some spinal pathology ? is surprising. Ligament involvement, fibrous sheet involvement.

The main cause for chronic neck pain is stiffness and pain due to sinus or infection of the Ent tract or lymph adenitis like that this pain usually worse in winters.

Second most reason for lumbar and sacral chronic pain is due to pure muscular ache due to confused inflammation attack in the back muscles.it will happen either due to strain in the back muscle causes confused inflammation to reach the back or sudden stretching of the back muscle after long time sedentary life style. This is happening to many people rather then real spinal bone and disc involvement.

Sciatica is again caused by C inflammation attack rather then impingement of the spine or crushing of the spine but again most of the MRI reports says there is nerve impingement then doctors says need for surgery? Sciatica with nerve compression will happen only if severe erosion of the spinal bones or injury or fall not every member who is having back pain is having some deep pathology within the spine.

All over the body the disease how it is occurred what is the cause nothing is known but orthopedic surgeon and neuro surgeon in India and Tamilnadu is removed this factor many years before most of the MRI will say some pathology otherwise, he is / was healthy and no history of trauma. SO, NO DIALAMMA? NO WORRY? CAUSE IS IDENTI-FIED I am seeing even the children's diagnosed as cervical bone pain due to spine bone pathology, so the pain?

Doctors read many dd regarding the back pain but they often find spinal bone pathology is the only common finding is the surprising diagnosis.

Since in homeopathy we will ask about all the complaints of the patient most of the patient age starting from 35 is having back pain? mild to moderate in nature. Dull and long standing.

Ankylosing spondylitis is purely having C inflam-mation. All other spondylosis is related with the C inflam-mation. The hyper mobility strain and sprain attract the c inflammation to the spine.

ANKYLOSING SPONDYLITIS :

Confused inflammation with final destructive stage as well as regeneration phase is marked here. The inflammation is eroding in nature .more then grad-ual erosion in the old age here the erosion fast and very earl-ier then expected (homeopathy simply name this kind rapid destruction under destructive miasm or syphilis). The usual osteo arthritis in the elderly takes nearly 20-25 years to see a great erosion and osteophyte formation.but here these erosion is so rapid as well as regeneration is happen in the eroded bone margin by fibrocartilaginas material then this matured as ossification resulting in fusion of the joint space causes multible bones fusion into single immobile bone.

TNF - GROWTH FACTOR , Macrophage ,T Cells and osteo clasts or found in the inflammation site.Stiffness is marked symptoms with pain in the back.slow immobility and loss of flexibility lead to severe impairement of day to day actitivity.

Uvitis is a extra articular future of the ankylosing spondylitis.colitis and inflammatory bowel disease is a most common extra articular future.

The suppressed inflammation from colon is reached to the spine and produce the inflammation then the iimune system activation causes the acro ilitis. It is not only the eye and spine involved more then that many other organs affected due to the wandering inflammation throught the body in homeopathy doctors are recommended to trace the affection of confused inflammation all over the human body parts rather then single parts.

Prevention attempt to distract and stop the inflammation is to be avoided.There are many medicines is there to controle and cure the early cases.

7.THYROID DISORDERS

An antibody will swallow all the dead bacteria and wasted tissues after the inflammation is over. This is considered as normal phenomena.

Doctors found thyroid destructing antibody they identify that. This lymphocytes, thyroid antibody [thyroglobulin anti thyroid antibody] are destroy the thyroid gland instead of destroy the bacteria.so they consider as new disease called auto immune thyroiditis.

They found some diseases originates in the same way antibody which swallows the tissues of the organ or some body part [so they name it auto immune hepatitis, auto immune arthritis,,,,,etc.

Now doctors having lots of waiting list disease yet to name auto immune disease but they are not having evidence [we have to prove that antibody is the cause for the disease this antibody having that organ or tissue within their antibody]

IS IT TRUE THAT FINDING ARE RIGHT OR WRONG.THE OBSERVATION IS WRONG. Actually, the antibody is having the power to swallow all bacteria as well as damaged tissue of our body and damaged cells of organs [liver, stomach, joints].

when circulating antibody swallows the thyroid tissues, they name it AUTO IMMUNE THYROIDITIS. actually the thyroid gland is in trouble for many years but doctors are waiting [or unaware] to classify and waiting for auto antibody to appear in the circulation.by the time all the glands is damaged so now it's a normal function of the antibody to swallow the dead thyroid.it is not special lymphocytes has come due to genetically induced to swallow the thyroid.it is a normal antibody all we have it swallows the damaged thyroid gland because it is the normal function of the antibody. The raising level of antibody titer indicates the damage is severe so that body appointing antibody to clear the dead tissue of the body parts.

We have to understand one clear facts in the mind that diseases are created not really occurred, so we are troubling the body beyond its tolerance limit so we have to expect something unusual can happen and consider this is normal in un highly unusual [abnormal normal].we are collapsing whole good system into worst and thereby we have to observe all things.

A inflammation is coming for save us we are closing and stopping that so that confused inflammation formed this is damaging the organs we name this is disease and again we give treatment again confused inflammation started this will further damage the organ now it's too much trouble to the body but every time body has an adaptive behavior having solvation

Yes, the antibody is created and send for killing the germs but unfortunately it has been not utilized so that antibody

is also not destroyed this anti bodies are hyperactive and join along with confused inflammation and produce severe damage to the organ.

The possible unemployment happen to immunoglobulin is by antibiotic using antibiotic kill the germs so there is not work for immunoglobulins if they not completed their task, they cannot withdraw from circulation this is the cause for antibody formation. I have enough proof that all over the body we have created lots of auto immune and auto inflammatory diseases without any auto antibody. The number diseases [I am saying all the diseases in general in the whole medical texts are auto immune and auto inflammatory disease only but when comparing that only less percent of disease only we have anti body for specific for the disease].

Antibody can come and join to the confused inflammation or real inflammation only if it is available in the circulation otherwise the damage to the tissue is happen only by means of confused inflammation chemical and cells.

Since we does not have any clue why and how the disease occur we are in search of finding anti body at least satisfy our self it was happen due to this but I am giving you 100 % cause for disease is either confused inflammation or broken feedback mechanism so don't waste your time to searching the cause in effect of the disease. THE CAUSE OF DISEASE IS DOCTORS AND ALOPATHIC PHARMACOLOGY.

Example By Thyroid Illness.

1.Simple Thyroiditis / Silent Thyroiditis ; no virus or bacteria-ESR normal, no thyroid antibody.

2.A dequervains thyroiditis : no virus or bacteria,ESR elevated,no thyroid antibody.

3.Hashimotos thyroiditis : no virus or bacteria, ESR normal or elevated thyroid anti body present.

Actually, in simple and dequervains thyroiditis, the gland is under chronic inflammation but not affected so severely so that we have never found any thyroid swallowing antibody, so they name it simple thyroid.to classify little more specific ESR elevated is dequerveins Actually speaking this is also a normal simple thyroiditis. and mostly or rarely the gland will be destroyed by the long-standing chronic inflammation and the lymphocytes will swallow that we name now as AUTO IMMUNE THYROIDITIS OR HASHIMOTOS THYROIDITIS.so this is the way they diagnose the autoimmune disease. They complicate this, wondering how this self-destructing lymphocyte comes.If the immunoglobulin present sure that will come and participate to the confused inflammation if it is not there then there is no immunoglobulin. (tumor is auto immunity,inflammation of thyroid is auto inflammation but you have worried about only immune cells is here so it is auto immunity ,then who called tumor to build a tumor within the thyroid any idea ?)

what is the cause of auto immunity prescribing anti biotic but they hide that.they say   No idea [they assume this is may be a genetic or something yet to discover] so all auto immune disease is under suspicion how it occurs by allopath's.

BUT MY OBSERVATION [Apart from viral or bacterial infection] there are only inflammation, there is no auto immune inflammation. What allopathy name as auto immune inflammation is nothing but severe organ or tissue changes of the same simple inflammation. [Distracted immunity].

I am explaining the inflammatory and immune cells are misdirected by wrong treatment of allopathy. But allopathy says activation of the autoimmunity is unknown or it could be due to genetic [modified genes].

Some gene polymorphisms contribute to several autoimmune
diseases, such as STAT4 and CTLA 4. All these gene polymorphisms/transcription/epigenetic combinations influence immune responses to the external and internal environment; when such responses are too high and/or too prolonged and/or inadequately regulated, autoimmune
disease results. -- HARRISON TEXT BOOK OF GENERAL MEDICINE.

Just go and read the character of the confused inflammation I have used and explained all this response why the inflammation and immune cells are behaving like this (the yellow marked lines are clearly explained in the confused inflammation cherecters)

When we say genetics then there is no need to worry about the present who is going to trace the genetics ? no such genetics read the explanation.

These auto immune theory explained well in scleroderma and vasculitis. The simple activation cellular and humoral immunity against the thyroid is initiated by the inflammation so based on the inflammation guidelines the immune system destructing the thyroid. So there is no genetic. The chronic disease and long time destruction is happening not again due to genetics or some other factor. All the true inflammation is guided and run by our body but the inflammation is distracted by any mode then the inflammation process will be stopped so the activated but distracted inflammation products remain in the body and keep producing the disease long time.

Inflammation preced before humoral and cellular immunity activation in the thyroid destruction we name it as simple thyroiditis but if cellular and humoral immunity activated then we name it as auto immunity. So, inflammation decide who has to be destracted so the immune system follows that. This is not the case in true inflammation both inflammation and immunity has the one target.

But I have clearly said the specific antibody formed against the germs is produced it means targeted attack. But the inflammation chemicals like histamine and bradykinin (chemokines) is also pored near the necessary site by release of monocytes and esonophil. Say for example if you have bacterial entry in the left arm the monocyte and esonophil will reach there and release the chemokin chemicals near there so the inflammation begin the left arm where exactly the bacteria entered upto this level if you not discovered anything against the inflammation there is no problem but just imagine what will happen if you take that chemokines is sprayed all over the body ? when you release the inflammation near the eye to attack the germ then inflammation start over there .if you relase the chemokine released inside the stomach then inflammation and immunity will be started over there. When you spread all over the body what will happen ? inflammation and disease will happen to all over the body and vasculitis and so many tumors everything you need you will have in the same time no need to go to genetic study.

but when we distract that chemicals into the circulation then now the bradykinin and histamine and inflammatory chemicals are roming within the circulation where ever it goes and produce the inflammation. When the inflammation is commenced then automatically either

confused immune or true immune disease also will be initiated is the cause for auto immunity.

I AM NOT USING THE TERM AUTO IMMUNITY ITS WRONG NAME, YES OF COURSE YOU NEED A PROOF THAT HOW AUTOIMMUNITY DEVELOPS. But I am asking you to classify under modified or altered or misguided inflammation / immunity, or distracted inflammation or immunity.

What is the necessity of such classification?

Of course, I see many subnormal chronic inflammations in the joints/skin/ thyroid,etc. which is not initiated by germs or other inflammation cause but it is happen. The body parts are become damaged by the misguided inflammations. so, put them under misguided immunity.

or we can keep like disprove that no germs or no antibodies then keep under misguided immunity/inflammation.

Thyroid swelling **[goiter]** and the tumor of the thyroid all will happen due to confused inflammation mostly it comes from the upper respiratory tract [nose, throat, tonsil,]. The lymphatic which carry the nasal cavity throat, oral cavity all is located in the neck near the thyroid gland helps in spread of the disease to thyroid glands.

Again, the **hypo thyroid** is the forrunner of the true thyroiditis evident to the doctors. Hypo or hyper thyroid indicates the confused inflammation has commenced within the thyroid gland treat the confused inflammation don't treat the hypo or hyper thyroid if it is self-adjusted with TSH secretion.

CLEAR THE CONFUSED INFLAMMATION FROM

THE CIRCULATION BY USING APROPRAITE TECHNIQUE OR HOMEOPATHY.

The lymphatics and the lymph node act as a good protective functions but when repeated anti-inflammatory and anti biotics administered it stops the protective functions even though it can work so that now the lymphatics and lymph node function as similar to blood vessels it carry lymph along with dead debris and confused inflammation this confused inflammation near the thyroid gland easily attracted in hyper functions of the thyroid especillay in growing period and in excess demand.

A healthy thyroid gland will meet the body need so easily it is rare to produce hypothyroid all the mal functions are happanining due to confused inflammation.

Prescribing the thyroid suppliments never prevent the thyroid inflammation and never cure the thyroid swellings. A thyroid nodule may undergo cancer cells when the stress is too much.

Prevent confused inflammation, remove the same if it is there save Thyroid.

Hormonal imbalance

Either high or low level of hormonal level is transient in an emergency situation or increased body needs.But it will come to normal after the body need is reduced. If the hormonal level is not return to normal for longer period need to be addressed properly and search for an confused inflammation in the particular gland.prescribbing simple hormonal supliments is not a real treatment.if the treatment is going on this way sure the computer will over take doctors that will give a feed back what can be done to the patient in this situation. If low then give supliment if hormone excess then reduces that. This is may not be right treatment identify the cause for excess or low hormone level trat and cure that.

8.GASTRO INTESTINAL TRACT

The suffering now a days is bit less then respiratory system due to

- improved water and food hygiene
- but parallel raise in eating excess spices and masala items fast food, processed and tinned food all will attract confused inflammation to the esophagus and stomach and it will induce the confused inflammation disease.
- Since health advice the people try to eat at regular time,since know that the cause is due to irregular diet pattern so eating at right time.
- but only patient is getting fear of confusing gastric pain as cardiac pain so meet the doctor often for his ailment since

the location of stomach and heart pain he experiences in the mid chest.

But most of the gastric complaints arise immediately after acute ailment, pain killers for many other complaints so taking allopathic medicine for the same.it means gastric complaints indirect due to allopathic medicine intake for other complaints makes more gastric complaints patient then real gastric disease.

When we take the allopathic medicine that irritate the stomach mucosa will invite the confused inflammatory chemicals and cells that will initiate the chronic inflammation inside the stomach.

WHEN THE PATIENT IS TREATED FOR ANY DISEASE ANYWHERE WITHIN THE BODY BY ANY ALLOPATHIC MEDICINE, THAT MEDICINE WHEN WE TAKE ORALLY THEN THE CONFUSED INFLAMMATION CHEMICALS WILL REACH TO THE STOMACH, LIVER, KIDNEY SINCE THEY ARE THE 3 ZONES PROMINENLTY INVOLVED IN ABSORBTION (STOMACH), METABOLISAM (LIVER) AND EXCRETION (KIDNEY) allopathic medicine. So, either the newly created confused inflammation or the old confused inflammation all over the body will mostly choose this site as choice of futre disease creation. So, *allopathic medicine act as great risk factor of the disease* and in that way the medicine also chooses the site for disease making by prominent acting site, for example thyroid hormone tablets choose and attract the confused inflammation to thyroid gland and make the disease. For example, antacid will choose the stomach as a site of action. So, the confused inflammation attracted towards the stomach.

People take home made medications more for stomach complaints then any other complaints taking some spices to relive indigestion and drinking soda to relive fullness of the stomach , try to take banana or fruits to relive the constipation etc. ,,,,,, so most of time, they postpone meeting the doctors. from very long time but recent days the trend is changed if the indigestion is starts, they rush to doctor and doctor will prescribe medicine or they will buy some medicine and consume since they know the name of medicine.

Some people will adjust to stay with gastric complaints since frequent eructation's, regurgitations, fullness of the stomach these complaints may not cause series discomfort. maximum people escape from over drugging by allopathy especially in GIT except anxiety person. There are other group of people fed medicine in general due to no much improvement after meeting many allopathic doctors and specialist.

But taking alcohol, tea, coffee addictions, depend on all time hotel and outside food, heavy work stress, delay in eating, skipping the meals, dieting, fasting, over eating, drinking contaminated water [less now a days]. This factor may lead to meet doctors for medicines . Since patient have some knowledge and they not giving much importance about gastric ailments. Stopping the medicine if they get alright. All this reduce the gastric disease less but this is limited only to the gastro intestinal disease but people suffering many diseases demand the patient to take many medicines other then gastric complaints causing the disease to the major organs.

Suppose the world is educated to meet homeopaths for their basic ailment then number of victims fall under gastric ailment will be extremely less. We can achieve even 100 % nil gastric ailment together some more habits changes .

ANTACID

Antacid – controlling acid secretion will clear all

gastric complaints? for fullness in the stomach, pain in the stomach, ulcer or no ulcer for all complaints, will try only one medicine that's called antacid. Doctors now a days found there is reason for gastric complaints, that is Helicobacter pylori, so they prescribe antibiotic. But still the antacid usage is not reduced it is increased due to popularity of antacid and many fold increase of other allopathic drugs and pain killers so there allopathic doctors try to give the antacid for protect the gastric mucosa. Increased consumption of antacid for all gastric complaints still in the raise ? since there is no effective allopathic drugs then antacid.

But antacid will help in grow the H pylori or it will kill the pylori ?. if any gastric complaints patient bye this drug [antacid] on his own and takes that as a remedy for any gastric complaints. who taught that? Many gastro endrologist depend upon antacid for basic relif of gastric complaints.

how the helicobacter pylori survive in heavy HCL secreting stomach mucosa?

Antacid will reduce the acid secretion over the period of time within the gastric mucosa that give the possibility of H pylori to grow without any resistance. H pylori gives the gastric irritation and ulcers and infections and allopathic doctors even suscpect it can cause cancer of the stomach.

GERD (gastro esophageal disease) & acid peptic disease/ Indigetion

What is the cause for GERD ? loss of sphincter control. Then what is the role of antacid here ? it prevents the hcl secretion eroding the esophagus. Then how will you treat the sphincter controle, is there any medicine for that? No medicine in allopathy, so they are calling to do surgery .

Will you send the cases when you don't have the medicine for gerd to other system of doctors for cure ? no ? why ? spincter is loose it can cure only by surgery medicine may not help ? how you deciding that ? Why the spincter is lost the control all of a sudden for many people ? no idea. We may say obesity. Then lean people are not having GERD ? we say alcohol ? then what about non alcoholics getting GERD ?

Trace the situation when the nerve stimuli relax the sphincter and dilate the sphincter beyond the limit ? that is when body decide to expel the food from stomach to mouth in disease condition [during vomiting].now the sphincters has to dilate widely then any other situation to expel all the food contents suddenly through a narrow sphincters and even it will be pushed by severe contraction of the stomach so it gives 2 options number one dilate the sphincter and two dilate the orifice of the diaphragm.

Ante emetic

How ante emetics will work and cause the disease.before that we must understand some basic facts. When we consume some spoiled food or poison then the sensor in the GI tract will understand that then the vomiting process starts 1. The total peristalisis will be turned opposite direction-Reverse peristalisis. The peristalisis helps to propel the food from mouth to stomach and stomach to till the anus. Peristalisis is a mild movement of the whole gi tract it is the one way from mouth to anus. Only when we do vomit then the peristalisis movements reverse then normal direction from colon to mouth. 2. Spinchters of the esopagus and stomach will be dialated more widely then normal 3.dialatation of the orifice of the diaphragm 4. Excess salivation in the mouth 5.we lost intrest in taking food and even water and it will go even to aversion to eat the food since peristalisis act great factor in inducing the hunger now that is opposite so we feel aversion to food & no hunger.6.stomach contract and pushes the content of the stomach to mouth, the whole content from 2-3 litters of the food will be ejected from stomach to mouth forcibly .7. intestinal content will be pushed and ejected towards mouth to outside. Now the person experiences unusual sensation like he never felt that the whole stomach and intestine is abnormally constricted to push the content this causes great uneasiness just before vomiting. 8.excess perspiration and weakness following vomiting .Felt great relief but this process may repeat again like nausea and constriction and gagging and vomiting then felt confortable like that. This uneasiness will be less for the people those who have chronic vomiting. 9. All the process will be return to normal like forcible pushing and contraction of the stomach and intestine will be normal then the uneasiness and nausea feeling will be less 10. Reverse peristalisis turned into normal peristalisis now the patient start feeling hunger and desire to eat. 11.The spicnters are closed properly 12. The diaphragm orifice is shrunk to its normal position. All this process and some other minor process happen due to protecting the person from the poisonas or germ in the food or other harmfull chemicals in the food. This process is automatic and self regulatory .

Now what will happen if we stop the vomting process in the mid by anti emetic without knwowing what is happening in the abdomen.

1.Reverse peristalisis will remain same.

2.the relaxed spincters will remain same. And diaphragmatic orifice will be widely dialated.

So, the person never feel hunger and always feel nausea sensation aversion to food.

The stomach and intestinal content including acid and other enzymes and bile moves forward and goes upto mouth causes mouth ulcers recurrent erucations of gas and this fluid. So that the stomach (bile reflux disease) and esopgaus (acid reflux disease) eroded and having severe ulcerations and even perforation of the stomach and esophagus. Severe indigestion will happen.

Indigetion :

Combination of the symptoms like uneasiness in the stomach and chest worse immedialy after eating ,feel fullness and tightness and pain contractions of the stomach. feel like food remain in the chest as if a stone for long time. Nausea feel is there worse after eating. So the patient felt better by vomiting from now onwards and better in empty stomach patient easily do fasting no hunger at all even can starve one day without any hungry feel.cooking smell will irritate and many sweets and food smell will causes vomiting sensation . Easy satity like the person eating one idly or one dhosa feel like the stomach is full connot able to eat again or if we force them to eat more then that vomiting sensation will start and vomiting also happen. Chronic cough and recurrent mouth ulcers and rapid discoloration and eroding of the teeth due to acid coming to the stomach. constand belching of some fluid or food and or gas. Belching of the food and the taste which he had it in many hours before like breakfast food taste till the night.

Over a period of time patient avoids many foods and become lean and lost the basic nutrition and nutritional deficiency will start within one or two months.frequant fainting spell and weakness and tiredness feel like lye down and aversion to do hose hold and office work.

There are many people will eat and try to meet many gastro specialist and drink liters of antacid and many other medications to come out of this complaint his hunger and pain will be temprorily recovered but not with spinctes and diaphragmatic opening.

Herniation of the stomach into thoracic cavity by wide open diaphragmatic orifice Hiatus Hernia.

when the medicine is prescribed to stop the vomiting will stop the vomiting process in the mid, so that the dilated sphincter is not been reordered to constrict [allow the food entry from gastric to esophagus – Regurgitation].

- reverse peristalsis will occur while vomiting, anti emetic will just stop the vomiting by blocking the nerves but this reverse peristalsis will be intact. Who will reverse the reverse peristalsis to normal peristalsis ? the reverse peristalsis reduce the hunger over all and feeling like vomiting all time but no real vomiting [nausea],acids and other contend from stomach will move towards the esophagus from stomach for longer time is the cause for GERD and this irritation in the esophagus will invite the chronic inflammation to esophagus so GERD with superadded inflammation and easily turn into cancer and this will create lot more other diseases. need a physiology knowledge to allopath, need basic understanding of the ailment. VOMITING is a physiological protective action by the body. don't interrupt it is because you are given more worst disease then this vomiting.

Oesopaghus is a connecting tube from mouth to stomach, most of the time the lower end of the esophagus will fall in disease including Gerd.

- Heartburn and regurgitation
- dysphagia
- chest pain.
- Extraesophageal syndromes with an established association to GERD include chronic cough, laryngitis, asthma, and dental erosions.
- A multitude of other conditions including pharyngitis,chronic bronchitis, pulmonary fibrosis,chronic sinusitis, cardiac arrhythmias, sleep apnea, and recurrent aspiration pneumonia have proposed associations with GERD.

Nearly 12.5 - 20 % (nearly 15 - 20 crore) of the Indian population is suffering from GERD. Gerd makes heavy anxiety to the patient as if they have some cardiac complaints. Patient kept long time allopathic medicines and need to frequent visit to doctors no much relief partial pain relive and patient looking alternative methods of treatment so frequently this is because most of the Gerd develops after allopathic medicines.

Over all 10-12 crore Indian population suffer from acid peptic disease.

Indigestion is most prevalent it starts from unusually too early age due to allopathic medicines. More then 25 - 30 crore Indian population suffer from indigestion and depend upon antacid the market sales of antacid will be excellent by the help of allopathic doctors. ANTACID WILL ANTE EMETICS WILL INDUCE THE DISEASE AND THE SAME MEDICINES WIL RELIVE THE DISEASE SYMTPMS TEMPORARILY.

Eating herbal product like pudhina,ginger,pepper, turmeric all will increase the symptoms of the chest burning and stomach burning so the patient from siddha and ayurvedha too rush to allopathy. Since homeopathy is hidden in many people mind they fall in allopathic hand again.

Spasm of the esophagus

You have medicine to reduce the stomach contraction [spasm] to normal? then why esophageal spasm, the spasm which is used to propel the stomach content into the mouth while vomiting is not recovered due to ante emetic in the mid so spasm of the esophagus [DES].

Pregnancy gives the high possibility of reflux acidity and herniation of the stomach. Recurrent painfull vomiting will demand regular intake of antacid and ante emetics so the person will have relaxed spincters and wide-open diaphragmatic orifice and increasing abdominal pressure by fetal growth causes pushing of the abdominal content causes herniation. Regurgitation facilitated and increased then other people since the fetus growth pushes the acid towards esophagus and produce GERD so easily. Pushes the intestinal juice and content easily to stomach.

Alcoholics will increase the possibility of acid peptic disease and reflux esophagitis by consumption of irritant to the mucus membrane so this disease exaggerated easily then others.

Childrens more prone to acid peptic disease since excess cold often end with vomiting ,slight raise of temperature also encourage vomiting recurrent stomach infection other infection causes vomiting . parents give the ante emetic frequently and so childrens are lost their appetite and early decay of the tooth.recurent mouth ulcers. Loss of the voice and asthma due to regurgitation of the stomach content into the lungs causes pneumonia and asthma.

In alcoholics and pregnancy and in some ulceration and erosive disease patient the spincters will remain open and peristalisis may not return to normal even if you not taking ante emetics this is because contineuse irritation signal from the stomach so that the vomiting signals may not be withdrawn fully.

role of helicobactor pylorai and development of acid peptic disease :

the acid peptic disease and gastric erosions can be easily triggered by antacid and ante emetics and consumption of excess tea and coffea , alcoholic many other pain killers and other allopathic medicines helicobactor is one among the risk factor for developing the acid peptic disease and ulcers. But antacid play a major role in growth of many other virus and bacterias within the stomach and intestine .

the mega real factor for inducing the disease in the upper gi tract is the confused inflammation the confused inflammation will be attracted very simple hyper activity but here there is great wound and ulceration happening due to acid entry and allopathic drug consumption within the lower end of esophagus and stomach so that the confused inflammation will reach easily to this part and create the disease more complicated and troublesome runining chronic course.

acid peptic disease will have all the symptoms of indigestion and additionally pain felt in the stomach and epigastric region. Worse after eating better by vomiting.

Cancer of the stomach and esophagus and oral cavity all is due to regurgitation of the acid and heavy antacid prescriptions and stopping inflammation of every patient nothing more then that.

So, prevention of the simple indigestion to cancer is easy if we try to regulate the allopathic prescription alone. So how will manage these situation and disease . use the homeopathy for all minor aiments and moderate ailments then automatically the new disease formation will be stopped. Since the people are educated well in regular intake of anti inflammatory and antacids, they have the habbit of taking medicine so that better alternate with homeopathy in that situation is the easiest way to prevent cancer of stomach and esophgus and oral cavity and I will give medicines and indications follow that to prevent all GERD AND ACID PEPTIC DISEASE AND CANCERS.

For vomiting – ipecac,pulsatilla,nux vomica

Indigestion – abis nigra, ant crudum ,nux vomica ,carbe veg ,lycopodiyam ,,, etc

Gerd – nux vomica ,ars alb , phosphorus.

Acid peptic disease – nux vomica ,graphities

So, the upper respiratory disease is preventable and if the disease is started before prevention then it will be cured by homeopathy medicines. Be happy but follow the procedure what I am saying since just reading and waiting for dis appearance of the disease is impossible, we have to spread the message to all and follow the preventive measures and utilize homeopathy for curing and help in BRINGING HEALTHY LIFE.

Inflammatory Bowel disease

There is a chronic destructive disease in the colon. severe annoying and disabling disease. The cause yet to identify [unknown] considered as auto immune disease. They are ulcerative colitis and chrons disease.

Now you might have an idea just say about what you newly learned and just apply that to this disease and comprehend what's going on rather then saying inflammatory disease. Just list the new research and try to fit with the IBD.

It is not an inflammation disease even though it is named INFLAMMATORY BOWEL DISEASE. Because inflammation never going to be chronic course, never produce great ulceration and destruction to the colon.

But named as inflammation due to evidence of finding inflammatory cells in the colon and tiny abscess in the colon. Sure, then it is a confused inflammation not a true inflammation.so name that as confused inflammatory bowel disease.

The scattered confused inflammation all over the body will choose the intestine and colon or and if the infectitius colitis is treated by allopathic drugs anti inflammatory, anti bacterial kill the bacteria but increase the possibility of confused inflammation within the colon then this inflammation will be attracted by varies trigger in the colon so the long standing inflammation happens and destruction of the colon is happen.

The inflammation which is remain silent in the intestine and colon get attracted any minimal hyper activity of the colon it may be an infection or diarrhea or even constipation or taken any medicine some new diet some artificial food additives in the diet, spices all will trigger confused vs real inflammation so there by slow increase in damage in the colon.

The inflammatory bowel disease, fissure, fistula, piles, recurrent diarrheas all type dysentery [except infectious] abscess in the rectal and anal region, tumors, cancer in the gastro intestinal tract diseases. will be produced by the CONFUSED INFLAMMATION.

Incidence And Prevelance Of Inflammatory Bowel Disease :

In india there are 2.5 - 5 lakh people affected with inflammatory bowel disease.nearly 3 lakg people affected in America northern America is having high incidence of the inflammatory disease next is autralia and south Africa affected least.

Prevention :

Inflammatory bowel disease is a most notoriyas destructive disease of the colon and intestine so we have to prevent this disease by not to interfere the inflammation. if the inflammation diverted and gives complications in the colon disease has to be identified and tackled with proper homeopathy medicine is BEST WAY OF PREVENTION.

If the disease started already if we use a homeopathy medicine then the disease will be cured by homeopathy. When the disease in the moderate stage also can be recovered by homeopathy but the advanced stage with eroded and destructed colon is difficult to recover and can be manageable.

Merc sol , merc cor, hydrastis, phosphorus etc will be the good remedy to recover the patietnt. It's a chronic long-standing disease need a proper analysis and proper constitutional remedy to cure better to consult best homeopathy doctor.

IRRITABLE BOWEL SYNDROME

Irritable bowel syndrome is an confused inflammation disorder only, the hyper mobility of gut pain and the fullness uneasiness in the abdomen all created by complications of the post anti inflammatory drug administration .when a person fall in dysentery or diarrhea treated with anti inflammatory and anti diarrheal drugs interrupt the regular automatic process of the body defense mechanism they forcibly stop the excess bowel activity. The excess nervous stimuli have to be withdrawn only by the brain but the brain orders blocked in the mid there by the sensation of urging and other signals yet to close it remain for many years.

During the diarrhea the colon get hyper motility, this motility helps in forcible expulsion of the stool into outside so by this time when we administer anti diarrheal then the motility is highly less will cause constipation. if the motility is stopped by medicines but once the action is over the augmented nerve signals start and keep hyper mobility will be the cause for IBS . His complication is not happening in everybody. This may again support by chronic confused inflammation. [WHEN THE PATIENT DESCRIBE THE IBS SYMPTOMS ALL THE COMPLAINTS SIMILAR TO INFECTIOUS DYSENTRY OR DIARHEA BUT THERE IS NO INFECTION NOT EVEN INFLAMMATION THEN WHY ALL SIMILAR SYMPTOMS BECAUSE ADMINISTERING MEDICINE TO STOP THE DIARRHEA WILL NOT RECOVER THE FUNCTION OF THE COLON FULLY WILL BE THE CAUSE FOR THIS]

This is due to the diarrhea initiated by nerve so the person having hyper mobility and urging to pass the stool is there , once the infectious agents are destroyed the purpose of inflammation is completed then automatically all the functions of the gastro intestinal tract will recovered like loss of hunger is recovered to normal to appetite and diarrhea is become normal and urging will be reduced.so totally patient recover

But when we interrupt this process by prescribing anti diarrheal and anti bacterial, Patient feel comfortable in fever, pain and number stool also will be less. but majority of the complaints remain same like feel nausea, no hungry, feel blotedness if we try to eat. The urging to pass stool will remain same and bowel movements are still high and patient start feel acutely all the bowel movement, he is become all time conscious over his bowel.

Here the medicine is removed the complaints but the body does not know this, so we can say more then confused inflammation here the remaining confused mechanism of inflammations [associated inflammatory symptoms] FEED BACK REGULATORY MECHANIS is not allowed to carry their function, so that the functions not been fully recovered by the automatic power. It is not much associated with panic but patient will panic due to the stool will come at any time.

There are many children's and adult will not recover their appetite after an acute illness. Prescribing antacid for every allopathic medication other then gastric complaint is more common and prevalence but this in turn make new gastric complaints especially secretion of the HCL.This prescription is forcible for everyone, every time when the patient prescribed painkillers simultaneous prescription of antacid is there. This medication for fever itself highly contradictory and in that again prescribing antacid is something hyper foolishness.

An acute viral fever patient has been collapsed made multi disorder how many mistakes here by prescribing anti inflammatory, anti bacterial and antacid.

1.Stopping fever will reduce the possibility of immune system wake up

2.Virus will be allowed to grow up.

3.Confused inflammation will arise and make future life disorder.

4.Stopping hcl secretion allow the new bacterial growth H pylori.

5.Antacid will have its own side effects.

6.HCL secretion sure will interrupt.

7.Anti bacterial will have its own complications and it is absolutely not necessary in viral infections.

8.recovering the functions of systemic loss of function is not recovered.

I HOPE RATHER THEN CURING, HELPING IN GROWING MANY DISEASES BY PRESCRIBBING UNNESSORY MEDICATIONS FOR THE PATIENT, THIS PRESCRIPTIONS IS MORE COMMON IN INDIA IRRESPECTIVE OF QUACK OR HIGH PROFESIONALS.

I don't understand what kind of benefit patient is getting by this treatment.

INFLAMMATION SYSTEM, IMMUNE SYSTEM + RESPIRATORY SYSTEM AFFECTED SURE, BUT IN ADDITION EVERY TIME PATIENT VISIT TO ALOPATHY CLINIC THEIR GASTRO INTESTINAL SYSTEM TOO DESTROYED AS BONUS OR GIFT FOR TAKING TREATMENT WITH ALOPATHY.

Nux vomica , Aloes ,Merc sol ,arsenicum album some of the leading remedy to recover the function of the intestine.

HEMORRHOIDS [piles]

Dilated rectal veins is called hemorrhoids. Why the rectal veins are bulged ? actually speaking till now the cause has not been identified but some factors will increase the possibility of the piles like pregnancy and obesity sedentary life style may be blamed as risk factor for piles but even a thin person, male , female all will affected the incidence is low below 15 years but the incidence is more common after 30 yrs.

Piles may be started during delivery ,less after delivery but the condition run for many years even after delivery.

Piles is not caused by any hereditary factor. Confused inflammation is attacking the rectal veins is the real cause for piles. A roaming confused inflammation cells will be attracted when the rectal veins pressure is more like sedentary life style, pregnancy, obesity, heavy constipation and strain to pass the stool.

Similar to rectal vein all through the extremity a woman getting varicose veins , bulge more are less it is subsided well and even the dilatation of the varicose veins will not happen in many women indicates nil confused inflammation or the inflammation seated strongly somewhere else in the body. If the confused inflammation is more in the women then she will develop sever varicose veins with bleeding and thrombus formation. A thrombai formation will be cleared by a healthy process but if the thrombai formed by confused inflammation then the thrombai will grow without any disturbance and make the disease.

More chronicity of the piles and varicose veins depend upon the underlying confused inflammations.

It is not pregnancy or obesity will induce the piles

if the women having confused inflammation has less toler-ance of the veins so that it allows to bulge beyond recover-ing limit and the confused inflammation strongly produce their effect within these dilated vassals especially more pressure, stressfull areas of the vessals [mostly rectum next legs and foot].

the same pressure in constipated person, sedan-dtry life style will invite the confused inflammation to rec-tum and damage the rectal veins produce the hemorrhoids.

Hemorrhoid is a confused inflammation disease of the rectal vein it is a more common disease in india and many other cuntry . nearly 1/3 of the suffering people taken for surgery few people having the recurrence even after surgery. More then 15 crore Indians suffering with piles dis-ease. There are 1 crore americans suffering with piles and more then 10 lakh new piles cases annually. No effective treatment in allopathy homeopathy will cure the disease in early and moderate hemorrhaoids late stage piles if the me-dicinal management is not helped then will be allowed to go for surgery. Americans spend 250 million doller for hem-orrhoid products.1.5 million prescriptions each year.more then 120000 surgical hemorrhoidectomies ,nearly 1.5 mil-lion colonoscopy each year in America.

Piles is preventable by simeply by allowing the in-flammation if we interrupt the inflammation then possibil-ity of the piles will be more if do sedanry life style and other risk factors for veins strains.

Sulphur,nux vomica,aesculus,hamamelis,acid nit will be some of the best remedy for hemorrhoids.

A inflammation will turn into confused inflam-mation and that will produce confused inflammation dis-ease these disease will shift easily and make another dis-ease if you try to suppress the confused inflammation disease .hemorrhoid is one of the confused inflammation disease the best way is to remove the confused inflammation don't try to satisfy the patient just prescribing some ointment externally or removing the pile mass this will shift the disease from anus to anywhere in the body it may not cease.

Fissure in ano

More common disease then piles , almost all the age and gender affected.most of patient feel that they have piles. Most frequently meet the doctors for the fissure then piles since piles is painless but fissure is having severe pain so that rush to meet the doctors. The pain in the fissure may remain hours together some patient experiences the pain round the clock till next time passing stoo. Due to the severe pain childrens afraid to pass the stool.

Confused inflammation near the anal regian makes the wound or cracks near the anus causes pain. The skin near the anus is dry and then cracks will have less pain and subsides no much recurrence . but if the fissure is happening due to rich confused inflammation background then the fissure is having severe pain and bleeding and having frequent recurrence surgery may not relive the fissure in this case recurrence more easily formed.

Fissure will be formed by same cause we can say mild to moderate congestion near anal region is the initial factor then if the stool passes in the anus then it causes cracks or skin peeling or abrasion with severe pain.

Large hard stool will make burning or pain few minutes it will cause cracks or ulcers near anus. The truth is the anal canal is inflamed already then even a normal or liquid stool will cause pain.

For developing piles need strong long raise of internal abdominal pressure or pressure inside the veins along with confused inflammation. but there is confused inflammation in the anal region but there is no intra abdominal pressure then these will cause fissure in anus. A hard stool will make the fissure will usually heal well may not cause severe pain and may not run in long chronic cases.

Standing long time as a profession like traffic police their veins slowly dilate and produce a varicose vein but this is marked and produce severe inflammation and ulceration is happen only those who are having confused inflammation. Other then anomalies [absence of valve and tumor or pregnancy obstructing in the course of veins causes the varicose veins otherwise all the veins getting affected with this confused inflammation and produce the varicose vein and bleeding and ulcerations.

Homeopathy medicines cure the fissure and prevent the recurrence formation. But prevention of piles will happen only if stop interfering the inflammation. Before taking the patient to surgery it is better to consult a homeopath since it is simply curable by homeopathy.

Surgery is may not be necessory in the fissure cases.

Rathania,nit acid , Sulphur ,graphitis are some of the importand fissure remedy.

Fistula in ano

A normal tissue will fight to the germs successfully with few fighting cells and recover fully without any structural abnormality with short duration.

When a person having many barrier in giving proper support to the injured or infected site leads to slow and delay in sending proper immediate fighting cells and healing cells so chance of easy multiplication of the germs and need lots of effort to fight and need of giant cell invitation to the affected area all causes an big abscess OR granuloma [sarcoidosis, tuberculosis] inside the anorectal area .The same barrier will affect the wound healing so that injured sites highly prone to infection so repeated abscess and bursting causes opening in both external and internal sites cause fistulas track. More ever the abscess if it is formed by true inflammation will heal without any medicinal support.

A.   confused inflammation will reduce the protective mechanism and help in encourage the bacterial entry and collapse the true inflammation carry out their functions smoothly so abscess stay unusually long time.

Unusually excess available lytic chemicals active phagocyting cells causes abscess formation, according to my observation every abscess is not a normal inflammation [physiological process] , it is abnormal confused inflammation process, it means abscess is created one.

No possibility of abscess or big boils to the humans, confused inflammation alone produce the big abscess. Any germs staphylococcus or streptococcus will be successfully killed and eliminated without great abscess formation. Abscess indicates excess lysis cells and profuse ready-made phagocytic cells.

An abscess turn into gangrene or severe septicemia indicates worst accumulation of confused inflammations all over the body causes severe distractions and severe long, systemic destructing confused inflammations.

An abscess is not a normal inflammation response more the abscess, spreaded bigger abscess indicates failure in controlling bacterial multiplications leads to excessive phagocytosis and abscess pure indication to confused inflammation.

Appendicitis

Appendix is a lymphatic organ which act as an immune protector of colon and intestine. If the person exposes infections in the colon, here appendix act as local protector it will identify that and clear infection from the colon along with inflammation and immune cells.

A Lymph gland is immune organ and it will take the germs to the lymph gland and destroy that and participate lymphocyte production.

But when we take the allopathic medicine [anti diarrheal, anti biotic, anti inflammatory] then the inflammation forcibly stopped, so the confused inflammation formed. This c inflammation will reach and settle in the lymphatic organ along with taking bacteria's and other dead materials via lymph vassals so the appendices inflamed and become hard and indurate and non functioning. Become the store house for infection prone to recurrent infection. So don't stop the inflammation and collapse normal immune system.

A non-functioning appendix act as a reservoir of infections in future possibility recurrent pain and infections is there this opposite function is created by intake anti inflammatory and antibiotic so that system collapsed and good functioning gland is non functioning.

[ANYWAY, THE PROTECTIVE MECHANISAM IS LOST WHY WE HAVE TO KEEP THE APPENDIS, BETTER WE CAN REMOVE THE ORGAN. IT MAY LOOK RIGHT BUT IT IS HIGHLY POSSIBLE TO RECOVER THE FUNCTIONS OF APPENDIS BY HOMEOPATHS.BECAUSE APPENDIS NEED FOR LONGER TIME TO PROTECT COLON AND INTESTINE].

A current trend is a surgeon see the appendicitis cases

and he plan to do surgery either removal or other procedure. It is not right and it is not legal to proceed like this, before planning a surgery get the opinion of both physician of AYUSH system. When you ask yourself (only discusing with allopathy and decides to plan surgery is something illogical and no law and it is criminalizam, of course you will say the disease is does not have medicine or it is incurable so you will plan for surgery and allopathy physician also will say the same, your system is a pre-planned system for earning money.

So, ask the opinion those who says that I can cure this. Every surgeon is passes out basic UG [MBBS], He knows that what is the possibility of the recovery in this case so compulsory need to get the opinion and no objection letter from AYUSH Doctors is mandatory, Since AYUSH doctors says he can cure and recover the appendicitis.

So, getting no objection letter from eligible person to object [AYUSH] is a law. It is absolutely unnecessary to get the no objection from anyway he is not going to object [allopathy] and not having any medicine to handle this situation is not eligible to object.

[kindly include this law in the forensic medicine under negligence section that a surgeon is compulsorily get the no objection letter from AYUSH doctors for doing any surgery] when physician fails surgeons can come and do his duty, is not a problem.

A liver and intestine and spleen will be affected in the similar way if the colon germs taken to the liver lymphatic system [Kupfer cells] then the germs destroyed over there if the liver is damaged already then lymphatic system failed in this time the entry of germs to the liver will easily makes severe fulminant hepatitis with rapid cirrhosis Or The confused inflammation spread via any other route will settles in the liver and spoil the lymphatic functions and leads to hepatitis.

A payer's patches in the colon function is to kill the germs in the colon but if the confused inflammation occupies in the payers patches it will damage the functions and lead to colitis or eroding or severe colon disease.

Spleen disease and enlargement is happening in the similar way when confused inflammation reaches the spleen the spleen due to its lymphatic functions but confused inflammation will slowly reduce the functions of the spleen causes spleen disorder.

So, for preventing such infections and related complication try to remove the confused inflammation from appendix , liver , spleen and lymphnodes and keep ready for fighting is right way preventing dreadable complications of the inflammation. Not recommended to remove the appendix in anyway.

9. OPTHALMALOGY

IMPAIRED VISSION ,LOSS OF
VISSION REFRACTIVE ERROR

When a person losing vision due to cataract and vitamin deficiency identified early and given better cure in earlier days by allopathy so that mass attraction is happen towards allopathy. But now a days allopathy doctors is happy in sales of the glass and people also habituated to wear glass. Almost most of the childrens in the school days wearing specks or using contact lens. There is no effective step to cure the condition almost 10 % of the childrens suffering with refrective errors. There is no effective way to prevent the disease since no idea how to prevent except some infection disease in some situation they know the cause of the disease but no effective medicine for solving the vision loss so it is again recommended for wearing glass.

Vision loss is a major disability (handicaped) but this disability is not been given importance to prevent even by world health organization. In many situations more then solving the problem allopathy doctors are using sales of the glass is importand then finding the cause and effective to cure the disease. Giving specks is eaqual to providing a stick to walking disability person but doctors are fixed in their minset that providing specks is the curative proced-ure for vision disability. Refractive errors are happen due to confused inflammation and due to that either stiffness or relaxation of the eye muscles it is easy to prevent con-fused inflammation and curable by homeopathy medicine referective errors also caused by other reason but related with inflammation and confused inflammation is curable by homeopathy medicine.

Just take survey of the people residing in the par-ticular region and see their effective treatment by assement of vision loss if the number of vision loss is prevented and cured then the doctor must be promoted and if the vision loss is more then disqualify the doctor working in the par-ticular locality since now a days making vision loss is more profitable then curing and preventing the vision loss so we have to take a corrective measures to solve this issues and we must demand the doctors to work for the benefit of the public.

Ophthalmic Disease Occurance

Cause of the ophthalmic disease other then infec-tion is and identified as auto immune disease remaining disease causes is unknown. So there is large number of disease is connot able to preventable and again auto immune disease origin also unuknown so the cure rate is too low . but now we discovered confused inflammation is the cause of the many unknown and auto immune disease. So , this discovery going to help us to prevent almost all major a minor vision loss disease I hope there is nill vision loss in future is highly possible.

So how the eye is getting the confused inflammation. When the nasal tract is getting the inflammation, we stop the inflammation by giving allopathic medicine so abundand confused inflammation is formed. This confused inflammation then easily attracted by face and having some skin disease in the face we immediately suppress that with the help of ointments and other allopathic medicines these medications is highly enough to run any disease within the eye. So, when we had any infection in the eye then this confused inflammations near the eye (face and nose) will be attracted and started troubling the eye then we use allopathic eye drops and medicines to stop the inflammation and together more confused inflammation formed now in total there is no effective single remedy to cure the disease in allopathy every medicine for used by allopathy is just give temporary relif or stop the inflammation and natural process of the protective mechanisam. Since allopathy doctors having same habbit like stopping the inflammation is a cure in his mind he do the same for everywhere the same he do in the eye then slowly the vision detoriarate but he says it is like using mobile or laptop cause for poor vision or long hours of working and eye strain like that all this explanation just for people satisfaction that is not applicable in the text book here there is no such explanation . watching TV and other mobiles and laptol never cause any vision loss it is rumor . adjusting brightness and sitting proper distance make a comfortable to eye but when we mis use this guidline never going to loss the vision.

Refractive errors

Myopia,short sightedness and astigmatisam are some of the refractive erros belived that anatomical defect and mal alignment causes this disease need specs. The eye ball is too big in childrens so the vision is fall infron of the retina so short sightedness and if the vision is focused behind the retina then the long sightedness this are all some basic facts.

For focusing the object exactly within retina need proper corneal convexicity not exces or not too less and making adjustability by lense with the help of ciliyari muscles and the nerve supply of the ciliyary muscles has to be intact. Obsolutely all this factor falls in trouble with confused inflammation that's why the vision complaints in the early life this is not just simple by big eye ball small orbital bone. The confused inflammation makes the spasm of the muscles and produce paresis weakness of the muscles make this change but the routine eye check up is what is the power and what is the corrective lens is the routine step so no thought of considering disease can induce the refractive errors.

Conjuntivitis / styes / corneal ulcerations

Conjunctivitis is caused by Virus, Bacteria, Fungus and auto immunity. Unhygine and poor personal hygine ,poor stand of living living with crowded population carry the risk of frequent conjunctivitis.

The infection within nasal cavity and regular intake of anti allergic and anti-inflammatory medicine for that will create more amount of confused inflammation cells and chemicals , thses c inflammation spread to face and eye and causes periodical congetion of the eye .when we observe infectious rhinitis patient they have only nasal congetion in the earlier days but when frequent attacks starts then nasal congetion associate with eye congetion and now onwards the trouble in the eyes starts in the superficial structure like styes + , itching in the eyes ++ , Redness of the eyes with pr even without congetion of nose . this redness and eye irritation and itching in the eye will demand the patient to rush to the opthalmolagist they started prescribing anti allergics eye drops now the supercial confused inflammation will reach to deeper tissues of the eye and started produce both superficial as well as deep ophthalmic disease including refractive errors uviyal, retinal lens all will affected slowly.

Recurrent styes , Frequent rednes of the eye's itchiness in the eye,dandruff in the eye lids is the very early and sure symptoms of confused inflammation presence. (for allopathy there is no protocol and warnining this is auto inflammation disease which is created allopathy medicines so they start prescribing the same medicine as eye drops). This is better good time for all the virus and bacterial growth. Since a congested conjunctiva will loss all protective powers so it will prone to infection frequently. Break the chain for infection the gigantic chain for infection is underlying confused inflammation.

I don't have better proof, which can be easily understood by a common man then nose and eye spread of inflammation. They crystal clear conjunctival and corneal part is so visibly red and itch and itch like anything so the sufferer will crush the eye all the time to optain relief. The same redness spread is happening everywhere to all superficial part of the skin but we connot able to see that because the skin is not transperant like a conjunctiva. But I have seen many men and women their skin is become red by minimal tap on their skin and redness in the skin by minimal sun exposure and scratch (DERMOGRAPHISAM). A micro invasion yet visible to naked eye.

The eye lid is having crust and itching and produce styes and ear is itching behind the ear is having crust and itchiness and eyebrows having itching and dandruff . The scalp is having dandruff and itching .The skin all over the body is dry and itches in the winter is the basic primary early sign of confused inflammation formation which is prominent in fold of skin (behind ear lob,in the neck ,in the elbow in the poplitel fossa in the eye lids,,etc) .what we have to do what we are doing. We have no idea how it is formed but we name this as atopic dermatitis or allergy. We say no idea how the atopic dermatitis (or else we will say it is due to hereditary and basic body nature etc). what else we do prescribe anti allergic this will give some basice relief and then come to same position after medicine so next level medicine steroid so now the congetion taken to the deeper tissues which is including within eye.

What we do to clear the itchiness redness and dandruff and styes ointments and anti biotics and anti allergics eye drops if it is not work out then stroid so patient will have regular conjunctival infection and congetion and refractive errors as a secondary superficial complaints flotes in the eyes there are tiny spotes in the conjunctiva and cornea which is white and block and brown spotes.

Uvitis and conjunctival and corneal congetion, corneal ulceration corneal opacity and conjunctival infiltrations and conjunctival and corneal micro deposites and growths started appearing (if sufficient confused inflammation and wound healing material is available) in the eye still the eye is giving chances to reversible deep changes in superficial structure of the eye this is secondary manifestation of the confused inflammation which is include the virus and bacterial infections.

The right way to prevent ophthalmic disease is not to create the confused inflammation (no paracetamol and no ant allergics) the right way to prevent primary maniefestation of confused inflammation is to eliminate that from body by prescribing appropriate homeopathy medicine . prescribing same antiallergics and anti inflammatory will increase the more deeper and larger spread of the confused inflammation (against the rule of inflammation the rule of body basic defence is surround the enemy and kill them in the particular area so that no much destruction of body parts spreading gives the possibility of more destruction of body tissues). The confused inflammation is not cleared from the body but stayes in the body and produce the complaints again by anti allergics and anti-inflammatory homeopathy uses the term suppression it means you need to eliminate the confused inflammation instead you are taken that more spread more deeper its danger you are seeding that into more deeper vital organ. The same story repeats here and everywhere .

In many auto immune and other chornic disease your explanation is like innate immunity is activated (macrophage) and T cell has activated B cells started activated compliment factors are activated and CD 4 and CD 8 cells are coming in the same way in many disease explanations but just answere me when the histamine and bradykinine and other confused inflammation sprayed AND spreading to all over the skin and deeper parts slowly from nose and respiratory tract in the skin surface may not trigger the sensor of the macrophage and T lymphocytes ? (it is the cause for induction of auto immunity - primary confused inflammation to secondary confused immune disease) because these triggers only the macrophage and Lymphocytes are activated in the view to support the inflammation stimulai without any germs. These is very very importand explanation for the auto immunity not just simple casual explanation. The macrophage act like bomb hidden in the land they will initiate the inflammation when any germ or injury is happened over there but the inflammatory chemicals crossing over there and making inflammation superficially will induce the activation of macrophage and lymphocytes and inflammation and immunity. Since there is no enemy and the confused inflammation which is triggered the immunity is not going to leave the site qcuikly the new inflammation created also is not going to remove this so the continuease long standing inflammation and immunity here liberation of chemicals and lysis everything happen thery started destroying this parts and gives symptoms like itch,pain,raise of temperature discoloration everything and everything. Steroid may stop the inflammation temporarily but will come immediate or later the steroid action is over.

Styes—pain,swelling and pus formation or will disappear without pus formation. It will be indurated and remain for long time for some people. (homeo medicine – belladonna, hepar sulph,silicia)

Conjunctivitis : redness,lachrymation,itchiness (prominent in confused inflammation very less in infection) photophobia ,pain and sensitive when looking into the light. Minimal scanty discharge if bacterial infection is more then prurulent discharge will be there. (Homeo medicine- Eupharasia , arg nit,thuja,belladonna ,pulsatilla,sulphur)

Uvities : pain and photophobia will be there. blurry vision.flotes in the vision.field (Sulphur , eupharasia ,merc sol)

Eye lid dermatitis (dermatitis) --- graphitis ,Sulphur ,petroleum.

Corneal ulceration --- merc sol , nit acit.

Tertiorry and penta confused inflammation disease

Retinopathy

There are many reasons explained for the development of retinopathy like diabetes, hypertension and many more reson one of the leading disease for vision loss.

The retinal vessals are damaged by the inflammation induced by diabetes and hypertension leading to vascular damage like leakage and hemorrhage and over a period of time the vascularity is obliterated now the new vascularity is formed and create vision loss. (allopathic explanation)

Deep seated confused inflammation initiate the inflammation process and damage the blood vessals and causes severe damage to vessals like breaking and partial recovery and regeneration of the blood vessals in some site and regeneration of the new blood vessals in some site like that any way the inflammation may not be successfully kill the enemy and save ourself since it is confused inflammation it will destroy the blood vessal slowly and create the symptoms slowly and make hemorrgahe and exudate and clotes and anurysam in some site all will happen. So gradual detoriaration of the vision is in the early days. Anastomosis and vascular dialatation is the normal response of the vascular block neo vascularization and that to it does not help in vision more then that make loss of vision is not a good inflammation function. Neo vascularization is due to regeneration part stimulation derived from suppressed wound healing or suppressed regeneration of the neovasularisation or suppressed regeneration of tissue somewhwere in the body could be the cause for neovascularization. Gradual narrowing of the blood vessal and initiation of the inflammation within the blood vessals years together is not a normal inflammation function that is confused inflammation functions due to deposition of fibrous cells and gelatin material make thick and narrow lumen. If the neovascularization is induced by the body natural inflammation process then that vasculature must be regeneration of the same vessal that will help in establish a vision. A planned perfect needed change allowed in the regeneration not just regeneration . a confused inflammation and confused wound healing will create a growth of their won choice wheather you like It or not. It is usefull here or not it will grow just like that. It is the confused inflammation cherecter.

Retinal detachement happen due to effusion so that the effusion detaches the retina and in some case fluid is loss happen so that vitrous is become concentrated. This concentrated fluid will cause sepration of the retina in some cases scar in the retina causes retinal dtachement and trauma to the eye causes retinal detachement except injury all other causes induced by confused inflammation so stop making confused inflammation.

- Feel like there or lots of flotes in the vision and then the central vision is lost and feel like flashes of light sensation repeatedly.
- blurred vision and central vision is lost can able to see only peripheral vision.
- impaired color vision
- Vision loss

Fluctuating vision.

Macular degeneration (MD)

Two type of (MD) dry and wet macular degeneration dry macular degeneration is happen due to deposition of abnormal material within this space and cause degeneration and vision loss .in wet degeneration there is a new blood vessal formation and causes loss of vision since new blood vessals and abnormal deposites all happen due to confused inflammation prevent this diseas by prevent confused inflammation formation.

Loss of vision.

Cataract

Opacification of the transparent lens is called cataract.is observed as disease of eye proper. But in my observation the eye diseases are almost always caused by confused inflammation. This chronic inflammation and infections and allergy easily transmit their confused inflammation cells to the eye and makes many diseases starting from simple conjunctivitis to severe blindness.

A long standing, silent or symptomatic ophthalmic diseases slowly, silently makes the cataract.

A healthy aging never produces cataract to produce cataract you need confused inflammatory cells in the body. A confused inflammation invites the cataract at the age of 30-40 itself.

cataract in the individual gives the clue to that person is having confused inflammation within or near eye.

cataract is curable by medicine and preventable if we arrest the confused inflammation.

It is highly possible to prevent all type of oph-thalmic diseases which causes vision loss and severe pathology. So be relax and happy .

10. REPRODUCTIVE SYSTEM & GYNECOLOGY

Fibroid or leiomyoma of uterus

- cause unknown.
- but observed fibroid growth helps estrogen.
- Myomas are rarely found before puberty and they gradually cease to grow after menopause.
- New myoma rarely appear after menopause.
- Fibroid having association with estrogen producing tumor and PCOD.
- Myoma increase in size during pregnancy and during treatment with oral contraceptive.

This are all some basic medical observation till date.

Discussion proper:

But it is easy to detect the cause of the fibroid both In the breast and uterus and other tumer of the liver, Since the breast and uterus has been developed much after the puberty so that exposure to variety of hormones estrogen, growth hormone and other hormonal stimulation causes hyperemia and proliferation of the tissue for development of genital organs. All this new development invites the confused inflammation to breast, uterus, ovaris and veginal canal so possibly many diseases will arise after puberty.

And again, when a woman undergoes pregnancy, she undergoes heavy hormonal changes that will also invite the confused inflammation to the female reproductive organs.

Estrogen causes increased blood flow to the myometriam of the uterus so that confused inflammation reaches to uterus produce varies inflammatory changes in endometrial and myometrial but these changes will be cleared due endometriam shed during menses and new endometriyam reformed after menses.

But myometriam is not like that. So, the remaining confused inflammation will attack the myometriam. The inflamed myometriam together with estrogen is responsible for production of leiomyoma's hypervascularity is responsible for equal increase in size of the myometriyam of the uterus but the location involved in confused inflammation is again hyperemic so that the confused inflammation area myometriyam gets duel support one is estrogen but estrogen suppressed phase of menstrual cycle this confused inflammation parts will have hyperemia so that tumor will grow all time. The growth within the mayometriyam will be just a transformation of growth order from endometriyam to mayometriyam. This may be facilitated by

during curratage like procedure and other surgical procedure like cessariayn section and suppression of the inflammation.

Once the menopause attained, the over all hyper
vascular changes and endometrial proliferation everything
altogether stopped so that now inflammation within uterus,breast,vegina all will not have any attraction of confused
inflammation so that the confused inflammation slowly
move other parts of body or else it will remain here itself.

Allopathy doctors accept this estrogen-based attraction of the tumer but what I am saying estrogen act as
a trigger for inviting confused inflammation but allopathy
doctors trying to convince almost estrogen is the cause for
fibroids but not have enough proof to say that but the impression of the text book is indirectly says that. Most of the
allopathic research is like that they always observe similar
and parlel incidence during the particular disease occurance. Some time this research will work out but most of the
time it distract the research direction. Here the observation is correct but need more understanding about confused
inflammation to complete the research about fibroid tumer
anyway the observation of allopathic doctors and observation of confused inflammation together will help in completing research, in finding the cause for fibroid.

A CONFUSED INFLAMMATION WITH NEO-
PLASAM MEANS, IT DOES NOT MEAN A TUMOR NECES-
SARILY DEVELOP FROM INFLAMMATION AND THEN TURN
INTO TUMOR.

I MEAN TO SAY A NEAOPLASAM ITSELF HAS IN-
CREDIANTS OR COMPONENT OF THE SPRAYED CONFUSED
INFLAMMTION. SO WHEN I AM SAYING INFLAMMATORY
ORIGIN IT DOES NOT REQUIRE A HISTORY OF TRUE

INFLAMMATION IN THE PARTICULAR SITE AND THEN TUMOR . A WOUND HEALING OR INFLAMMATION ABOUT TO RENOVATE THE EPITHELIYAM OF THE WOUND NOW IF WE APLY THE EXTERNAL APPLICATIONS THIS ORDER TO REGENRATE NEW CELLS DILUTED AND SPRAYED CIRCULATE ANYWHERE IN THE BODY WILL CREATE A NEW TUMOR WHERE EVER IT STUCK AND HAS THE FAVORABLE ENVIRONMENT.

BUT THE CANCER IS MOSTLY HAVE THE HISTORY OF INFLAMMATION IN THE PAST AND THEN THAT INFLAMMATION CELLS TURN INTO CANCER.

Why this explanation since a tumor is pure building up of natural new tissues and so no possibility of tunring into cancer but the cancer is develope from inflammation site (and from destructed tissues) is having inflammation base with damaged tissues so there by turned in to cancer. Most of the tumor is having simply growth with lakcing of other inflammation and destruction site so there is less possibility of turnining into cancer.

There are many time suppressions of the inflammation during women life time but these confused inflammations induce the disease in the later life mostly within the fallopian tube and ovary and cervical and veginal canal since the endometriyam shedding reduce the possibility of disease occurance due to confused inflammation. So the disease sows its domination either ebove the endometriyam (fellopiayn tube and oveary) or below the endometriyam cervix and vegina).

Ovary is similar to uterus undergoes monthly release of the ovum. Ovary is again exposed to varies hormonal influences so that there is high attraction of the confused inflammation to the site so that it creates lots of chronic inflammation diseases inside the ovary like pcod,ovariyan failure and there by infertility.

A diseased ovary and ova produce lots of congenital disorder to the child. But more the ovum under function lesser the disease because no hormonal actions so no attraction to confused. If ovum is not functioning then automatically the confused inflammation cells will move to the nearest organ which makes the attraction and produce the disease over there.

Estrogen not having control effect upon the inflammation [but indirect] but it takes all the confused inflammation over estrogen dominant region or part of the body. It is not from puberty to menopause the women is not having any inflammation at all or not having any disease anywhere in the body. They shifted inflammation within the genitals as well as all over the body gets high affinity to estrogen dominant parts. But it does not mean the inflammation for female will happen only to estrogen dominant parts it happen all over the body but worst inflammation effect upon the female reproductive organs because body natural construction is happening after many years of birth will sure trigger the inflammation to the site [and of course we might underwent lots of allopathic treatment for many illness during child so that we have huge confused inflammation in the body]

A sharp raise in endometrial cancer from 40-70-year women indicates confused inflammation domination upon the non shading endometrial [no menses].

A similar effect upon the breast is happening the age incidence of the breast cancer is raises from 40 to 70 years. [due to dominant effect of the confused inflammation a long-standing confused inflammation within the breast will undergoes stress which makes the cancers?]

More or less another organ which is develop after long time from birth is prostate in male. Having most possibility of tumor and cancer development.

Hypertrophy of the prostate with hyper vascularity will invite the confused inflammation to the prostate but the age-related atrophy gives the stress to the chronic inflammation cells causes cancer.

A uterus , prostate, breast not necessarily become chronic inflamed organs but if the confused inflammation is there in the body then sure these organs will attract that. [others need natural changes or triggers to attract the [Conf Infl] like exposure to sun or chemicals or over work, getting wet in the rain,,,] but here the normal physiological growth is attracting the cells and act as a triggers.

Since there is a monthly cycle and number of hormonal influence and pregnancy altogether female has bit low disease incidence of common disease the time between menarche to menopause all the hormonal influences reduced then women over taking the men in disease incidence. but man, disease incidence is more or less equal in genitals as well as remaining body.

Comparing to women men has to undergo less possibility of disease and cancer occurance but he is taking more chance equal to women due to his habbits (ciggeret smoking,alcohol consumption , choosing hard work option,driving etc).

a menses and pregnancy, cesarean sections, lactations all are remove the confused inflammation cells forcibly from the women body to outside so that a multipara's women get relief comparatively then nulli paras [no child] women. It is not completely free from disease but there is a possibility of less effect of intensity of the disease.

CERVICAL CANCER & Human papilloma virus (HPV)

Human papilloma virus (HPV) AND ENDO-
METRIYAL CARCINOMA , HPV makes the endometriyam and
cervical mucosa is undergoing constant chronic inflammation. After the menopause the confused inflammation may
shift from genital to other areas since the HPV the confused
inflammation is remain inside the uterus and veginal canal
and produce the inflammation in these organisms for longer
time before undergoing as cancer. The age-related atrophy
makes this chronic inflamed surface is become the site of
cancer.

A longer time thrival of hpv inside the veginal and
uterine wall is indicate absolute failure of immune and inflammatory system, a doctors are never made an attempt to
recover the immune system to normal to clear this virus, it
is so simple target for the virus to clear this but it is not happened due to confused inflammation and failed immune and
inflammation system by repeated anti-inflammatory and
steroid. Suppose if the women inflammation system is good
enough to fight and eliminate the virus any way we may not
allow that we rush to the doctors say there is a complaints
then he will prescribe medicine to suppress the disease.
So this hpv invite lots of confused inflammatory cells and
chemical inside the genital organs of female and produce
cancer.

Pelvic inflammatory disease and other chronic
pelvic and female genital diseases are occurring due to
chronic confused inflammation. As we discussed earlier inflammation has its own role to protect human if we allow it.
When we interrupt then number of diseases will come will
stay for longer time and shift from place to place within pelvic organ and produce disease or move to other parts make
diseases.

A local application for skin disease of vegina and

anti inflammatory and antibiotic given for treatment of the leucorrhea will produce confused inflammation and produce many long-standing diseases to uterus, fallopian tube and ovary. This confused inflammation breaks the protective mechanism of the vegainal canal and allow the germ entry inside the female reproductive system and urethra and bladder.

Globally There are 5,25000 women affected in the cervical cancer and nearly 2,65,000 women death due to cervical cancer in one year. In india nearly 1,20,000 women affected each year almost 60000 women died of cervical cancer.

This cancer is not affecting before the pubertal age and again this tumer is more common in women who is undergoing early marriage. The prostitute and the women those who have multi sex partners are having high possibility of this cancer. Those who not maintaining good hygine over the private part is having high risk of cancer. those who had warts near the veginal canal is having bit high risk of cancer then those who do not. The person who is under hormonal pills are having high risk of cervical cancer . this observation made already by allopathic doctors.

But the doctors are not satisfied with observation and research made till date since there is no identifiable cause for the cancer cervix they say it is not possible to prevent it.

But keeping the veginal part is clean and taking vaccination against the HPV and detecting the cancer in pre-invasive stage or erlier then worst final stage can prolong the life of the patient.

Prevention is possible now since the cause of the disease is identified confused inflammation. So, prevention of most danagerus disease is in our hand. Together now awareness of hygine and HPV VACCINE AND NO CONFUSED INFLAMMATION then 100 % possibility of the cancer free world.

Taking homeopathic treatment for acute or chronic disease of the all gynocological illness prevents the possibility of the confused inflammation productions is very very importand.

BREAST CANCER

48 Women affected in 1 lakh women in west Europe. 19 women is having breast cancer per 1 lakh women in south Africa. Comparing to developed country under developed country the rate of incidence is less but the survival after diagnosed cancer case is better in developed country then under developed country.

In india nearly 1.45000 new cases recorded in the same year nearly 70,212 women was died by breast cancer in 2012.

A women conciving very late age ,taking hormonal pills and early puberty and too late menopause all this type women is having high possibility of breast cancer.

Obesity is considered as one of the cause for cancer,

Self examination.

Mammogram and other scanning make the

After the research the cause for the cancer is identified exactly rather then vague and in aqureate guess work like cancer is caused by distracting the inflammation and it causes many confused inflammations within the breast like fobroadenoama and adenosis. When sufficient confused inflammation disease present inside the breast in this situation the growth option is optained by the chronic inflamed breast tissues turn into cancer.

Prostate cancer

is caused by a confused inflammation which is remaining in the prostate together with prostatic hypertrophy [PIA-PROSTATIC INFLAMMATORY ATROPHY, PROSTATIC INTRAEPITHELIAL NEOPLASM] CAUSES CANCER OF THE PROSTATE. a geographical high incidence in some part of the world and low incidence some part is basically determined by the demand related hypertrophy of the prostate like sexual excess and taking many medications to improve sexual life all these factors are help in constant hyperemia of the prostate which will invite the confused inflammation cells to the prostate. an only organ which is getting hypertrophy even in extremely old age with confused inflammation causes the prostate cancer.

Prostate cancet death was high before 1990 but the number of prostate cancer death is less now.more the age advances more the possibility of cancer death. Cancer death rate sharply raises from 55 to 80. Nearly 1500 men will be died of prostate cancer around 75 years but it is less then 200/ 1 lakh during 55 years.

More are less a women closing their hypertrophy and hyperplasia of the genital parts at the age of 50 that is the time when prostate start enlarging so a men having over all diseases now focused to prostate it means prostate hypertrophy having attraction to the confused inflammation so that inflammation is starts and produce the chronic confused inflammation and neoplasm.

But when compare to women men hypertrophy is negligible and again the hypertrophy is happening very slow, long process it may begin around 45 and complete hypertrophy is around 60 or 70 somebody complete it around 80 years.

Somebody starts hypertrophy around 60 and matured hypertrophy around 75-80.

So, this will not have a great attraction to the confused inflammation in the elderly. if there is equal strong stimulus happening somewhere in the body then it may move over there like constipation or smoking, excess spices

But still hypertrophy of the prostate and prostate cancer incidence indicates excess sexual indulgence and taking strong medications invites the confused inflammation over there.

11.DENTAL DISORDERS

•   All the Tooth's erupting after birth and all the tooth's fallen and new tooth erupting again in childhood itself is one of the trigger factors for oro dental disease or disorders related with tooth eruption, Since the confused inflammations remain all over body will be attracted to the oral cavity. During dentition.

•   exposure to crowded population in school encourages possibility of high respiratory tract infections and importantly they undergo repeated allopathic treatments so this unscientific treatment makes the nose, lymph nodes around the neck and jaws in the chest all the glands and basic protective functions are lost in early life makes the high vulnerability of the disease in general. since all the protective organs of upper respiratory tract failed in too early life persistent chronic disease are started troubling from childhood itself.so the confused inflammation moves and change the locality here and there from nose, eyes, mouth and tooth then chest like that. This upper respiratory tract infections gives the possibility of dental disease in the teeth but these disorders run chronic courses to till adult and old age until all the tooth are decayed and removed.

• All the oro dental disorders are confused inflammation only.

• the teething trouble in the childhood like slow in eruption and mal aligned tooth are happening due to hard gums [due to confused inflammation] the tooth finding to difficult to penetrate and erupt.

• bleeding gums, sensitive tooth, gum abscess, ulcers in the mouth all created by confused inflammations. chronic rashes appear inside the mouth is caused by confused inflammation in association with generalized skin disease or as a local eruption.

• **The warm food. The cold drinks, the spicy foods, the smoking, the betel nut chewing, irritating chemical drinks [alcohol] all factors invite the confused inflammation from all over the body to mouth.**

• This confused inflammation cells easily taken by nose and sinus and produce chronic inflammation Most of the patient with chronic nasal infection almost always having caries tooth. Most of the oral diseases easily shifted from nasal and sinus mucosa and produces variety of the disease. Nose to mouth and mouth to nose wise versa according to the situation.

• All of sudden people will have severe mouth ulcers and chronic aphthous ulceration for many years usually associated with sinus complaints.

• Gum bleeding is the chronic silent complaints patient will bleed and bleed every time when they brush, they not notice it or they think it is normal due to heavy brushing causes or its normal like that patient imagine. And most of the time the bleeding gums has to be ruled out from bleeding disorders so unnecessary blood tests for homeopathy it is easy job to cure. This gum bleeding direct the physician or dentist to sale vitamin c tablets patient drinks so many citrus fruits to avoid bleeding. If it is solved or not, it was cured by homeo or some other doctors is not problem, but they have understood the relation between nasal disease and oral disease is importand. since the gum bleeding may stop automatically when sinus complaints worse.

• Gum boil, gum eroding, epulis all the disease is happening due to confused inflammation.

12.LIVER DISEASE (HEPATOLOGY)

S ave liver it is very importand organ.
Since the liver is doing all metabolic functions. A diseased liver may not produce effective metabolic activity so that lots of metabolic disorder will come to the people including cholesterol and diabetes.

More then this, it is not necessary to prescribe heavy long-time doses to spoil the liver even few 2-3 days allopathic prescriptions and new chemical entry will attract the confused inflammation to the liver will cause severe long-time damage by that confused inflammation.

Normally insulin is helping to store the glucose inside liver but when the liver is diseased then muscles is the only option for store the sugar. The insulin will be normal and the glucose also will be high in the liver damage related diabetes in type 2 DM.

Liver is the important organ for cholesterol metabolism the cholesterol is converted into bile salts and then secreted as bile. Fat also formed as phospholipids and lipo protein. All these functions are collapsed and cholesterol metabolism is altered so that excess cholesterol in the circulation and formation bile and phospholipid and lipo protein formation is reduced.

liver damage in childhood will makes severe malnutrition, liver is wonderful organ for many functions including plasma protein synthesis and clearance of the ammonia. When the liver is severely damaged then the formation of plasma protein is failed so that the immune functions is lost.

Liver damage interfere the storage of the vitamin D, B 12, synthesis of the vitamin K.LIVER also helps in metabolism of allopathic drugs and detoxification of chemicals and many hormones in the body.

Prevention Of Liver Disease By Current Medical System

The number of liver disease is too much and destructive diseases are many but the dominant medical system (allopathy) in the world is struggling to save the liver and liver disease since there is no effective curative medicine no effective recovery medicine when the liver is affected with disease. No much proper medicine for both known etiology as well as unknown etiology disease. Then what is the role of liver specialist here ? no idea.

We say sweetest things and act very smart but actually we do nothing here then earning money. No effective medicine for many hepatitis including auto immune and some viral hepatitis ,no remedy to cure the liver damage like cirrhosis and other liver destructive disease. No curative or preventive medicine for prevention of tumers and no curative remedy or preventive medicine for cancer of livre ? then what is the role of specialist here once the liver is fall severe sickness then the liver is destructed the specialist will remove the liver and help in fixing new liver. Then what is the role of preventive medicine here ? to just count how many members are had liver failure , how many of them is going to have drug induced liver failure in future is the role of preventive medicine here. Why the world health organization not giving any warnining to allopathy doctors to reduce unnessory allopathy prescription and not to supporting ayush medical system and alternative medical system to reduce the drug induced organ failures.

Nearly 4.5 to 9.5 percent of the global population suffering with cirrhosis (30 crores to 65 crores of people is affected with liver cirrhosis in the world) the disease under estimated since there are many individual livings without signs and symptoms. According to national statistics in the UK liver diseases is the 5 th importand common cause for death.

The liver disease is increasing by year by year.

-S.K.SARIN,MD,DM(Department of hepatoly– New delhi)

-Rakki.Maiwal.MD,DM (Department of hepatology ,institute of liver and biliary science – New delhi)

Allopathy is there in the opposite direction in preventive medicine of the liver, since they are not able to prvent the disease and again they are creating liver damage by 2 way one is by prescribbbing allopathy drugs is having heavy worst destructive issue this is direct effect the allopathic medicine is fully metabolized in the liver and it is having harmfull effect in the liver tissues but they hiding the truth and the second leading problem created by allopathy is creating confused inflammation this will destruct liver indirectly . But the allopathy doctors are hiding this truth and say alcohol, virus and other reasons. Instead of curing and preventing liver disease is created by allopathy doctors DENOTES STRONGEST NEED FOR ALTERNATIVE AND AYUSH TREATMENT .

Saying preventive medicine and allowing allopathy doctors to create the disease is the highly objectionable.

How The Disease Originating In The Liver :

India is consuming allopathic drug very egarly and fond of eating allopathy medicines for every minor and major and avoidable situation. No much education about bad effect of allopathy medicine. The allopathic medicine consumption age is starting from day 1. The current situation is almost all Indian childrens especially in urban areas consume allopathic medicines for almost all common cold viral flu. Pracetamol and cold medicines are the top most medicines consumption. I hope paracetomol is a liver tonic and preventing all kind of liver damage according to hepatologist and pediatrician ?. there are many commercial preparations for fever killing. Many Indian house having paracetomal syrub just raise of temperature you have to consume the paracetomol. No much education to controle the infection and good approach to cure the disease but stop the fever. Paracetamol taken as a preventive for fever and educated by many spcialist and allopathic doctors. So, by the age of 10 many childrens liver are spoiled. Taking paracetomol and cold combination for everything.

Direct counter prescription is a fascion in india to

buy some anti pyretic and anti histamin and painkillers all are educated by allopathic doctors in india they never taken any single step in controlling unnessory prescription. There is no education about drug related complication and preventing disease the only target is boost the pharma product nothing more then that is happen here to sale that drug we need some specialist.

The exact problem is prescribing medicines for self curing disease is the major fault doing by Indian allopathic doctors. Educating the public to do the same to increase the medicines sales.

So now the liver is damged enough will attract the confused inflammations. The confused inflammation mostly recived from the gastro intestinal tract and also from respiratory tract. Prescribing medicine for stopping diarrheal disease and medicine for stopping gastric infections leads to production of lots of confused inflammation so easily reaches liver. So now the liver is having both medicines induced livre parenchymal damage and confused inflammation induced liver damage. This liver is prone to easy infections that infections again interrupted by allopathy medicines anyway here they will not allow the infection to continue they prescribe medicine and stop the inflammation process so the virus will stay with us life long.

There are 2 addictions created in the city one is liquer addiction and another one is allopathic drug addictions. The alcohol addiction people know this is bad to health but allopathic drug addictions people may not know this harmfull drugs like they know but they forgot the side effects of allopathic medicines in the recent days including allopathic doctors.

HEPATITIS

VIRAL AND AUTO IMMUNE HEPATITIS

Hepatitis A virus affects yearly 14 lakh people .this disease will escape from physician knowledge since the mild symptoms and signs .death rate is too less. less then 1 %. The disease spread by feco oral route . defecating near the water source causes water contamination. Hand hygine play a major role in preventing hepatitis A. A person working in the kitchen having less hygine habbit will carry high risk of hepatitis A.

Washing the hands now ant then with soap and using the water after proper boiling and chlorination will prevent the disease. Vaccination available.

Signs and symptoms is mild only .loss of appetite and mild jaundice and stomach pain will be there for few individual .asymtomatic cases are high.

IgA and igG IMMUNO GLOBULIN AND LIVER function altereations will help in hepatitis A Viral diagnosis.

HEPATITIS - B

Most dangerus viral illness and it is one of the sexually transimited disease. Since this virus remain silently without symtoms there are 2.5 crore wolrd population suffer without knowing they are hepatitis B positive patient. Few individual recovers with mild symptomatic case death rate less then 1 % but nearly 40 % of the patient associated with cancer and 30 % hepatitis patient associated with cirrohosis.

The virus remains in the blood,semen,saliva,veginal secretion so this is spread by sex and blood transfusion and to doctors and health care workers while handling blood.

So there is a strict cheking is made with precautions like presurgery hepatitis b screening and before blood transfusion the blood is screened for viral illness especially hepatitis and Hiv.

Hepatitis b vaccine is available ,practicing safe sex, pre surgical precautions all will prevent the Hepatitis B virus prevention.

But additionally, stop prescribing allopathic medicine for the viral illness. Since the prescriptions aimed to stop the fever not aimed to kill the virus so confused inflammation will form and that is the reason for chronic viral illness and causing cirrohosis and cancer. Here the cause for cancer and cirrhosis is not simply by virus this is because of confused inflammation and breaking chaing of recovery by anti inflammatory and steroids. The allopathic medicines are damaging the liver and hepatitis is used as a excuse for hiding the side effects of allopathic medicine complications.

Hepatitis - C

This virus spread from mother to child or the through blood transfusion. Both acute chronic diseases induced by this virus nearly 1.5 crore people in the world is affected with chronic hepatitis c virus infection.Nearly 50 % of the hepatitis c virus patient is turnining towards developing chronic hepatitis viras c infections.

Allopathic doctors are having anti viral medicine for the hepatitis c.

Loss of appetite and jaundice and abdominal pain is a acute manifestation of the hepatitis c.

Clinical Symptoms :

The *prodromal symptoms* of acute viral hepatitis Constitutional symptoms of

anorexia, nausea and vomiting,

fatigue, malaise, arthralgias, myalgias,

headache,

photophobia,

pharyngitis, cough, and coryza may precede the onset o of jaundice by 1–2 weeks.

alterations in olfaction and taste.

A low-grade fever between 38° and 39°C (100°–102°F) is more often present in hepatitis A and E than in B or C,

rarely, a fever of 39.5°–40°C (103°–104°F) may accompany the constitutional symptoms.

Dark urine and clay-colored stools may be noticed by the patient from 1–5 days before the onset of clinical jaundice. *clinical jaundice*.

The liver becomes enlarged and tender and may be associated with right upper quadrant pain and discomfort.

Splenomegaly and cervical adenopathy are present in 10–20% of patients with acute hepatitis.

Rarely, a few spider angiomas appear during the icteric phase and disappear during convalescence.

During the *recovery phase* , constitutional symptoms disappear, but usually some liver enlargement and abnormalities in liver biochemical tests are still evident.

Complete clinical and biochemical recovery is to be expected 1–2 months after all cases of hepatitis A and E and 3–4 months after the onset of jaundice in three-quarters of uncomplicated, self-limited cases of hepatitis B and C (among healthy adults, acute hepatitis B is self-limited in 95–99% while hepatitis C is self-limited in only 15%). In the remainder, biochemical recovery may be delayed.

Some Of The Importand Medicine For

Homeopathy medicine for complete ,early recovery of the hepatitis is (nux vomica,bryonia ,eupatoriyam ,chelidoniyam ,lycopodiyam ,pulsatilla ,nat psulph, merco sol) indication given in the prevention of communicable disese.

Chronic hepatitis

Hepatitis B in immunocompeteant individual makes severe acute hepatitis and less then 1 % only developes into chronic hepatitis. This observation is the importand point which I am frquantly stressing if the person able to produce better inflammation then they will kill the virus and no chronic hepatitis.

Chronic hepatitis happens only when acute inflammation is stopped then all the inflammation function carried out that movement is stopped so there is no recovery from the inflammation no virus killing since the stagnation of the inflammation slowly damage the liver paranchyma and produce a cirrhosis and then cancer of the liver.

This is the basic facts in the hepatitis from childhood not having enough immune power to clear the virus or the inflammation was stopped forcibly without knowing that the fever is happen due to hepatitis (This is normal in every infection and inflammation to stopping the fever by medicine so the hepatitis is stopped in the mid and the inflammation is remain as confused inflammation and the virus is also remain without killing) . Prescribbing anti viral may kill the virus but the confused inflammation will take the liver into cirrhosis and then to cancer.chronic hepatitis B is run from childhood is causing severe cirrhosis and cancer of liver .

When the virus is allowed to stay inside then that virus is replicate and make severe disease infectivity and severe damage to the liver. Not happening to everybody. virus is replicating in many individual viruses is not replicating in many individuals. virus present with hepatitis e antigen and hepatitis e antigen abcent hepatitis.

Patient is often complaints of malaise and develop now and then acute exacerbation ,slowly the lung paranchyma is destroyed and then finally lung is cirrhosis and then the ascitis and varicel bleeding and emaciation then few individuals goes to cancer of the liver.

When a virus is infecting in the liver it produce acute hepatitis is the real facts and again if the virus is re infect and again periodically reinfect it was produced hepatitis this is again the usual response but how we can say the cirrhosis and cancer is produced in the liver by virus ? we have two observation one is viral infection will cause hepatitis and we found these virus is not fully eliminated and we found the cancer and at the same time still the virus present this is just a normal observation but how we can say surely virus is produced cancer. and that to only the patient those who have virus from childhood not others ? this observation needs a proper interpretation.

The road and car and the dead body will present always in accident it does not mean the road was did a accident purposefully or with intension to kill someone. When we prescribe the paracetomal without what caused this fever from that day itself the problem started so the virus is identified by the body and tried to kill that we are collapsed the infection by anti inflammatory and other medicines , this virus will remain life long without killing and will cause hepatitis then again and again we are trained to stop the inflammation so confused inflammation created and causes cirrhosis and cancer confused inflammation has the power to create the cancer. Virus is present here that's all.

If enough chemicals are available the confused inflammation will produce cirrhosis then the cirrhosis is turned into cance only if sufficient and necessary chemicals is available to induce the cancer. The role of the virus here act as a risk factor to bring the confused inflammation to the liver.

Auto immune hepatitis

Auto immune liver disease is the basic common chornic inflammation of the liver. It can be triggered easily due to heavy intake of anti inflammation and antibiotic so there is great number of confused inflammation and heavy immune globulin against the liver. These confused inflammation easily attracted by liver cells either by subsequent liver infections or regular intake of some of other allopathic medicine so now this confused inflammation will initiate the liver damage by confused inflammation once the inflammation started that will trigger the humoral and cellular immunity (this is achived by confused inflammation chemicals which is present and damaging the liver causes initiation of the humoral and cellular immunity). The liver damage is highly increased by excess consumption of the allopathic drugs this is the real cause for heavy liver damage and loss of basic protective functions.

But these immune receptars can also triggered by inflammation chemicals which is coming from somewhere else or in the same site . when a histamine or bradykinin or other pro inflammation chemicals come in contact with burried receptors then inflammation easily triggered then humoral and cellular immunity starts so easily and so simply. Allopathy doctors know very well that the histamine bradykinin and other proinflammatory chemicals actually act as a chemotactic factor there is no dought about these chemicals can induce this lymphocyte and macrophage but they do not know the possibility of roming unwanted readymade inflammation (confused inflammation) there may not be any more objection from allopathy by accepting my point of view.

Here the allopathy doctors believe that abnormal sensitivity is happening by inborn genetic abnormality. They also giving justification like this auto immune hepatitis present along with auto immune thyroiditis and rheumatoid arthritis and this auto immune hepatitis associated with many auto antibodies like that.

The simple reason behind the liver infections is breaking the protective power of the human by allopathic medicine,removing protective organisam in the nose and throat causes easy reach of the infection to the git and liver within the

liver again the protective mechanisam is collapse due to re-current unnecessary intake of allopathy drugs. This causes damage in the liver so that the infection and the confused inflammation easily invited to the liver and stay unusually longer time without any ressitance and produce many liver diseases.

So, when you plan to prevent the liver disease and save the liver from infections you have to choose and learn simple medicine which does not harm the liver is the first step.by doing this even though if the infection is there it may not affect as severe as now.

Choosing simple medicine ? what is that ? homeopathy is top most harmless non toxic and non chemical medicines and acu pressure and acu puncture is another simple harmless medicine.

Choose a doctor who is trying to preserve your body parts rather removing it now and then and making you vulnerable to infection all time.when the door or entry route is guardless no protector then every offending agent come inside the body without any resistance.so preserve tonsil,adenoid.keep healthy nose and mouth.

Taking antacid is another way to escaping the germs from stomach to all over the body.antacid is taken not only for gastric complaints it is taken for all the allopathic prescription so that chance of stopping antacid is increasing.so choose medicine other then allopathy for your ailment is right way to protect liver and other organ damage.

Observation prevention and treatment for auto immune hepatitis:

Once the patient is infected, they started clinical

symptoms of hepatitis it better to consider homeopathic medicine,since to reduce the long-time recovery phase.

Since many patients under allopathic medicines if the clinical symptoms sure with confused inflammation so that instead of saving the patient confused inflammation will destroy the liver so it necessary to have the homeopathic medicines.

Hospitalization and observation need in all the cases.

When homeopathy handle the case possibility of deveolpping confused inflammation is zero so that future liver damage (tumor or chronic liver disease,cancer) is nill.as well as no confused inflammation in future from this infection.

So, the necessity of PREVENTING CONFUSION INFLAMMATION IS THE MAIN AIM. THE PRODUCTION OF CONFUSED INFLAMMAITON GIVES GREAT BURDEN AND IN PREVENTING THE INFECTIONS. Since if we fail in preventing infection the infection gives the mortality and morbidity is the head ache but now I am saying even if you recover from the infections you may have future chain of diseases due to confused inflammation.So , prevention of infection gives double protection one is prevention of infectiuse disease and second is prevention of non communicable disease.

Suppose if you allow disease to recover naturally then the possibility of confused inflammation will be nil. But this allopathic era everybody is having confused inflammation with their body so it is necessary to take treatment with homeopathy this treatment is again gives double benefit no 1 is curing the sickness and number 2 is removing the confused inflammation.so that if the person taken homeopathy treatment can be allowed to natural recovery but any way with observation.homeopathy believes confused inflammation need a long time treatment to remove the miasmatic backgraound (confused inflammation).

1   A Patient treating infectinos with *allopathic medicine* causes confused inflammation.If the patient having confused inflammation,if he undergoes treatment for infection by allopathy is having chance of

1. Escape of infective agent (except bacteria).

2   the inflammation is going to be incomplete it give the way to cancer and source of future infection.

3   confused inflammation doubled now due to stopping present inflammation.

4   functions of the present organ or tissue suspended is not recovered hence possibility of either clinical or subclinical development of diseases or syndromes or single symptom disease is going to develop.

5.give the way to development immune complex ,auto immune and altered immune disease.6.allopathic drug direct side effects.

6.a.A patient never undergone any allopathic treatment *allowed for natural recovery* will prevent non communicable disease.but will not remove the confused inflammation in case if the patient is having confused inflammation before the infection.

6.b.A patient with confused inflammation with acute infection under *homeopathy treatment* will recover from infections as well as reduced confused inflammation so prevent non communicable disease.

8.A patient with confused inflammation suffering with infection is taking treatment with *ayurvedha, siddha, unani, naturopathy* having hopefull recovery but not sure about preventing confused inflammation formation and not sure about eliminating the confused inflammation since when comparing to allopathy siddha and ayurvedha medicines are highly less side effect but it never act like a infection instead of that this medicines attempt to heal or treat the complaints directly so that it may support the preventing extensive liver damage to less but never support to remove the confused inflammation.if any medicine act like infection and stimulate the body to remove that then only the body will try to remove the confused inflammation if any medicine do that function then the working principle is homeopathy.the benefit of utilizing ayurvedha,siddha,unani and naturopathy single benefit like it will help to recover the current infection or liver injury.

> 5.   A patient taking treatment with *acu pressure, acu puncture and others like pranic healing and touch therpay* regarding   handling the infections and power removing the confused inflammation need to included based on observation.

Homeopathic therapeutics :

If the confused inflammation is strongly making disease somewhere in the body then the infection within the liver will be unmixed with confused inflammation so natural recovery or recovery with homeopathy is possibly recover from infection alone.so need medication for the non communicable disease after recovering from the acute infections.because we have to make sure no confused inflam-

515

mation within the body and this non communicable disease not having gurantee that all the time it will not mix with acute infection.

ALCOHOL AND LIVER DAMAGE

Alcohol injure the liver and stomach very badly and help the damaged to tissue to become cancer.alcohol is playing major role in inducing liver injury and cirrhosis and finaly liver failure take the many people life away due to drinking alcohol. Need a controle effect to reduce the liquer sale.

- Alcohol play a mojor role in poverty.a family depending upon the single person ,that single person fall in alcoholisam brings the poverty to the family.
- Alcoholisam reduce the personal ebility of the person and reduce the working skill as the alcohol addiction is become more.
- Alcoholic psychosis and neurological syndromes is another burden to the individual.
- Alcoholisam destroy the many family peacefulness.
- Alcoholisam is known great killer of the individual and makes great uncomfortableness to his family and surrounding.

The modern life style slowly includes the drunkanness to a woman as well as teen so this will cause early diseases family dishormoney and many pther unwanted issues in the family as well as in the society is expectable.

Allopathic drugs and alcohol plays majaor role in producing disease. Need to be controlled. It is waste to write anything about the preventive medicine, if there is no controle in these two major diseases producing agents.Dont say anything we prevented this disease or that disease, every-thing is humbag if you not stop these 2 factors.

CIRRHOSIS OF THE LIVER

Are you going to observe the chronic liver disease patient , then observe how the self curing disease has been distracted as chronic disease (why the disease irrecover-able by body on its own). Read the dominant inflamma-tory chemical which is doing the pathology here. Which stage of the inflammation or immunity is here involved in pathophysiology?

Identify and define the cherecter of the inflamma-tory chemicals and immune cells like modality (worse and better factor,pseudo cause ,,,, etc).

Identify other symptoms along with the present dominant liver inflammation symtoms to be observed.sim-ultanease associated symptoms present in the body irre-spective of disease diagnostic symptoms.

Prevention Aspect :

Thinking that disease is incurable giving some medicines as for as possible just like managing is not fall under any prevention. The current allopathy is not taking any preventive care in chronic disease it means the disease will progress but the doctor will ease some didtrssiong symtoms but patient thinking that doctor is curing his dis-ease or patient educated this is not curable disease.

So the acute disease has come and that disease is distracted now he is in chronic disease what kind of preven-tion we can do here. Yes we can make many prevention even now.

517

curing the sickenss in total makes the highest happiness to the patient and reduce the economic burden and it will bring make the smile in the family.So this is going to reduce necessity of frequent hospitalization.yes it is going to reduce liver failure and other complications yes it is going to reduce the burden of organ transplant and some time prevent the possibility of cancer,prevent the possibility of death so a doctor must aim to cure.

A Doctor must aim to cure the patient it is possible.if the liver damage is more the chronic congetion (inflammation is removed) but the liver paranchyma damaged is not recovered it means possibility of the recurrent infection is more so prevention is directed towards preventing furdher infections is importand.

There are medicine in the homeopathy to eliminate the carrier state of the hepatitis but when the medicine works it bering the fever and all acute haptitis symtoms taking anti pyretic will abolish the cure so the patient will be in the same stage (carrier stage will continue again)

Inflammation with necrosis of the liver paranchyma.

As we discussed earlier there is no chronic disease. when we allow the natural recovery of the acute illness the disease will clear itself without any remanence but here we administer the medicine to stop inflammation so the infections is remain silent and stay here produde *chronic hepatitis* and all the virus coming here after settle here and destroy the liver along with their immunoglobulin since the immunoglobulin never kill the virus since confused inflammation and liver damages by medicine causes better space for viral multiplications and need heavy immunoglobulin to kill the virus.

When we stop the inflammation at the time of after immunity development then the possibility of the *auto immune hepatitis* will form.The third variety of the chronic hepatitis with unknown etiology since there is no proof is there no immunologic evidence or virus or any other chemicals so its fall under hepatitis of unknown etiology and belived again it is auto immunity because when the disease progorss evidence of immune mediated cell damage.

So, all this 3 major classification of cell damage is caused by simply inflammation process alone. But allopathy consideres this is a nature of the body and inheritance this is not true.

The virus is there but not producing any symptoms because we administer anti inflammatory simply for every fever and the patient is having habbit taking anti inflammatory for all the simple reasons.So this unscientific prescription gives the way to 2 possiblity one is virus escapes from the killing in the inflammation process so virus is stay inside the body and produce hepatitis.

Number 2 is virus is induce the immunity but we again not allow that to complete so that the uncontrolled auto immunity destroys the liver.when we allow the immunity to complete its course then this immune cells will destroy the appropriate virus and after the completion of the viral killing the immune cells will be withdrawn from the circulation or stop the furdher production.when stopping immune cells and clearing immune cells and immune complex from the body then there is no possibility of immune destruction within liver and extra hepatic auto immune disorders and the third possibility is there is no immune complex disease.

What he think about chronic viral hepatitis he observe virus will enter and stay without doing anything (he accept this theory) it means he did mistake and that is the reason the virus stay without resistance but he study in different way a hepatitis may come and stay without doing anything and he name this stage as carrier stage.he hide or forgot his unscientific treatment is the cause for Hepatitis carrier state.he never question how the viras is remain inside the body without any inflammation or any protection.

Then he observes in some patients it develops symptoms due to inflammation why and how this happen he does not enquire and he accept this and he name this is as *active hepatitis.* The inflammation has to save us why here the destruction and necrosis of the liver paranchyma ? no question.

When sufficient confused inflammation within the liver then it starts destroy the liver this damage are purely carried out by the confused inflammation not because of the virus.so that is why the liver is damaged and produce mild to moderate jaundice and weakness and loss of appetite.when the damage approached toward cirrhoisis of liver then ascites and oedema will develop.when the cirrhosis is worse then it gives the complication of the varicel bleeding ,enchepalopathy,liver failure,,.

Then he sees the auto auntibody in the circulation in some cases, so he now accepts and belive this antibody is formed against the virus but he never asks himself the antibody has to destroy the bacteria not the liver why the liver cells are damaged ?.he observe this and he try to give varies medicines for above named diseases and thses medicines are spoiling the patient and many of them where dead and few of them survive with less active phase of the disease for some more days.here the antibody is forming to kill the virus alone but he never allow to kill the virus. The second normal possibility is the antibody is formed somewhere and reached here and destroys the liver and destructive material is formed by the body itself to remove the dead tissues.

second leading cause is alcohol consumption and both of these cause invites the confused inflammation towards liver.THE LIVER IS UNDER GREAT TROUBLE BY ALLO-PATHIC DRUGS MOST OF THE LIVER DISEASE SECONDARY DUE TO WEAKNESS CREATED BY THE ALLOPATHIC DRUG-S.IF THE ALLOPATHIC DRUGS CONSUMPTION IS NILL OR AT LEAST LESS THEN THERE IS NO LIVER DISEASE AT ALL.

Liver is involving in all metabolism it helps in control fat, protein and vitamins and mineral metabolism. similarly, all the medicines have to metabolized in the same organ only. Massive unnecessary allopathic drugs prescriptions will damage the parenchyma of the liver.

Next to upper respiratory tract and extremities liver is the one among the common organ for confused inflammation disease. Drug induced cirrhosis is common disease. People are consuming more and more allopathic medicines for every ailment.So they fall in severe liver damage unnessarily.There is no effective treatment for cirrhosis in allopathy again they do not allow the patients to take treatment with other systems so LIVER TRANSPLANT is unavoidable.

Alcohol consumption and allopathic drugs will severely damage the liver so that Many diseases. There are four factor which is gives the severe liver disease which is there for many adults like

- alcoholism,
- allopathic medicine,
- hepatitis and
- confused inflammation altogether produces severe liver disease like hepa-

titis, liver cirrhosis and cancer of the liver.

Extensive liver destruction and regeneration is carried out by confused inflammation.Hepatitis (viral, auto immune and chemical and toxins induced) ,alcohol consumption all will damage the liver cells and leading to cirrohosis of the liver fully with underlying bas of the confused inflammation. Cirrhosis of the liver is nothing but liver failure if the liver failes automatically it affects general metabolic system failure and circulatory failure it means heart failure.

Presenting Complaints :

- Itching
- Jaundice
- Ascites and generalized edema
- Varicesl bleeding like blood vomiting
- Earlier liver swelling then followed by shirinking of the liver size
- Symptoms based on loss of liver function like easy brusing

Prevention of the cirrhosis , written more then enough in the previus chapter. Prevention of the liver failure is massively depending upon reduceing allopathy medicine and stopping alcohol consumption.

Learning and educating how to prevent infections like hepatitis and other infections hygienic food preparation, good drinking water. Maintaingin hygiene in sanitation and safe sex and avoiding drug abuse. Reducing allopathic medicine and using alternative system of medicine allowing the inflammation to controle the infection and removing the confused inflammation by using appropriate remedy all are having high marks in preventing chronic liver disease.

Carcinoma of the liver

Observation and clinical verification given by allopathy.

- Hepato cellular carcinoma arises from chronic hepatitis B,chronic hepatitis C infection.
- Chronic liver disease,cirrhosis is play major risk factor for liver cancer.viral hepatitis and alcoholisam is top leading cause among this risk factor.
- Aflatoxin produce liver injury,potant liver cancer.
- Metabolisam and genetics associated with hepatitis c is willson disease and alfa 1 anti trypsin deficiency.
- Hemochromatosis (iron over load)
- Hepatitis vaccination reduce the number hepatitis B related liver cancer.

According to allopathy public consume allopathy drugs life long from day 1 of their birth to till end of life will never cause any cancer. Allopathy says even the herbal medicine causes liver injury and damage liver paranchyma but not much discussion under cancer and allopathy drugs relation.

No one included allopathic drugs can cause liver injury and cancer.

Enough discussion we done already. How the liver tissues are damaged how we have to prevent chronic liver disease.we list once again here all again.

Liver cancer is possible to prevent since the cause is known and many of these casues easily preventable much earlier then it turns into cancer.

Dont take allopathic or any pathy medicine to stop inflammation so stopping inflammation will help the spread of infection and virus and bacteria will multiply.

Stopping inflammation lead to unrepaired injured inflammation sites this will lead to chronic disease this chronic diseased damaged tissue will turn into cancer . if the growth signal recived by a damaged tissue then the damaged tisseues will grow as a cancer.

Stopping inflammation causes heavy distraction of the inflammation so the distracted inflammation will be wandering inside the human body will ofcourse choose the liver as a prime choice due to heavy allopathic medication from birth to death of current generation. So this is the cause for *auto immunity/ auto inflammation* within the liver, liver tissue damage, then cirrhosis and turn into carcinoma of the liver.

When the liver is so easily and so quickly get into a chronic distracted or confused inflammation / immunity and this liver changes ideally very negligible it takes longet time to reveal the true clinical evidence.But this liver tissue changes causes loss of basic protective functions of the liver so it is easy for viral or any othe infection get multiplicaitons (replications) and growth within the liver without any resistance.

The cause is known but there are no effective medicines in the allopathy so they handle case unusually longer time to give minor change again they belive their drugs all are major risk factor for the liver cancer. It means the cases sure it will turn into cancer but no effective medicine in allopathy again allopathic medicine is the major risk factor for developing cancer in an non alcoholic patient. A TOP MOST HIDDEN BUT OPEN CAUSE FOR CANCER OF LIVER allopathic medicine.

Choosing the medicine which is not act upon the liver will prevent nearly 75 % liver disease.because all the allopathic medicine act upon the liver causes parenchymal damage of the liver.

When you not stopping the Inflammation will be the great help for reducing major liver disease and choosing the medicines other then allopathy in case liver disease patient will prevent further liver damage and get rapid recovery or the liver cell possibility to turn cancer will be less since the injured or damaged liver cells will undergo stress when you take allopathic drugs speed up the liver cancer then other medication hence CHOOSING NON ALLOPATHIC MEDICINE IS MANDATORY FOR LIVER AND KIDNEY INJURY PATIENT.

Loss of appetite, jaundice, loss of weight ,abdominal pain and then weakness fluid accumulation in the abdomen and legs. Liver and spleen enlargement all are signs and symtoms of the cancer of the liver.

Unusually longer time is available to prevent cancer of the liver so better to prevent then cure. Reducing alcohol , reducing allopathic medications preventing confused inflammation formation etc will prevent the hepatocellular carcinoma taking hepatitis b vaccination prevent the cancer risk.

Abcess within liver

When the bacteria and paracyte enter into the

liver then it will develop liver abcess read it and practice as said into the text no comprehensive idea how and why.An abcess within the liver or lungs or the kidney is not a normal inflammation response to a germ. The confused inflammation is the cause for abcess.

When the liver is full of confused inflammation then the entering organisam invite the confused inflammation and the normal inflammation lead to abnormally prolonged inflammation the destruction of the tissues is more and need more inflammatory cells so that excess accumulation of the dead bacteriyam and dead tissues so that abcess formation.

So here the prevention is again to reduce the confused inflammation or remove the confused inflammation otherwise abcess formation unavoidable.

When the liver is not having any confused inflammation and it is having good fighting power then liver cells easily fight with the bacteriyam or parasites and destroy that organisam very easily. We have basic defect in understanding what is happanining within the body. Since we belive when the course of the disease heals themselves, we belive the same organisam causes modereate course we name the same disease if it is severe .we does not understand something is beyond the organisam and the immune system is happening. More severe the abcess more profuse confused inflammation the recurrent infection and these infections.

Injury to liver , rupture of the appendix , perforated bowel ,,,etc . gives high possibility of the abcess.these are all some exception then what said.it means heavy pouring of the infected germs into the liver then abcess formation possibility is high even to the normal liver.

Clinical Future.

- chills

- vomiting

- fever

- right upper abdominal pain

- sudden dramatic weight loss

- diarrhea.

Prevention is the prime aim in the abcess of the liver, so we are going to prevent the abcess by breaking possility of confused inflammation formation and supporting to the body to continue their job (killing the germs) by prescribing best homeopathic medicine – silicia ,hepar sulph ,merc sol , graphitis,,,,,,etc. this homeopathic medicine will cure the abcess.

13.MIND

There are many classifications for psychological disease, but in homeopathy there are 3 important classifications 1.disease originate in the body treated improperly and this disease shift to brain and produce psychological illness.2.disease originates in the mind treated improperly shift to body 3.Psycological diseases originate due to bad habits faulty preach, inhabitant in a immoral back ground.

The first 2 classifications are clearly indicating the shifting nature of the confused inflammation . It means if you treat in an improper way then the disease in the body shift to brain and produce series psychological disease. And again considering only psycological disease and missing whole disese caused by confused inflammation is considered as one sidedness.

Similarly, a disease in the brain [mind] caused by confused inflammation treated improperly so that it moves and produce bodily ailments.

Both psychological as well as bodily ailments appear in most of the cases if they treat the strong medication of the bodily or mind disease then the disease shift to one side either bodily ailment or psychological disease. so, it considered as one-sided disease.

14.CENTRAL NERVES SYSTEM

PAIN / NEURALGIA

How Neuralgia Occurs?

a pain which is caused by injury to the tissues will invite the natural treatment by inflammation but stopping this inflammation by means of anti-inflammatory or antipyretics causes huge collections of confused inflammatory chemicals scattered all over the body will give great many neuralgias which is lack in evidence of proper support like long standing neck pain in children's and young healthy adult and severe unresolving back pain yet there is no great erosions or structural changes in many cases occurs.

When blocking arachidonic acid conversion into prostaglandin result in pain or fever relived temporarily. By this action inflammation terminated. But the injury is still there will keep send more arachidonic acids dumped and sprayed all over the body so this arachidonic acid is now readily available all over the body, without any injury. Now onwards, minimal pressure, just a strain in the back, abnormal posture all will induce the arachidonic acid. But basically, this acid has to come if there is injury and again only limited to the injured site not widespread. Since there is excess chemical and this chemical start pain signals to nerve when they get mild stimulation like pressure, temperature changes and so an.

Minimal cold exposure will bring the neck pain. minimal sun exposure will bring the head ache. Taking cold drinks will bring the tooth ache, exposure to ac room will bring the ear pain etc ,,, and etc.

Keep that in your mind, only pain, it is not going to bring the whole inflammation, only neuralgia. So , the doctors never imagine that the pain is a inflammation remenents, this is not just pain not just neuralgia.

Pain ,redness ,swelling ,fever all are signs and symptoms of the inflammation here only the pain appearing so this pain will annoy the patient and he will suffer . there is no purpose in this pain actually the inflammation pain has the purpose yes, it is going to heal the injured tissues but here only pain that pain will torture the patient life long. The pain indicates we did mistake we have created confused inflammation.

Pain and pain everywhere pain. there was a time ,when the person is absolutely healthy, he was having pain with fever so its signs of inflammation it was the normal body functions, he will be alright within one or two days. But we are not ready to wait. We took anti pyretics and analgesics. Now he is suffering with pain and pain for many years. Allopathic doctors also exhausted by selling eye glass for head ache and belt for back pain, doing so many surgeries and sold all their medical products but no cure.

That pain and fever is produced by immune system with aim, the aim is clear the enemy and cure the injury. But what will happen when you blocke the inflammation ?. The aim / purpose of the inflammation now scattered aimless confused inflammation. It will produce this kind of symptoms alone. This confused inflammation may not go to initiate strong real inflammation. Eventhough it produces real inflammation again you are going to prescribe the anti inflammation medication again – pain killers [dumping of the arachidonic acid and sprayed all over the body will started produce pain or fevers] realize what you are doing

You have thousand and thousand disease in your hand but no idea how it occurs but I am just opening your insight see that how the disease occurs. who is the cause for that ailments ? I don't have any disease which is unknown origin, now I have discovered cause for all disease. All are originated by prescribing against body protective functions.

Any chronic pain (other then accident or birth anomaly related) all are fall under confused inflammation chemicals alone.

I am discussing the cause of the disease, the cause for the diseases are allopathy medicine not only now the whole text describes and criticize the allopathic treatment.

BECAUSE ALOPATHY IS THE CAUSE FOR ALL DISEASE. Throw the allopathic pharmacology use better pharmacology.

Chronic fatigue syndrome, fibromyalgia

Terminating the inflammation prematurely causes accumulation of cyclooxygenase, this cyclooxygenase is hypersensitive to external and internal strong bodily movements will produce excess generalized malaise and body pain. The fibromyalgia syndrome coupled with confused inflammation [neuralgia] causes severe generalized body pain. It is vague not able to define and put in particular categri of nuealgias and patient may not respond well even with painkiller it keep changes. The description is too much and many . back pain shoulder pain, to day back pain tomarrow head ache day after tomarrow it may be stomach pain. No much tenderness to elicit a diagnosis or abnormal sensitiveness in particular sites in the shoulder and in the back muscles. Nuraligia it self is partial diagnosis this fibromyalgia may not fit into that category of the mayalgias and general classifications which we have currently.

Eating too mnay medicines meeting so many doctors undergoing so many invetications in labs and scans. Usually patient comes with heavy bundles of MRI and ultrasound reports. Patient has no progress.

Most of the patient precisely says their ailments started after any fever and some infections from then onwards the complaints.

Most of this patient diagnosed as psychological illness and even this fibromayalgia and irritable bowel syndrome all this kind of disorders are considered as pscyco-motor disease (involving mind and body). Allopathy doctors consider this as abnormal over sensitivity of the pain and conscience of the of their bodily ailments.

But this is purely confused inflammation disease.

HEAD ACHE

How headache comes (machanisam of head ahce) :

A head ache is not something neurological it is purely inflammation (confused inflammation) in origin. But every doctor thinking and believing head ache is related with central nervous system in origin.

Head ache is one of the most frequent common complaint for which patient visiting to the clinic and hospitals.Patient now a days educated to take direct allopathic pain killers to relive the pain and learn slowly what causes head ache so that they accustomed to live with head ache.Head ache will be the universal complaint and I hope all the people affected once in their life time

As we think and doctors believe either migraine or headache in general is not a disease. The aspect of popular opinion is differing from reality. It means head ache or the neuralgias considered and approached as separate cause and separate disease is not true. The pain is arising from excess chemical called *prostaglandin* in the circulation is inducing this. This prostaglandin is produced due to usage of pain killers to stop fevers or inflammation in the early life causes the excess accumulation of prostaglandin.

So when a inflammation is commences it gives pain, raise of temperature (fever),swelling and loss of functions all of this. but due to distraction of the inflammation inducing chemicals. Only pain no fever only pain no swelling only pain no loss functions all happen due to this pain is not something normal bodily reactions when we have injury we may experience pain but here there is no injury but there is a pain. this altered pain sensation is recived by circulating excess pain inducing chemicals ,this pain is disproportionate then the real injury or tissue damages or even we can say pain will be there without any tissue injury.

A normal injury will have the pain, this pain will invite the healing cells and chemicals and heal the injury so no pain, but pain throught the life is not a normal response. When we expose to cold, we have the pain, when we expose to sun heat we have the pain, when we get over stressed then we have the pain, it means we have excess pain stimulating chemicals which was derived from distracted inflammatory chemicals that is easily triggered by varies external stimulai and gives the pain.

A migraine or head ache is caused by pain inducing confused inflammation chemicals.

Types Of Head Ache :

1.TENSION HEAD ACHE

2.MIGRAINE

3.CLUSTER HEAD ACHE

4.BENIGN PAROXYMAL HEAD ACHE

5.HEAD ACHE ASSOCITED WITH OTHER DISEASE

6MEDICINE OVER USE HEAD ACHE

Tension headache

this is the very common head ache.

the pain is usually constant and generalized but often radiates forward from the occipital region.

pain described by the patient as tightness, pressure or a band round the head or pressure at the vertex

pain will be continuous for weeks or months without any interruption.

patient continue the work with the pain, patient feels better when doing work or diverting their mind.

pain is less severe in the early part of the day pain worse as the day goes on.

patient will take many painkillers without much changes.

The head ache often associated with anxiety, depression, over stress.

Management With Homeopathy :

tension head ache is very simple head ache there is no deep-seated pathological condition behind that so the affected person no need to worry about much.

affected person learn to over come the stress
(by stress reliving exercises, relaxing outing, entertain themselves in sports, doing yoga) & learn to live happily & positive thinking and approach)

homeopathic medicines are reliving the headache and prevents the recurrence of the attack.it reduces the stress and make the individual to withstand the stressful situation.

(lac defloratum, silicia, spigelia, natrum mur , nux vomica ,argentum nitricum ,,,,,,,,,,,,,,, etc)

100 % cure is possible in the tension headache.

Migraine

head ache is a very common symptom. how we can say the head ache is migraine.

1.paroxysmal head ache(periodical head ache) one side or some times both sides.
2.vomiting
3.focal neurological symptom(like blurred vision)   if these 3 symptoms are present in a person then it is a classic migraine. but however, in majority migraine is presented like paroxysmal head ache with or without vomiting,but no focal neurological symptom.   course of the migraine-affected person feels tiredness and irritability,then the aura will come (some unpleasant subjective sensation like seeing zig zag lights,unpleasant smell,or confusion etc,,this aura premonitory the individual that he is going to get the head

ache) then severe throbbing hemicranial head ache with photo phobia and vomiting.head ache will be ok after the vomiting,but some body will not get relief even after vomiting.

during the head ache patient prefer to be in quit,darkened room,and go to sleep.there is often the migraine will run from the family.in some individual migraine will come during menses time,after taking cheese,chocolate or red wine.

even if the person is having stress the migraine will come at the end of the stress so migraine attack common in the beginning of the holidays or the week end.
homeopathy and migraine: surprisingly the standard medical textbook describe the migraine in the very similar way how the homeopath approach the patient in all other disease like how the head ache will starts what exactly the sensation and what are all the factors makes the head ache worse and better.

homeopathic medicines completely cures the migraine with very short span of duration since the migraine is very severe and the symptoms or freshly remembered by the patient so the co operation from the patient side will be good so the elimination of the migraine also very simple.homeopathic medicines prevent the genetic tendency.

the caution to be taken when the head ache is always in the same side (right) it never moves on other side or never comes on left side not even a single time then patient need to evaluated and then treatment is directed on this direction. sensory symptoms or common then the weakness of the limbs if the patient complain that then the diagnosis might be hemiplegic migraine.

WHO (World Health organization) view about

head aches:

Key facts

Headache disorders are among the most common disorders of the nervous system.

It has been estimated that 47% of the adult population have headache at least once within last year in general.

Headache disorders are associated with personal and societal burdens of pain, disability, damaged quality of life and financial cost.

A minority of people with headache disorders worldwide are diagnosed appropriately by a health-care provider.

Headache has been underestimated, under-recognized and under-treated throughout the world.

Barriers To Effective Care.

Lack of knowledge among health-care providers is the principal clinical barrier. Worldwide, on average only four hours of undergraduate medical education are dedicated to instruction on headache disorders. The minority of individuals with headache disorders worldwide are professionally diagnosed; 40% for those with migraine and TTH, while for MOH it is only 10%.

Poor awareness extends to the general public. Headache disorders are not perceived by the public as serious since they are mostly episodic, do not cause death, and are not contagious. The low consultation rates in developed countries may indicate that many sufferers are unaware that effective treatments exist. 50% of people with headache are estimated to be self-treating.

Many governments, seeking to constrain health-care costs, do not acknowledge the substantial burden of headache on society. They might not recognize that the direct costs of treating headache are small in comparison with the huge indirect-cost savings that might be made (eg, by reducing lost working days) if resources were allocated to treat headache disorders appropriately.

Medication-overuse headache (MOH)

MOH is caused by chronic and excessive use of medication to treat headache.

MOH is the most common secondary headaches.

It may affect up to 5% of some populations, women more than men.

MOH is oppressive, persistent and often at its worst on awakening.

Taking homeopathy medicine will prevent the head ache from the beginning this will help in preventing the pain killer induced gastritis,kidney and liver disease. Headache is the one of the major reasons for taking pain killers.

Guillain barre syndrome

Rare confused inflammation disease but it has been accepted as post-inflammatory or post infections disease. But the doctor's name it is an autoimmune disorder.

The confused inflammation cells attack the nerve cells, and damages so there is group of symptoms. arises. these syndromes observed after the infections so that doctors identify this is as a post effect of a viral illness or autoimmune disease.

(But almost all the diseases are happening in a similar way but doctors missing the connection with the previous disease. since the complication disease arises many years after the main disease so it is not possible to suspect the past disease with present ailments.)

But here the history is clear that the present suffering arises immediately after the recent past illness.

Prescribing anti-inflammatory medicine causes spraying of the pro-inflammatory chemicals all over the body to attract the immune cells and misguide them as the nerve is the enemy that causes nerve damage by the immune cells.

Allopathy explanation excess cytokines and interleukins are inducing both cellular and humoral immunity. They target the nerve sheet as an enemy and attack and damages the entire nerve and cause paralysis and sensory abnormality. This is explained as autoimmunity.

I am explaining the cytokines and other pro-inflammatory chemicals are normal natural inflammatory mediators of the past inflammation or immunity they distracted from the circulation roaming all over the body and stimulate the humoral and cellular immunity to act so they attack the nerves.

The cytokine or other inflammation / immune-stimulating chemicals are excess in the body (?) is considered as some genetic malformation or some other unknown factor but I am saying this is wandering chemical mediators of the past infection or inflammation. So, it is not an autoimmune disease this is the immune and inflammation distraction induced disease. This disease is one of the good examples of confused inflammation disease since past illness and present disease is happening in a short duration.

Clinical Symptoms

paralysis and sensory loss and reflexes are diminished.

low blood pressure or hypertension.

A preceding gastrointestinal infection like diarrhea and vomiting or some cold and flu-like illness.

Prevention of the disease possible by stop prescribing any medicine against the infections and inflammation. what will be remedy if the person catches the disease there are good homeopathic medicine for handling this disease but it is unideal to expose ourself as a trial since it is series life-threatening disease suppose if the nerve cells of the heart and blood vessel seriously affected heartbeat and blood pressure everything collapse so the patient will die. So prevent the disease. once the disease started then difficult to cure by any system.

Myasthenia gravis

One of the confused inflammations disorder this inflammation destroys the neuromuscular junction so that paralysis occur.

Explanation by allopathy : The neuromauscular junction is damaged by antibody. Acytyle choline receptors are destroyed by antibody but lymphocytes and antibody against the acetylcholine is not known.   belived that thymus may be the cause for production of self destruction antibody. Since the thymus is swellon and having tumor sometimes, so that it lost the power of preventing self destruction.

Explanation by me : destruction is due to presence of huge antibody which is available excessively due to prescription of antibody so that the confused antibody will be stuck anywhere or attracted by over active sites and creates the disease.Hyperactivity of thymus due to long continused excess production of antibodies and regulation and training of thymus so that hypertrophy. (continues antibody production ? due to no completion signal from a antibody produced already so that continues antibody production is heappening. All this happen due to completion of work by antibiotic so body assumes that the germs not killed).

Doctors must respect the doctors doing work already.So internal doctors producing antibody, allopathy doctor prescribing antibiotic so this antibiotic killed the bacteria , so now antibody not having work is roming within the circulation and produces many damages.

Missile is produced to destroy if bacteria is not there now (killed by anti bacterial) so it will be destroying our body. Yes, it was sended with education not to destroy the body ok but the body cells are behaving like enemy due to endo toxicity or antigen circulating within the body (in anti bacterial kill the bacteria but not remove the antigenic property of the bacteriaya) is attached to the body cells like nerve cells or blood cells or any tissues within the body.

But most of the time it is not just a antibody only directly destracting the body tissues there is always induction of the inflammation and immune system and started destroying the body tissues. This is just trigger the immune system by inflammation system.

The usual trigger of the inflammation or immunity always there is an enemy or germs (virus or bacteria) then inflammation activated and then the inflammation is activating immune system. So in every immune and inflammation disease we are searching the enemy like bacteria or virus because that is normal inflammation and immune system so there is no such enemy or germs that's why many disease is fall under unknown etiology but inflammation will induce immunity is happening here that every doctors know that but again the question is why the inflammation is coming that is distracted from past inflammation. So, either cellular or humoral immunity activation in all the auto immune and other immune and inflammation disorders are initiated by circulating confused or distracted inflammation. Here the same incidence is happenining.

Diplopia ptosis and weakness and tiredness is happening especially after continues work the complaints worse in the evenining or after heavy work better by taking rest.

Preventable by stopping anti inflammatory medicines. Stopping inflammation and distracting the inflammation.

Seizure & Epilepsy

Globally 5 crore epilepsy patients are there. Every year 50 lakh new cases diagnosed.non of the cases is cured so the burden the burden increases every year. Since there is no cure for epilepsy in allopathy.

Epilepsy is one of the non communicable,chronic,neuralogical disease.

Abnormal and excess stimulation of the nerve cells causes seizures. The cause for the epilepsy in space occupying lesions and other. But the true cause behind this seizure are confused inflammation even in tumor and space occupying lesions. The first and basic significant symptom confused inflammation entry is sezure. The insignificant vague cns involovement is twitchings and tremblings,numbness and tingling sensations, giddiness, ,,,etc.

Most of the people highly scared of convulsion and epilepsy even highly educated people are much scared about epilepsy. One among the top most reason for taking long time medication and in some individual life long medicines in allopathy. febrile fitz cases demanded to have anti epileptics throught the childhood period by few allopathic doctors.

If the child is suffering with febrile fits then the parents are scared both for fits as well as for the fever, So, for every single degree of fever elevation parents give the paracetomol syrub to the kids and antibiotics top most reason for over drugging (Any disease which demand the hospital admission of the child makes the parents panic so they over drug the child to prevent another hospital admission, because of this they stop all inflammation prematurely before it complete the work not only the patient all the allopathy doctors in the same stress when the patient comes they have to prove the efficiant doctor by stopping the inflammation when the febrile symtoms are not stopped then the doctor considered as he is inefficient so doctors prescribe from the day one strong antibiotic and steroids and heavy anti pyeretics to gain the confidence of the patient).

When the confused inflammation reached to the brain if possible, to create the local disease then it makes the local disease like abscess or tumor or any other disease and produce local [focal] epileptic seizures. generalized seizures happen due to histamine or inflammatory chemicals sprayed all over the brain and get simultaneous accentuation to produce epilepsy.

Loss of sleep , excess brain works or excess bodily work causes to trigger the confused inflammation reach the brain so that either it will produce epilepsy immediately or it make the epilepsy when other suitable time.

Sun stroke or exposure to heavy sun heat invite the confused inflammation to the brain. The first episode of fainting may invite the confused inflammation to the brain but the real epilepsy may come here after for many triggers not necessarily the same it can be any slight exaggeration of the brain functions like over study, loss of sleep , skipping the meals, over strain in general, fevers, infections, injuries, cold bathing, sun exposure any unusual or even usual events make the generalized epilepsy.

We can compare dermographism or generalized atopic dermatitis to brain involvement of histaminase.it means in dermographisam or the genralised skin inflammation is giving the clue to the spread of the confused inflammation all over the body skin surface in the same time the confused inflammation can also spreaded all over the brain and meninges. Some time both brain (mind + central nuralogical affection) and bodily ailmens produced by confused inflammation or if the trigger is strong enough to produce the diseae in the body then the confused inflammation moves from the brain and produce local disease . or if the stimulus strong enough in the brain then bodily aimlents shift from body to brain all the confused inflammation produce the ailments in the brain.

The development of the disease have almost always local pathology like if it is in the brain then nuron and axons and local immune system produce the symptoms if it is with the body then blood cells or some tissues are damaged or some organ tissues are damaged , and generalized immune system also activate but in all the case the trigger almost always confused inflammation.

The excess histamine induces the local skin disease (folds of the body parts) when the disease helped to grow further by prescribing antihistamine then whole of the skin in general affected. In the similar fashion the histamine and other inflammatory chemicals sprayed all over the brain and it will create confused inflammation which is producing generalized seizure.But it is not like a meningitis, epilepsy most insignificant then meningitis, like some discoloration in the skin (which is confused inflammation).

Sensing that epilepsy is going to happen by the patient is called aura (this aura other then brain symptoms explain association of the presence of confused inflammation or / and presence of confused inflammation in the particular location of the higher centers in the brain like visual hallucination or auditory hallucinations indicates that the presence of confused inflammation in the occipital visual area or temporal auditory area.

Epilepsy will develop so earlier and quicker than any other neurological disease since immediate suppression of the cold the histamine or other inflammatory chemicals spraying happening in both body and brain, so possibility of prevention is less. But it's easy to cure. The prevention is highly possible if stop using anti-inflammatory and anti allergic drugs and other unscientific medication.

Generalaised epilepsy develops due to inflammatory chemicals spareyed over the brain.focal epilepsy developes due to development of structural diseases by distracted inflammation or trauma.

Epilepsy Caused By

PRIMARY-Confused inflammation disease
secondary -asscited other disease again indirectly caused by

confused inflammation (like tumor abcess) truama,bleeding disorders,asphyxia etc.

Prevention Of The Epilepsy

At present there is no cure for epilepsy. Prevention of birth injury with precaution and avoiding accidents prevents the epilepsy (less then 15 % epilepsy) Remaining all the epilepsy is caused by bad inflammation directly and indirectly.

Homeopathy medicine will prevent the epilepsy related with bad inflammation and also prevent all the future nurological disease.prevention is possible upto 90 %. The 10-15 related with congenital and accident related death.

MULTIBLE SCLEROSIS [MS]

Multible sclerosis is more common in America, Australia and is less common in Asian country. Probable observation and explanation for this ailment is less sun exposure increases the risk of vitamin D - 25 Deficinancy this is blamed as the risk factor for development of this disease.

MS is more common in femal then male the reason belived is female using sunscreen creams or lotion prevent the proper sun exposure so this is favores the MS.

Earlier exposure to virus infection lesser the possibility of the MS and upper-class people is having more possibility of MS ? this observation says hygiens and away from infections increase the risk of MS.

There is another survey in the twins is giving many observations.

If we keep observing in varies probability ,then we will have so many useless observations. yes, like age sex geographical.But the main core cause for the disease limit our unnnessory unusual explanation and disprove our false belives. Yes.

Multible sclerosis is one of the distracted immune disease.

The t cells and b cells presence in the multible sclerosis is considered as the T cell stimulation is happen just for induce this multible sclerosis.this is not true since the T and B cell activation could be in any disease to attack the virus or becateria since we have medicine to disttact the continuity of the inflammation and immune funtions.But in multible sclerosis damage of the myeline sheet is , the distracted inflammation will start damage the mayelin then the inflammation stimulate immunity T and B Lymphocytes takes active part in this myeline destruction.

Involving TNF and OTHER interlukins will be in the same way.

The remission and relapse is the usual in many chronic Distracted inflammation / immunity due to this INFL/IMMUN will easily distracted by the strong another stimulai and run away to induce one more disease or if the stimulai is not strong enough to make the damage then the disease will stop then if the stimulai enough then the disease will continue.

In psoriyasis the remission and relapse are happen in summer disease will be in relapse and if the winter comes the disease will start again here the external stinulation is the winter cold.similarly the multible sclerosis is getting remission and relapse.

My dear doctor there are disease in the body there are disease like process in the body we have to understand that first.

We observe generally some criteria for each disease like cause,course,recovery,complications, pathophysiology and pathology like that we assume every disease is happenining in the same way so that you think that there is cause for every disease so you are failed to identify that so that waiting or doing research based this. The direction is wrong so the result may be wrong or right you may not go to find it because your search is like that.

First of all, multible sclerosis or asthma or psoriyasis or rheumatoid arthiritis etc diseases are not a true disease so we connot expect every protocal of the normal disease here. Then how to handle this disease read the cherecter of the distracted inflammation and then do observation and then observe all other perameter or protocol for each disease separately.

For example, psoriyasis or multible sclerosis or not a true disease so we observe one typical finding here the location of the disease is cns and more specifically myelin sheet.just right cause is not necessary since this is a Distracted inflammation/ immune disease or simple write cause is Distracted inflammation / immunity is the cause.

An infection is a true disease or if really a deficiency or toxins or excess chemical ingetion and related diseases are true disease ,it means a body will protect from these dangers and produce true disease mostly success if the offender is strong enough then recovery delaye (true chronic disease) or patient death.

What we have in hand (multible sclerosis or asthuma or rhuematisam is not a true disease all of this disease has been arises due to distracting the inflammation it means from disease to another disease) we connot keep this is even as a complication. why because complications again a true disease in most of the cases.the disease arising from dist infl/immune is having clear cut cause the cause is DIS-

TRACTING THE INFLAMMATION /IMMUNTY don't search for the cause again.(only verify what I am saying is true or not).

Understand this D infl / imun may have power to produce any disease within body .it is the greatest surprice for me in the early my observations yes the distracted neutrophil or inflammation chemicals get stimulated and produce disease either in skin or bone or in the brain or in the genitals.This observation is highly importand because we study and expect different cause for different disease and we study in detail of the anatomy of each organ of our body because we can trace the cause but here I distracted inflammation in the nose can give disease in the brain or anywheare in the body.

We are observed and studying very limited harming agent as a risk factor like smoking or alcohol or eating cholesterol and actually we missed to trace many external environment and internal factor influencing this distracted inflammation and causing disease.it means the real risk factor is not taken for consideration for example Doctors can consider a contaminated water makes the cold but patient drinks the pure highly purified but chill water can make head ache and cold is not been observed and added within the medical text a person drinking pure mineral water but the hot water can able to produce cold or head ache is not been included within the medical text book but patient is observaing this facts and keep complaining about this but the allopathy doctor always having in his mind that what you drunk is a contaminated water nothing more then that.

I have explained highly purified cold water can attract this distracted inflammation and immunity and produce the disease or cold attack this is actually a risk factor for cold.

A modifying factor for a disease has to be

observed. The pathology and pathophysiology of the distracted inflammation has to read in different way then normal pathology and pathophysiology since pathophysiology of the normal disease can explain the influence of the germs and body simultaneasly how makes the destruction in the tissues and we observe it but in contrast in the distracted inflammation or the immunity how the protective inflammation / imun alone makes the destruction dont name this dieases as auto immune name the disease doctors induced auto immunity.first of all don't use the word immunity and destructing immunity this makes strong conviction of the doctors to blame immunity as a enemy.all the pathology and pathophysiology now narrowed as or limited to only about Distracted inflammation and immunity.why we have to study special way then normal study since pathophysiology of the distracted inflammation has some unique character which is again a good research you already did but the research but interpretation is wrong (your beliving inflammation and Distracted inflammation is same) so there is no idea for many disease why this is happen why the atopic dermatitis always choose flexor as a site of origin and you don't know why there is remission and relapse many disease (distracted inflammation). Unless you think this is as distracted inflammation your research will not be succeed. You have completed many researches and having lots of discovery but only one thing is missing that is called wrong interpretation and wrong understating is collapsing your observations.

Keep prescribing external applications and distracting the inflammation where ever they surface causes more deeper organ damage.infact the D infl disease having tendency to develop disease in both side both in brain and body but we keep prescribing the medicines for bodily diseases especially skin and respiratory illness causes complete shifting of the disease towards brain or only central nervous sytem disease in the middle and old age people.

Multible sclerosis : cause : Distracted inflammation / immunity.

Targeted organ and tissue : mayline sheet of the nerve cells.

Basic pathology : mayaline destruction and regeneration of the mayeline sheet with sclerosis.

Basic cells present : T cell and B cell . Present explanation for the destruction of the myeline is the myeline protein is act as a antigen for the T cells so that T cell induce the inflammation over there.

My explanation : T cell and B cell both or distracted immune cells.They are get attracted towards mayline cells by antigen property attached with mayelin sheets (this is favored by anti bacterial since bacteria killed but not completely removed from the circulation) or eroded and destroyed by the inflammation first then the immune cells induced and attacks mayaline sheets attacked by T AND B CELLS.

Since body never invite the immune cells to attacke our own body cells the distracted immune cells will be guided any over activity rather then waiting for true virus or bacteria. (THE PRIMARY LEARNED BEHEVIAR IS HIGHLY APPLICABLE FOR A TRUE INFLAMMATION/IMMUNITY. ONCE THE CELLS ARE DISTRACTED FROM THE MAIN FOCUS THEN THESE CELL (IMMUNE) ARE READY TO DAMAGE THE BODY CELLS THIS IS BECAUSE THE TARGETED ORGAN IS REMOVED BUT THE CELLS ARE NOT WITHDRAWN SO THEY ATTACK THE TARGETED ENEMY OR BODY CELLS NOW .THE ONLY THING NEEDED NOW IS NEED ANTIGEN OR ANTIGEN LIKE PROPERTY.

Aim of management : stopping the auto destruction and eliminating or withdrawing the all distracted inflammation from the circulation (this will prevent another auto immune disease.

Why management ? because no idea what disease it is and who is the cause for it not detectable and the belive that inflamm/immunity is doing that so having medicines to controle so allopathy controle and manage that rather then curing it.

Clincal Future

Diplopia,dimness of vision,blurring of the vision,tingling sensation,hyperesthesia ,depression,sexual weakness,Muscle spasm,bladder dysfunction is there, memory loss, difficulties in excutive function,weakness ,,,,, etc.

What is the new management plant for multible sclerosis?

Since we identify the cause we can cure these rather then managing the disease.

Who sended these cells is recommended to withdraw these cells so that sure there is no further damage of mayaline sheet damage.what else ,if the homeopathy medicine rightly stimulated the regeneration will happen without any break or sclerosis so there by the healing will happen normally cure is possible?.if the nerve damage and sclerosis is too heavy and irreversible then we can only prevent the furdher damage of the axon and prevention of auto immunity further that's all.

PREVENTION OF THIS DISEASE IS BY AVOIDNG INTERUPTING INFLAMMATION AND AVOIDING THE LOCAL APPLICATIONS FOR SKIN DISEASE AND RESPIRATORY ILLNESS.SECONDARY OR TERTIARY LEVEL OF PREVENTION IS CURING THE SICKNESS BY HOMEOPATHY MEDICINE AS EARLY AS POSSIBLE AND PREVENTING AUTO

IMMUNE DISEASE.ALLOWING SUN EXPOSURE WITH AL-LOWING SKIN DISEASE TO SURFACE AND INVITING THE CONFUSED INFLAMMATION TO PRODUCE DISEASE IN THE SUPERFICIALY THEN DEEP VITAL ORGANS.

Parkinson disease (PD)

Allopathy point of view of parkinson disease:

Parkinson's disease (PD) is a neurodegenerative disorder that affects predominately dopamine-producing ("dopaminergic") neurons in a specific area of the brain called substantia nigra.

- one million people in the United States and ten million (1 crore) people worldwide affected by this disease.

- The Centers for Disease Control and Prevention (CDC) rated complications from PD as the 14th cause of death in the United States.

- It is possible to have a good to great quality of life with PD. Working with your doctor and following recommended therapies are essential in successfully treating symptoms by using dopaminergic medications. People with PD need this medication because they have low levels or are missing dopamine in the brain, mainly due to impairment of neurons in the substantia nigra.

•   Scientists are exploring ways to identify biomarkers for PD that can lead to earlier diagnosis and more tailored treatments to slow down the disease process.

•   Incidence of Parkinson's disease increases with age, but an estimated four percent of people with PD are diagnosed before age 50.

•   Men are 1.5 times more likely to have Parkinson's disease than women.

•   Medications alone cost an average of $2,500 (Aproximately 2.07 lakh INR/ year) a year and therapeutic surgery can cost up to $100,000 per person.

Information gathered in the official web page of - Parkinson foundation – USA.

Clinical future

- Tremer when at rest
- stiffness (rigidity) due to this stiffness over all movements is slow (so impairement in gait and balance.

- speech difficulty (soft low voice)
- masked face (expression is less in face)
- stooping
- non-motor symptoms include: apathy, depression, constipation, sleep behavior disorders, loss of sense of smell and cognitive impairment, this disease progress in to dementia.

My View Of Parkinson Disease

One of the neurological disease due to confused inflammation but usually gives their symptoms in the elderly so we have enough time to prevent Parkinson disease.

Risk is more in Rural living and exposure to pesticide drinking well water (?) all this observed could be a risk factor but not found true cause. The neurologist thinking it could be due to genetic or environmental or both.

The degeneration heppaning here similar to end part (destructing and apoptosis of the damaged cells) of the normal inflammation process. In this disease the major pathology in short is degeneration. Brain Cell death is the final degeneration, like apoptosis and mass cell death is happenining. So, this degeneration cause loss of dopaminergic nurons in the substantia nigra, this neuronal loss is also occurred in locus ceruloses, raphy nucleus. This neuron loss causes loss of control over the movements so tremer and stiffness.

The cause for Parkinson disease is till now unknown but the pathological future observed as a degenerative disease, degeneration of the brain parts (like substantia nigra,putamen, globus pallidum ,,, etc).

A true inflammation will never give only degeneration, if the inflammation degenarates then sure regeneration follows then there is no disease at all. But it's a confused inflammation disorder so only degeneration.

A simultaneuse pathological changes happen in most of the cases in the brain and body but mostly the exposed parts get quick attension for remedy even tiny mm level spotes in the skin get medical attension quickly even though it is not giving any symptoms no pain no itching. If that brain changes not having any symptoms then that will be ignored by many times by both patient and doctors. This is the reson the Parkinson disease get medical attension only after complete degeneration.(pain,cunvulsions and unconscitiousness, numbness all will get quick attension by a patient then tremer most of the time patient post pone meeting the doctors but the current trend is changed)

So, this is one among the ignored degeneration disease of the brain.

Why inflammation ? what is the other finding here to say this is inflammation how we will say this is inflammation.why some poisoning or some other complaints.

Distracted inflammation with degeneration producing chemicals So degeneration chemicals carried through the blood vessals and attracted within the basal ganglia and substantia nigra so there by slow and gradual degeneration of the neuron and producing clinical symptoms in the late age or in the middle age. dont suspect something may or may not be. give priority to strongly what we did. This is like research we distracted inflammation and imunitty all the people in the world and now we are studying what happen to them .

ok . we are not sure weather the patient is exposed to environmental toxin or not similarly not sure about the genetics but we did distraction of inflammation and the degeneration and regeneration all is a part of inflammation. IF POISONING IS DESTROYED SOME PART THEN BODY MUST

REGENERATE THE PART AFFECTED AND REMOVED IT WHY IT IS NOT HAPPEN WHY THERE IS NO PROTECTIVE FUNCTION HEPPEN HERE.BECAUSE THE THE DESTRUCTION OF SELF NEVER BEEN STOPPED BY THE BODY AND NEVER BEEN REPAIRED BY THE BODY.

So, screen the people more early age for neuran degeneration.there is good homeopathy medicine for curing the neuron damage in early degenaration.

AVOIDING THE MEDICATION TO DISTRACT AND STOP THE INFLAMMATION WILL PREVENT THE PARKINSON DISEASE.Eliminating the confused inflammation will prevent the disease.

Most of the neurological diseases are happen due to shifting confused inflammation from nose or ear or from scalp or face inflammatory diseases.avoid giving unscientific treatment.if you do this inflammation sure will shift to the brain and do many diseases.

Self medication or taking help of specialist are increasing especially for cosmetic and ent diseases repeated strong administration fo drugs and will not allow the disease surface in the skin of face is so common now a days any small pimples and scars or the pigments worrying the people so they try varies pharmacy products or meet the doctor they hide it then only they rest.

Allopathy is so keen in observation and they study ultra micro study in studying all basic subject like anatomy physiology and pathology and patho physiology but these things is not reflecting in the treatment. Totally unscientific approach for the treatment do anything to hide the disease hide it that's all is the final aim. Due to this attitude everything is collapses.

DEMENTIA

simple diagram explains the brain and psychological disease possibility.

Distracted inflammation in the head & brain shifts to body and make the disease so the people will have less possibility of brain disease and dementia.

This picture explains more distracted inflammation from all over the body has moved to brain is having high possibility of brain and nerve cells disease and high possibility of dementia in future.

World Health Organisation EXPLNATION AND PREVENTION PROGROME FOR THE DEMANTIA.

· **Although dementia mainly affects older people, it is not a normal part of ageing. Worldwide, around 50 million (5 crore) people have dementia, and there are nearly 10 million new cases every year.**

Dementia is a syndrome – usually of a chronic or progressive nature – in which there is deterioration in cognitive function (i.e. the ability to process thought) beyond what might be expected from normal ageing. It affects memory thinking, orientation, comprehension, calculation, learning capacity, language and judgement. Consciousness is not affected. The impairment in cognitive function is commonly accompanied and occasionally preceded by deterioration in emotional control, social behaviour, or motivation.

Dementia results from a variety of diseases and injuries that primarily or secondarily affect the brain, such as Alzheimer's disease or stroke.

Dementia is one of the major causes of disability and dependency among older people worldwide. It can be overwhelming, not only for the people who have it, but also for their carers and families.

Signs and symptoms:

Early stage: the early stage of dementia is often overlooked, because the onset is gradual.

- Forgetfulness
- Losing track of the time
- Becoming lost in familiar places.

Middle stage: as dementia progresses to the middle stage, the signs and symptoms become clearer and more restricting. These include:

- Becoming forgetful of recent events and people's names
- Becoming lost at home
- Having increasing difficulty with communication
- Needing help with personal care
- Experiencing behaviour changes, including wandering and repeated questioning.

Late stage: the late stage of dementia is one of near total dependence and inactivity. Memory disturbances are serious and the physical signs and symptoms become more obvious.

- becoming unaware of the time and place
- having difficulty recognizing relatives and friends
- having an increasing need for assisted self-care
- having difficulty walking
- experiencing behaviour changes that may escalate and include aggression.

Common forms of dementia

There are many different forms of dementia.

Alzheimer disease is the most common form (60–70% of cases)

vascular dementia.

dementia with Lewy bodies

frontotemporal dementia

The total number of people with dementia is projected to reach 82 million in 2030 and 152 in 2050.

Treatment And Care

There is no treatment currently available to cure dementia or to alter its progressive course. Numerous new treatments are being investigated in various stages of clinical trials.

However, much can be offered to support and improve the lives of people with dementia and their carers and families. The principal goals for dementia care are:

early diagnosis in order to promote early and optimal management

optimizing physical health, cognition, activity and well-being

identifying and treating accompanying physical illness

detecting and treating challenging behavioural and psychological symptoms

providing information and long-term support to carers.

Risk Factors And Prevention

Although age is the strongest known risk factor for dementia, it is not an inevitable consequence of ageing. Further, dementia does not exclusively affect older people – young onset dementia (defined as the onset of symptoms before the age of 65 years) accounts for up to 9% of cases. Studies show that people can reduce their risk of dementia by getting regular exercise, not smoking, avoiding harmful use of alcohol, controlling their weight, eating a healthy diet, and maintaining healthy blood pressure, cholesterol and blood sugar levels, Additional risk factors include depression, low educational attainment, social isolation, and cognitive inactivity.

Social And Economic Impact

Dementia has significant social and economic implications

in terms of direct medical and social care costs, and the costs of informal care. In 2015, the total global societal cost of dementia was estimated to be US$ 818 billion, equivalent to 1.1% of global gross domestic product (GDP).

Impact on families and carers

Dementia can be overwhelming for the families of affected people and for their carers. Physical, emotional and financial pressures can cause great stress to families and carers, and support is required from the health, social, financial and legal systems.

Human Rights

People with dementia are frequently denied the basic rights and freedoms available to others. In many countries, physical and chemical restraints are used extensively in care homes for older people and in acute-care settings, even when regulations are in place to uphold the rights of people to freedom and choice.

An appropriate and supportive legislative environment based on internationally-accepted human rights standards is required to ensure the highest quality of care for to people with dementia and their careers.

My View Upon The Dementia

Dementia is like brain failure, that also end part of the all the inflammation and destruction damages the brain slowly and produce the dementia. So, preventing the dementia is is not possible or the hard task. It is possible and easy to prevent Parkinson and vascular diseases by alloaing the inflammation and removing inflammation remenents. So, it is possible we can prevent dementia. The future projection of dementia burden is completely possible to destroy. It means we can make a zero-dementia case in future then present heavy dementia possibility.

So, when we prevent all minor and major ailments of the brain disease then there is no dementia. Like in kidney failure we should not worry about the kidney failure and how to treat it more then that we have to treat the disease which causes and initiate the kidney failure. So, we are not giving the possibility of the failure of any organ more then worriying about the treatment and prevention of orgon failure. Clearing confused inflammation is the best way of preventing all the disease possibility sub acute and chronic inflammatory / auto immune disease so that no dementia in future.

The dementia related awareness given by WHO stress us to take inititive towards dementia. WHO observe only or majorly allopathic standpoint and homeopathy is having many good remedies to prevent the dementia and the diseases which causes the dementia?

Most of the time either public or the even the doctors will be curies what remedy will cure dementia. This education again we trained from allopathic medicine consumtion. so that if you say one medicine, they will try to use that medicine as a triel if it is not helped then they through that.

Just read the given point this will help how we are going to prevent and treat the dementia.

Prevention Of The Dementia :

Dementia gives the more then sufficient time to prevent the disease. our duty is to prevent the diseases in general so that dementia will be prevented. like preventing alzmeirs Disease,vascular disease and frontoparital disease.

It is something new we are going to read then the basic pathology which is causing the disease,which we have read many time in this book   Distracting the inflammation and immunity as well as the wound healing is the cause for dementia so strictness regarding the treatment plan is very importand.when the inflammation is allowed to carry normal then less possibility of distracted inflammation diseases (alzmeirs disease,vascular disease,,,,,)

If the inflammation is distracted already has to remove from the body.

Allowing the distracted inflammation to create skin disease and removing distracted inflammation without any external applications especially ear, eye, facial , scalp disease highly limit the possibility of the brain disease limit the metastasis of the bodily disease towards brain.

Since brain is the most protected body parts most of the wandering distracted cells choose all over the skin and joints and external body parts first then brain ,if the brain is having any inflammation or distracted inflammation disease then we have to support the true inflammation to carry out successfully and we have to remove the distracted inflammation from the brain is the aim of the treatment.

Any head injury and brain damage invite the confused inflammation to the brain so need to remove the confused inflammation. Preventing confused inflammation and removing that will prevent alzemier as well as Parkinson disease, atherosclerosis.

Reducing the smoking and reducing and stopping

alcohol usage and other substance abuse will minimize and help in preventing atherosclerosis and other psychological disease and brain diseases.

Exposure to allopathy drugs going to reduce massively will reduce drug induced nerve cells damages sure will prevent known and unknonw brain cells damages in future.The same cause will prevent the early kidney and liver damages so that there is less possibility of internal toxicity and following internal organ failures including brain damage.

Most of the early brain and psychological disease curable by homeo medicine. this will reduce the possibility of the brain disease and dementia in future.

RIGHTLY CHOOSEN HOMEO MEDICINE WILL CURE THE EARLY BRAIN DISEASES SO THAT IT WILL PREVENT DEMENTIA.HOMEO MEDICINE WILL HELP IN PREVENTING AND TREAT EARLY DEMENTIA CASES AND POST PONE THE RAPIDITY OF THE DISEASE.

The diseases are metastasis from one organ to other organ and the diseases are caused by distracted inflammation and immunity nothing more then that I hope we now have the enough knowledge about how to prevent the disease. Regulating inflammation of the brain and regulating inflammation of the skin and regulation of the inflammation of the kidney etc are not different all are same.Doctors don't panic to handle brain and central nervous system.all we are going to just regulating inflammation and immunity that's all.

The history of repeted external applications and strong allopathic medicines will

15.BLOOD DISORDERS

aplastic or proliferative disease of the blood cells.

When the confused inflammation attacks the blood cell producing organs (bone marrow and lymphoid organs) causes more cell production due to that congetion within the bonemarrow and tenderness.But this hyperfunctins followed by less cell's productions if the confused inflammation still attacks severely then the blood cell production will be exceedinly low.

    1.   The bone marrow attack of confused inflammation will be marked in the childrens since there is a possibility of high and recurrent infections so need to produce excess cells (hyper functions).

2.			The bone development will be marked in childrens so that bone and bone marrow part is busy with hyper perfusion of blood so that childrens prone to get more bone and bone marrow disease then adult and elders.bone infections like osteomyelitis and even blood related cancers are more in childrens.

3.			The childrens are reciving too much of allopathic medicines (is act as a chemical exposure causes stress to the confused inflammation sites will easily turn into cancer sites).but allopathy doctors diverting the world as if the child is exposing ionizing radiation and so many chemicals and genetics this and that as cause of diseases and cancer.

The top most cause of blood cancer is Confused inflammation , confused inflammation created by allopathic medicines.

If the blood cells producing organs been infiltrated by excess fibrous tissues or waste material causes slow under production to nil production and necrosis of the bone and tumor of the bones.

Demand and supply related fast production since the confused inflammation in many situations abnormally demand to produce more blood cells which is due to hypersensitivity, the scattered confused inflammation chemical get sensitivity to environment or touch or food so that every time when the person exposure to dust the confused inflammation gives the signals as if the enemy is enter inside the body so that particular inflammation cells will demanded to send excessively. Since the confused inflammation scattered all over the body so that this will have possibility of frequent and widespread sensitivity so that brain will receive repeated and unexhausting demand to produce excess blood cells.

Abnormally excess blood cells including immature cells in the circulation ? Considered as malignant.

When a foreign body or germ entry will initiate the inflammation so that cells within the circulation as well as stored white blood cells all will be accumulated to the site of infection and then generalized due to multiplication of germs.So, there by any germ or noxious agent entry will lead to excess accumulation of blood cells initially near the spots then all over the circulation in case the germ spreaded. this is a normal response.

When a confused chemo tactic chemical sprayed all over the body is started responding abnormally to all noxious as well as even normal external factors so that continues stimulus to produce massive cells as well as this will not going to stop and it is continues.This abnormal blood cells within the circulation in prolonged period causes varies diseases yet with fully matured normal but excess blood cells within circulations.

If this situation is continuing then the bone marrow cells attract confused inflammation all will lead to heavy stress to produce cells in excess for longer period causes malignant transformation leads to production of abnormal immature blood cells of the demanded type initially later all type of cells.

In other situation inclusion of confused inflammation cells into the bone marrow causes chronic confused inflammation of bone marrow causes production either excess blood cells or less to nil blood cell production.Splenomegaly may be due to over function to destroy this excess blood cells as well as need to work more to face excess germ entry due to poor immune status.THERE IS HUGE COLLECTION OF BLOOD CELLS WITHIN THE CIRCULATION YET THERE IS NO PROTECTIVE FUNCTIONS (BECAUSE IT'S A CONFUSED INFLAMMATION)

Lymph node enlargement is due to massive entry of germ inside the body so that lymph system works hyper then normal caused swollen lymph node.

There are specific cell proliferation is happen in some condition is explainable like interruption in particular of the inflammation, say for example neutrophil is ordered to produce excess by brain now we stop the inflammation so then brain may not receive the feedback that neutrophil work is complete so it will keep produce the neutrophil life long until reciving a feedback response. so here the inflammation terminated prematurely so that neutrophil production is excessive and ever ending causes leukemia especially neutrophilic predominant.

Similarly, excess lymphocytes will happen.

Immune related Anemia, Thrombocytopenia

•   Diseased bone marrow failed to produce effective blood cells leads to low blood cells count. BONEMARROW FAILURE.
•   Chronic Increased lysis in the spleen due to long standing chronic spleen inflammation.

Hemorrhage and hemorrhagic diathesiss :

Hemarrage, spontaneous bleeding occur in nose,piles,intestines due to varies resons,but the top most cause behind this bleeding is confused inflammation gives bleeding in many situation , especially early stage of inflammatory chemicals, that will make vaso dilatations and vessel wall damage and bleeding.continuese presentation of this one stage alone gives the impression as if the bleeding disorder.A chronic confused inflammation of the nose gives the bleeding from the nose.gives the bleeding now and then but there may not be any progression like a inflammation in some cases but may progress into next stage of inflammation but throught the inflammation it remain as if it gives the bleeding.

Many ulcers bleed profusely, many skin eruptions warts bleed profusely or oozes due to confused inflammation super added with that.

When this stage is marked then bleeding happens in many places, like bleeding in nose, rectum or excess menses called hemorrhagic tendency.

When the low platelet also will produce the similar effect. [low platelet count is due to confused inflammation.

Anti phospholipid
antibody syndrome

When a injury is happening, bleeding will be there, this bleeding is arrested by means of clotting mechanisam with the help of platelet. When we apply any external medicine then the chemical involved in the clotting allowed inside the circulation then this makes *intravascular clotting.*

The accentuation of this chemicals during the hyper liberation of the pregnancy hormone induce the intra vascular clotes.

The presence of antibody against the phospholipid is invitation of the confused antibody which was readily available already is joining here to involove in this disease process.

Prevention :

Avoid applying and prescribing any external application, try to controle bleeding only in an emergency by applying mild ligature then applying ointments or medicated lotions. If it is mild wound then allow bleeding to stop automatically.

16. DIABETES

Nearly more then 60 crores (600 million) of world population having diabetes. Every year the number of cases is increasing gradually, in India nearly 2.5 lakh death annually. Nearly 12 lakhs to 22 lakhs people died of diabetes all over the world each year. The estimated number is too less then reality since there are massive group of people under diagnosed in the rural population . The urban people undergoing for frequent diabtes check up.

" Why the public and health sector and well wisher are cautious about diabetes. The top most reason is the fear about the complications of the diabetes like kidney failure. This fear is advertised in a fantastic slow and strong emotional way, like most popular persons lost their legs, leg was amputed due to excess sugar that person was not had their sugar tablets so he lost his legs and even he or she is dead this was the time in tamilnadu the anti diabetic tablets was sold like anything after making fear regarding the disease". so, the public are highly scared and most of the people are started consuming their diabetic tablets very regularly."

" Since there are lots of people are suffered with kidney failures our great quack [allopathy] even though does not know anything about the cause of disease including diabetes, he is very precisely announced to the world that diabetes is the cause for kidney failure " [kidney failure is caused by confused inflammation and confused allopathy induced auto immune disorders]

" when ever you are going for any surgery, he will ask your diabetes level, then he put you on heavy drugs to control and then he will do surgery. In this way he is made a fear about the diabetes and he helped pharma company to sale the diabetic tablet ".

Diabetes has to keep parameter for curing the confused inflammation. It is not going to do great harm then confused inflammation all the complications of diabetes are not created really the diabetes; it is created by confused inflammation.

When you suffer with any excess infection, he will check diabetes and he will inform to you that your sugar level is 400 to 450 that's why the infection. He will demand you to continue the diabetes tablets. Heavy infection and septicimea is always caused by confused inflammation. confused inflammation is always caused by allopathy doctors is the true reason, a infection is does not heal well the body struggle to controle and eliminate infection all caused by confused inflammation alone.

Diabetes will cause vision loss;diabetes will induce gangrene ;diabetes will produce cellulitis like that he is making so many intelligent stories about diabetes and scared the public in that way he asked entire universe to become allopathic pharma company slave. Nearly half of the elderly Indian population is suffering with diabetes and consuming diabetes tablets.

But the MBBS AND MD AND THE DIEBETIC SPE-CIALIST AND ENDOCRINOLOGIST does not know why the diabetes. No, one is trying to cure the diabetes. They will only manage the diabetes. It means the sugar level will be kept in controle with some medicine if some one is not responding to the drugs; they will be kept under insulin seriously the patient kept under insulin and uncontrollable diabetes teaches many things to the allopathic doctors but he refuses to see that lessons. He closes the chapter of dia-betes, by prescribing anti diabetic tablets, but the uncon-trollable diabetes is saying I am more then that but he is not listening that.

He is in the delusion that he saves the kidney failures by prescribing the anti-diabetic, he is saves the eye by prescribing anti diabetic, he prevents infection by prescribing anti diabetic. How it's the delusion ? the number of kidney failures gives the success rate, how beautifully he controlling and save the kid-ney ?, almost all the diabetics consuming the anti diabetic tablets but people fall in kidney failures increasing like anything.

" It means the confused inflammation is damages the the pancreases and peripheral tissues kidney and eye all over the body it makes the disease. This is the reverse research against the allopathic opinion he believes diabetes is causing the infec-tion that is not true. Confused inflammation is causing all the changes like cellulitis, gangrene, periphral neuritis, kidney fail-ure he utilized this chance to earn money." Diabetes is like a shield to protect and ecuse his mitake. Diabetes is most dangerus and make many sicknesses then why don't you prvent that " ? why you are not attempting to curing that. ERADICATION OF DIABETES IS POSSIBLE USE HOMEOPATHY MEDICINE

YOU HAVE TO BE IN DELUSION NO OTHER-WAY.YOU ARE NOT A PROFESSIONAL YOU ARE A SLAVE YOU ARE PREPARED TO SALE PHARMA PRODUCT YOU ARE DOING THAT EXCEEDINGLY WELL. SO, I AM GOING TO APPOINT DOCTOR FOR SAVE THE PEOPLE. BE PREPARE.

Type - 2 Diabetes

Entire world is in Allopathic era, it means you are handled by great quack, and surrounded by this qualified quack. So, we can ask ourself till we are not diagnosed as diabetes ? since allopathy doctors are doing many wrong treatment and unscientific approach to treat the disease high possibility is there to get diabetes.

1. I Have said that type 2 diabetes is due to poor utilization of the insulin due to misguided inflammation in the body. So that to supply enough sugar to that hypo glycemic cells, the pancrease is demanded to produce excess glucose. Here we can see in the blood excess sugar is excess but this is a adaptation to a demand (hypoglycemia of the peripheral cells).

2. Another cause: I cannot accept the observation that initial INSULIN excess so that it will destroy the remaining insulin secreting cells so that permanent complete or less secretary failures of insulin.

But THIS WILL HAPPEN ONLY WHEN THE INSULIN SECRETING CELLS ARE DAMAGED BY THE CONFUSED INFLAMMATION NOT NECESSARILY NEED GREAT PROOF OF THAT INFLAMMATION IT MIGHT HAPPEN SILENTLY. Similar to simple thyroiditis.

3.Confused inflammation of liver disease and pancreas disease CONTRIBUTE THE DIABETES MELLITUS.

My theory here is pancreatic cells are destroyed

due to chronic misguided inflammation. Then what is the proof ? what proof we have in simple thyroiditis [No ESR elevation, No antibody] minimal tenderness in the thyroid that's all. Even it is tough to elicit this tenderness in the pancrease. this inflammation may not be sufficient to make exocrine function failure. The beta cell inactivation is happening extremely minor confused inflammation changes. That is also partial working of the beta cells of the pancreases.if the pancrease is severely affected by confused inflammation then it gives the clue to us like auto immune thyroiditis with auto auto antibody in this auto immune pancrease is also having proof with auto antibody against the pancrease.

At least you have accepted there is an inflammation in thyroid which will come even without any inflammatory marker but I am observing number of misguided inflammatory disease which is yet to add.

I can give a minor proof that crp elevation in some obese diabetics. but it is not due to obesity. I have never come across in the physiology that obesity will produce inflammation so that elevation of crp (inflammatory marker) elevation. The researchers found crp elevation is supporting my theory but the thing is as they dont find any active inflammation they may blame fatty acids induce inflammation.

Increasing confused inflammation all over the body , reduces peripheral circulation by depositing micro dead cells and other waste materials along the blood vassals, silent vasculitis and destruction of the insulin receptors all will happen within the blood vessals and tissues, then diabetes develops as a demand related supply.

The peripheral tissue damages easily assed by the confused inflammation to the peripheral nerve causes peripheral neuritis. The micro vasculature failure and micro neural failure together create tissue damages cause disruption of self regulating mechanisam so that sugar level is increased in the circulation.

Type 1 and type 2 diabetes both are auto immune and inflammation disease only but the type 1 causes direct rapid and dominant action of the immune and inflammation cells targets directly to the pancrease insulin secreting cells so there by sugar level is increasing, but the type 2 diabetes confused inflammation mostlly targets all over the body tissues and micro blood supply and neural supply of the peripery and too some extend central organs it is highly slow process and directly related with severity of the whole body tissues. So, event though the peripheral damages are starting around the early childhood days diabtes diagnosed mostly early 40 peaks at 50-60 and then gradually increases.

Assessment Of Confused Inflammation In The Body By Diabetic Respons :

Sugar level stagnation at one point (usually less then 200 post prandial sugar level) responding well with anti diabetic drugs all indicates confused inflammation too less- mild case.

Slow and steady increasing sugar level elevation sugar level now and then high respond with medicine.occasinal need of insulin. Orgaon complication expected but mild and after long period of diabetes detection.   (indicate confused inflammation significant level)

Not responding with anti diabetic demand to more insulin therapy Severe complications rapid destruction of kidney and other parts indicates the confused inflammation is more.(severe confused inflammation within the body.

So, type 1 develops at any age especially in childhood and teen but type 2 is developing incidius onset too late age especially after 40 and diabetes is a MARKER OF CONFUSED INFLAMMATION. But this changes connot able to prove since it's a generalized and widespread can easily proved when the patient has typical chornic disease like ckd and gangrene in the extremity and visual impairement. (most exact cause)

4.Administration of sugar product other then oral route (iv administration of the sugar) will confuse the feed-back and controle mechanisam of the sugar metablisam will lead to initiation of carbohydrate metabolisam disorders. (refer failed feedback and controle mechanisam chapter) . (rare cause but don't try to give saline when there is no need)

5. Stopping the inflammation at the mid causes inability to recover the hyperfunction of pancrease. when the person suffer with hypoglycemia in fever and gastro in-testinal disease like vomiting and diarrhea the brain sense that demand the pancrease to secreate the excess glucose to meet the demand but one the patient recovered from fever and gastric disturbance if they started eat normally then the brain will sens that and withdraw the stimulation towards pancrease so that now the pancrease will produce normal insulin to controle the sugar metabolisam but when stop the inflammation OR other disease without consider-ing many supportive functions underneath the disease then pancrease functions left unrecovered so that excess sugar level in the blood.

6. Increasing functions of the pancreas in turn at-tract the confused inflammatory cells to the pancreas causes confused inflammation attack of the pancrease – chronic pancreatitis mostly targered attack of the islets of langar-hans cell in the pancrease over a period of time slow inflam-mation of all the cells of pancrease.

The treatment of diabetes has to be two way if the

serum insulin is absolutely normal then we have to search inflammatory foci and treat it and another step is to reset the inflammation in right direction all this is possible in HOMEOPATHY.

In this case anti diabetic is not necessary we have to keep the elevated sugar as a diabetic marker. if the sugar level is increased or decreased will gives as a clue to effectiveness of treatment. the cure is highly possible.

another way if the sugar level is high but the insulin also is less then it indicates fault is in pancreas also so we have to prescribe medicine to prevent further damage of pancreatic cells as well as
insulin poor utilization (here the anti diabetic remedy either in allopathy or in other system needed). The treatment out come is
judged by normal insulin level or stable low level [it means it does not further deteriorate].

1. Allopathy doctors has to send the pre diabetic and gestational diabetics and early diabetics to homeopathy doctors. you are requested not to give any anti diabetics to the patient. HIGH POSSIBILITY IS THERE TO PREVENT AND CURE THE DIABETICS.

2. If the insulin is normal but the sugar level is high this case ideal case to cure.

3. either this case is cured or not all the diabetic patient has to be compulsorily treated by homeopath this is because the insulin resistance is because of silent bad inflammation. This inflammation will damage the kidney, eye and all other tissues in the body in future.

Either the sugar level is normal or high the patient will sure will develop all the complication he listed in diabetes this is because of silent confused inflammations running in our body. That inflammation has to be solved to cure the inflammation.

YOU HAVE DONE ENOUGH TO THE PATIENT AL-READY IN THE NAME ANTI INFLAMMATORY. SO DONT TRY TO PRESCRIBE AGAIN ANTI INFLAMMATORY and medicine against the basic physiological function. THAT WILL GIVE AGAIN GREAT MANY NUMBER OF DISEASE.

The allopathy quack is doing always doing the same routine similar to thyroid disease. The thyroid disorder will be caused by something else he will not treat that but he will manage the thyroid. Similarly, diabetes is caused by confused inflammation he will not treat it but he will do some other job like managing the diabetes disease will progress as usual and will damage the kidney and eye and nerve easily even with anti diabetic tablets.

So MBBS .MD, MD diabetologist and Endocrinologist All is for cheat you and get the money from you. He never attempts to treat you. He is managing.

Managing is unavoidable in emergency situation not all through the life.

Your complaints will remain same he will sale the medicine, he is appointed for that only. If you suffer severely, he will admit you and earn money if you suffer more severely, he will do surgery and earn money. If you suffer more then that he will admit you in ICU and earn money. Keep in your mind he never treats the basic cause of the disease till now he will send you safely to burial ground.

He feared if you cured or treated then he will loss the earnings. You are the potential customer he doesn't want to loss you. You have to be present and keep give money for him till end of your life.

TYPE 1 DIABETES MELLITUS :

Diabetes mellitus due to nil production of the insulin this is belived that destruction of langharhan cells by some specific antibody. langharhon cells are present in the pancrease this secretes the insulin loss of this cells causes no controle in the sugar metabolisam so diabetes.

The infectious diseases of the gastro intestinal tract / food poisonings treated with allopathic medication causes development of distracted inflammation / immunity this chemicals and cells will reach the pancrease and produce the diseases causes TYPE – 1 diabetes mellitus.

Pretty much sure distracted inflammation and immunity causes this so prevention is easy if we stop stopping the inflammation before it is completing.

PREVENTION IS HIGHLY POSSIBLE BY PREVENTING THE ALLOPATHY MEDICINE FOR ACUTE ILLNESS of GASTRO INTESTINAL TRACT AND REMOVING THE CONFUSED INFLAMMATION FROM THE BODY BY PRESCRIBBING APPROPRIATE REMEDY.

So, prevention of diabtes is highly possible. There is no more diabetes in future be relax.

17. URINARY TRACT DISEASE

Global Burden Kidney Disease (Copy And Pasted From Who Official Website Without Any Alteration):

Although often considered a comorbidity of diabetes or hypertension, kidney disease has numerous complex causes.5 Importantly, such disease has an indirect impact on global morbidity and mortality by increasing the risks associated with at least five other major killers: cardiovascular diseases, diabetes, hypertension, infection with human immunodeficiency virus (HIV) and malaria. For example, the Global Burden of Disease (GBD) 2015 study estimated that 1.2 million deaths, 19 million disability-adjusted life-years (DALYs) and 18 million years of life lost from cardiovascular diseases were directly attributable to reduced glomerular filtration rates.6,7

The GBD 2015 study also estimated that, in 2015, 1.2 million people died from kidney failure, an increase of 32% since 2005.7 In 2010, an estimated 2.3–7.1 million people with end-stage kidney disease died without access to chronic dialysis.8 Additionally, each year, around 1.7 million people are thought to die from acute kidney injury.9 Overall, therefore, an estimated 5–10 million people die annually from kidney disease. Given the limited epidemiological data, the common lack of awareness and the frequently poor access to laboratory services, such numbers probably underestimate the true burden posed by kidney disease. It is therefore possible that, each year, at least as many deaths are attributable to kidney disease as to cancer, diabetes or respiratory diseases, three of the four main categories targeted by the 2013 action plan.2,10,11 In addition, the estimated number of DALYS attributable to kidney disease globally increased from 19 million in 1990 to 33 million in 2013.12 In 2016, the DALYs associated with chronic kidney disease, along with those associated with cardiovascular disease, cancers, diabetes and neurological disorders, were found to have increased significantly between 1990 and 2015.6 A report from the GBD 2016 study highlighted the important omission of focus on chronic kidney disease and suggested that "the SDG agenda offers at best a minimal platform for drawing attention to the health care and monitoring needs of [chronic kidney disease]."13

Kidney disease is associated with a tremendous economic burden. High-income countries typically spend more than 2–3% of their annual health-care budget on the treatment of end-stage kidney disease, even though those receiving such treatment represent under 0.03% of the total population.14 In 2010, 2.62 million people received dialysis worldwide and the need for dialysis was projected to double by 2030.8 Globally, the total cost of the treatment of the milder forms of chronic kidney disease appears to be much greater than the total cost of treating end-stage kidney disease. In 2015, in the United States of America, for example, Medicare expenditures on chronic and end-stage kidney disease were more than 64 billion and 34 billion United States dollars, respectively.15 Much of the expenditure, morbidity and mortality previously attributed to diabetes and hypertension are attributable to kidney disease and its complications.12,16

The burden of kidney disease is increasing day by day not reducing but the cause is directed towards there is no much awareness or no early diagnosis and no effective treatment available like that, but the truth is that there is no effective treatment for preventing and curing kidney disease in allopathy that's why the burden is increasing. WHO says that in 1999 to 2013 nealry 30-40 % increase in kidney disease and related death? The top most hidden reason by doctors and people are casually knows that allopathic medicine is become more popular widely used now a days and readily available and everybody knows that allopathy medicine is having heavy complications and kidney will be damaged. There is no medicine to cure the kidney disease by allopathy is the major reason. Why a greater number of dialysis center ? why there is a greater number of kidney transplant centers ? because no medicine to cure in allopathy.

When we have war with neibour country you will buy a land for burriyal gorund and you will build the more hospital for treating the solidier or you will buy good weapon and show intrest how to compate and win in the war.

The doctors are educated to save the patient life and reduce the mortality and morbidity but the in-practice doctors are learned to kept patient under long time morbid and finally death all is related with money. And only money . world health organization should not encourage the allopathy for kidney disease. Don't hide them and there mistake you need to warnt this malpractice sure if some one warn the issues then allopathy doctors will regulate their practice.

World health organization provided nearly 16 guidlenes (sustanabel deveolpement goal- SDG- 1 TO SDG -16) but following this gosl strictly never give great success since not discussed with curative aspect never discussed about reducing allopathic drugs not discussed or encouraged about implementing alternative system of medicine for handling this kidney disease.

- The allopathic medicine which is excreted through kidney invites confused inflammation present all over the body to kidney.so that a deep vital organ (kidney) so simply getting disease in an unusually early life and commonly.There is very less chance to get kidney disease.the urethra and the vegina then bladder then ureter then the kidney,it means the kidney is located extremely safe more or less equall to heart. Then how the kidney disease is so common.The all and sole reason for inviter of confused inflammation cells all over the body is allopathic drugs which is excreted through kidney.

Usually the disease will strart from the periphery and reach to the center the URINARY TRACT has both end disease the kidney will attract the disease and spread from kidney to ureter and bladder and urethral or veginal diseases treated by allopathic drugs will make confused inflammation and then the disease spread to urethra to bladder and ureter and then to kidney.

•   The roaming confused inflammatory cells choose the site to create confused inflammation in place where birth anomaly or post inflammatory strictures or partial closed pathways of urinary tract and develop chronic recurrent infections.
•   Phimosis and para phimosis will be the cause for recurrent infections in children's and
•   urethral stricture.
•   Testis, prostate, uterus development DURING PUBERTAL AGE invite the confused inflammation cells to these parts from urinary tract. Causes many pathological diseases and produce infertility.
•   post inflammation treated with strong anti inflammatory and antibiotics,
•   sex with infected person cause infection urinary tract infection.
•   cathetrisation and keeping the catheter long time will attract the confused inflammation towards urinary tract.
•   stone in the UTI and post injury after stone crossed over the ureter.
•   other procedure like insertion of stone removeing catheters,
•   all delivery (child birth) related injury in case of female attract the confused inflammation towards genitals and cause urinary tract infection.

•   Once the profuse confused inflammation present in the genito urinary tract causes disease exaggeration even after sex with non infected person.(the pressure or frictions here act as trigger for attracting confused inflammation)

In other case the established chronic disease will get worse after sex with non infected person (so search of infection will be failed but all the signs and symptoms of PID or UTI will be there).

Most of the confused inflammation cells in the body will reach to the nose and recurrent cold will be there but here the urethra and bladder get recurrent infections so demand to prescribe anti inflammatory drugs will cause profuse confused inflammation which will settle down in the Genito urinary and pelvic organ will produce early kidney disease then other childrens.

• The sexually transmitted disease or otherwise any infections in the urinary tract will have better chance to multiply easily , any trival injury in the Genito urinary tract will not heal as simple as easily it takes longer to recover from one attack of inflammation to other inflammation .The medicine used for treating urinary tract infection will produce more confused inflammation chemicals and confused inflammation so that the confused inflammation cells slowly started inflame all Genito urinary tracts either silently or with symptomatic they will be develop easily kidney failure.

Keeping private parts clean and neat ,reducing intercourse , avoid taking allopathic medicines gives the improvement minimally but having another strong trigger somewhere else in the body to attract this unwanted cells deposits [immune complex, fibroblast, gelatin, confused inflammation cells] along with good hygiene, sexual abstinence will leave the urinary tract freely and shift the location towards stronger triggers.

Almost all allopathy drugs have to be excreted through the kidney so that it will attract the confused inflammation cells to kidney so that acute renal injury will happen mainly confused inflammation partly with allopathic drugs.

Chronic confused inflammation will create chronic kidney disease happen when the confused inflammation having rich of fibrous and gelatin material or more destructive confused inflammation chemicals so that slowly the kidney loss its function and finally, stop functioning maximum need dialysis or organ transplant.

Either subacute or chronic kidney disease all are caused by confused inflammation cells migrated from all over the body to kidney or from Genito urinary tract to kidney. so learning the basic structure of the kidney and searching cause for kidney failure within the kidney will give failure in the treatment of kidney disease. The wrong treatment given by doctors for cystitis has produced lots of confused inflammation which is giving trouble after many days , or decades now. The wrong treatment given for UTI many decades back now giving chronic kidney disease. So prescribing medicine to stop inflammation [ANTI INFLAMMATORY,STEROIDS] and infection in the Genito urinary tract will damage the kidney function . NOW YOU UNDERSTAND HOW THE KIDNEY FAILURE OR THE CHRONIC KIDNEY DISEASE ARE HAPPENING SO HERE AFTER PREVENT THE KIDNEY FAILURE DON'T ALLOW THE KIDNEY TO HAVE CHRONIC

SIKNESS AND LOSS THEIR FUNCTION.

Don't believe don't spread Rumer as if people suffering with chronic inflammation.Trully there is no chronic in inflammation only acute disease rarely sub acute. If the inflammation is become chronic it is confused inflammation created by DOCTORS.A healthy person accoding to my observation will not develop chronic disease.

Kidney stones are formed in the sites of confused inflammation. This type of stones formed even if a person sitting in ac environment [less possibility of dehydrations but stone formation]. No much history of dehydration, sophisticated life style but kidney stones.

Testis, prostate, uterus development DURING PUBERTAL AGE invite the confused inflammation cells to these parts from urinary tract.then the sex also will invite the confused inflammation to private parts. Causes many pathological diseases and produce infertility. if the trigger is strong enough within the urinary tract then the confused inflammation shifts from these organs to urinary tract it interplays and produce many diseases. Many times, the inflammation shifts from rectum to genitor urinary tract. Like after acute diarrhea or dysentery, piles or fissure then similarly strong allopathic drug again push the urinary tract infection to gastro intestinal tract so the disease alternating each other through the life time.

Acute kidney disease

There are many diseases produced by confused inflammation within the kidney.this confused inflammation causes many tissue injuries is causing both acute and chronic kidney diseases.

- antiphospholipid antibody syndrome,

- malignant nephrosclerosis,
- thrombotic thrombocytopenic purpura
- scleroderma,
- atheroembolic disease.
- renal artery dissection,
- thromboembolism,
- thrombosis,
- renal vein compression.

As usual many drugs, antibiotics, chemotherpauritc agents including some contrast material, radiation material nepritis also produce severe kidney damage and causes renal injury and failure of the kidney.

There are many few other conditions also produce the acute kidney disease like obstruction and reduced renal flow and burn related fluid depletion,toxic ingetion and then injury septicemia.

Early symptoms of acute Glomerular Nephritis include:

- puffiness in the face
- urinating less often
- blood in the urine
- extra fluid in your lungs,abdomen.
- High blood pressure.

Prevention of acute kidney disease :

There is a effective treatment is there for the removel of confusd inflammation so by doing that and curing the predisposing cause for akd will prevent the akd.

The prime aim is to prevent the confused inflammation formation and there by preventing micro and macro vascular disorders so there is no possibility of acute kidney disease. All the vascular disease and blood disorder how it happens and how to prevent this diease is discussed in the previuse chapters. All this disease including scleroderma is formed by confused inflammation alone this disease has kept under unknown etiology now the cause is detected. So, prevention is sure and success rate will be good in future by homeopathy. The cause for producing confused inflammation and cause for kidney disease is by allopathic medicine alone so there is no possibility of reducing kidney disease by allopathy at all.

When the confused inflammation is not there then there is very less possibility of the need of the antibiotics or other cancer related medications too.

Chronic kidney diseases
(Kidney failure)

Allopathic drugs can cause kidney failure , the awareness about the kidney disease and allopathic drugs was there in most of the people. diabetes and hypertension, auto immune disease some genetic disease like polcystic disease cause chronic kidney disease (renal failure). So other then genetics remainining causative factors largely preventable.

Patient is having disease we supported to cure the patient. What is the benefit of the cure ?. His kidney may not go to damage in future, his liver will not spoil by homeo medicine or by homeopathy aproach. The necessity of long-time medication is stopped. The necessity of long-time domination of the natural function of the body by allopathy medicine will be prevented.

A patient will recover with homeo medicine and I can abel to certify my patient will not get any auto immune disease ,tumor or cancer ,no liver and kidney failure.

This is going to be the best service of the Doctors TO THE SUFFERING PEOPLE. BUT THE CURRENT SPECIAL-IST trend changes everything FOR EVERY DISEASE BUT NO CURE SO THE DISEASE WILL REMAIN LONGER AND WILL GIVE MORE MONEY, THIS ATTIDUDE NEED TO BE CHANGED.

So, when we are not interfering normal inflamma-tion and immunity there may not be no chance of auto im-mune and auto inflammation disease to the patient so possi-bility of kidney disease is highly less and nill

The hypertrophy and the subsequent sclerosis of the kidney is not something gradually happenining as the sequence of the kidney failure. This is simpley an transfere of confused inflammation (constructive part of the inflam-mation). It means the inflammation cells and fibroblast and gelatin material and immune complex and all these cells are deposited over the kidney so the function of the kidney is detoriarated slowly. Who dumped these cells in this place by our wrong prescription so now we have to intimate this to body so the immune system will clear this from the kid-ney so the kidney failure will be prevented ? But we have to take the steps to remove this inflammatory waste before too much damage is happen and before the kidney going to be irreversible changes.

The doctors identify the kidney failure nearly 10 – 15 years before the patient death and 4-5 years previus to dialysis but what is the use in early diagnosis. There is no effective medicine to cure and stop the damages within the body no idea about how the immune complex and inflammation is destroying the kidney but allopathy not having any medicine to cure or eliminate the immune complex and inflammation and toxins just waiting and observing and how the kidney destroyed and patient fall to initially dialysis and taken to kidney transplant. Cause is not known is the primary defect and there is no medicine to prevent,cure and recover the kidney from failure and from chornic kidney disease is tha status of allopathy.

1.   We have enough time to save the kidney eventhough we have reciving after the inflammation distracted and reached to the kidney and failure started.

2.   We are not going to give allopathy medicine here we are recommending something else to recover the failed kidney like homeopathy naturaopathy acu pressure or acu puncture system to recovery.

Signs and symptoms of the chronic glomerular nephritis

· blood or excess protein in your urine, which may be microscopic and show up in urine tests

· high blood pressure

· swelling in your ankles and face

· frequent urination in the night.

· foamy urine, due to excess protein

· abdominal pain

signs and symptoms of kidney failure

excess accumulation metabolic waste product within the blood due to impaired kidney function causes many signs and symptoms.

- fatique

- lack of appetite

- nausea and vomiting

- insomnia

- dry ,itchy skin

- muscle cramps at night

Urinary tract infections and its management was discussed under communicable disease and homeopathy management.

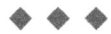

PART-5

1. New medicine

    2. Dynamisation

    3. Case taking

    4.Scientific assessment of cure

1. DISCOVERY OF NEW MEDICINE & NEW MISSION

W e have discovered confused inflammation. so, that we have to discover new medicine for all this confused inflammation disease or else we have to choose best medicine among the existing medicines, to remove the confused inflammation.

Alright how that medicine prepared to clear the confused inflammation ?. How we are going to recover the lost functions ? what is the name of medicine ? like anti confused inflammation.

Till date we don't know the cause of disease so, prepared medicine (Allopathy medicine) for the purpose of reducing or just trying to minimize the destruction of cells or tissue damage. So, more or less the medicine prepared to stop that particular harming agent. We never know that the harming agent is a part of inflammation and we don't know about its cherecter (it may shift and never die until body withdraw this).

We have an idea that enemy is harming us so we prepared to manage that attack but we come to know that our body protecting system malfunction is the cause.

1. So, if we stop using inflammation and immune collapsing medicine then there is no disease at all – PREVEN-TION IS 100 % POSSIBLE.

I am not simply giving target like we have to clear all the disease in 2050. I am sure that disease is arising not by inimical force ubt it is created by our own body immune system so that sure we can prevent disease in future. the mission is highly possible.

To achive this we need to popularize this book and educate all non communicable diseases are created by some medicines alone so by stopping this medicine alone (chap-ter 5) we can achive success .

Preparing vaccine and preventing disease is cur-rent trend stopping medicine and preventing disease is going to be a new trend and easy way to prevent disease.

2.If, we learned to repair the collapsed in-flammation and immune system then person is ready to fight for future – Maximum possible to recovery of collapsed system (95-100 % possible).

What is the success rate of cure at present in curing the disease is less then 5 % this is because we don't know the who is making disease, we are managing the dis-ease by the time the disease may shift their place so we as-sume that we are cured the disease ? Homeopaths and other ayush system trying to give cure the cure,but the percent is not much when comparing to the burden of disease this is because huge number if patients are holding by allopathy itself.

But we know the cause of the disease and we know if we remove the confused inflammation then the person is cured. it is not a great task to give the better cure percentage. Now we know,asking the patient not eat sugar and salt may not cure the bp and hypertension. asking the patient under strict less pottasiayam diet may not cure kidney failure, we know very clearly what is causing the disease and we are not going to give many list to the patient to follow diet and exercise we are not going to depend upon the patient to get minor success we are just clearing the confused inflammation from the body and we will cure the disease and we will certify that there may not be any more disease to the patient. We are going to educate the public all the diseases are curable and we are also equally going to cure the disease. Sure, the mission of disease-free world is possible.

Since we know how the disease arising, we are never going to allow the disease to mature and we are not going to wait until disease is mature enough to surgical harvest. Since we are well educated what is causing the disease so we will clear before it is going to make deep seated disease. Yes ofcourse if the disease is progressed to severe damage then the possibility of reovering the disease to healthy state is difficult. This was the routing now a days it means eventhough the disease is slowly maturing and producing severe damage also we have to keep observe it and announce it to the wolrd, since we don't know anything about the disease. But the discovery of confused inflammation disease gives excellent prognosis to all the disease it means all the acute and sub acute confused inflammation disease is completely curable by medicines so no possibility of choronic disease and no severe irreversible pathology disease in future. I mean all the superficial acute,chronic disease present today is curable. And all the chornic disease is curable except the disease is progressed to worst tissue damage (This incurable cases nearly 25-30 % of total disease in the world,luckily after 2050 there may not be any chronic non curable cases since we are not going to allow the disease to chronic irreversible disease). Absolutely no orgon failure and absolutely no orgon transplantation necessary in future.

So, the mission is possible disease-free world is possible.

And now, what is the right system of medicine to remove the confused inflammation and achive the cure ?

Allopathic pharmacology is failing like anything in preventing, recovering, controlling the Non communicable disease. But now we are very clear all the disease is caused by confused inflammation alone. So, treatment target is removing confused inflammation. There is no such medicine in allopathy to remove confused inflammation and recover the function.

Before jumping to homeopathy medicine lets us discuss one more popular medicine which is giving better success and it is very similar to homeopathy that is vaccination.

Vaccination preparation is so simple the causative agent has to be identified and then it is inactivated then given to the needed person. So, the immunity will develop against the particular bacteria or virus. Now medicine is ready for prevention. So, this is effective but the vaccination has a limitation like we cannot prepare vaccine for a non infectiuse disease. Vaccinations may not work in non communicable disease.

How the vaccination working ?

Vaccinations is prepred to prevent the infection disease like disease caused by virus and baccillai. How we can prevent this. When any person attacked with any germ then the particular person davelopping the protection power to the same infection in future. but most of the time the infected person was died but those who recovering from the virus is having good immunity to kill the same virus, if he is re expose (learned immunity). infections are giving fearing mortality and morbidity in the olden days. Since no good immunity due to poverty and unhygienic living environment. slowly people learned to hygienic environment but still patient lose the life due to infections. But there are many persons recovered from the infections are developed immunity to the same infections it means he is not affected by the same infection in future ?

So, if a person exposes to the measl virus in this year he is recovered normally is having good immunity to measals heare after he will not have measals again if at all he had measal infection the virus is killed by ready made immunity was there already in his body against the measals.

So, the researcher does not will to loss the patient life and expose them to a natural sickness since loss is more so they prepared dead virus and asked to consume / injected, these virus to a normal person and observing what happenes. The result is good yes now the person having good immunity to the particular virus. This is the story behind the vaccinations.

The basic truth is every time when a person expose to particular virus or bacteria sure the body will prepare the medicine and kill that virus but during that time if the person immunity is slowly devolpping after entry of the virus during this time if the person is under poverty not having good nutritious food then he connot able to prepare himself good immunity against the infections and having many close contact he will die and before that he spread that infection too many people. So, to prevent death and spread of the disease vaccination is utilized. Any way the person will prepare medicine to kill the virus but we don't want to take the risk so vaccine.

Either vaccine virus or the natural virus infection both is tackled in same way like body will identify that and induce the inflammation and the immune system to found the virus and prepare special cells to kill the virus (but the virus is dead and never going to harm us in vaccine virus) so immune cells will kill the virus if it is present now and also will kill the virus if it is come in future also.

There are many importand virus are tackled easily by preparing vaccines. In recent days. But vaccines are less virus are more. The problem in vaccine is we have to give the vaccine to a maximum people to save them is the major draw back otherwise the vaccine discovery may not be fruitful. Due to this reason vaccines are limited to few major viruses all other viruses allowed to natural recovery and symptomatic approach. PRACTICALLY SPEAKING THERE IS NO NEED OF VACCINATIONS SINCE WE ARE AFRAID OF SOME DISEASE LIKE PNEUMONIA ACUTE LIVER AND KIDNEY INJURY BRAIN DAMAGES we are feared and preparaing vaccine for all acute infections. But I have explained enough how the pneumonia occurs and we have enough good medicine in homeopathy no need to worry. Not all the people will develop pneumonia and we are giving chances to develop pneumonia (all are discussed in the same book as well as in infectious disease and homeopathy management). Pneumonia,septicemia and other fearing complications and death is due to again confused inflammation background alone so if we remove that then there is no fear about the worst complications of the disease and no need of vaccination. If the person expose to infection has to handle the homeopathy no need to worry about the death by infections.

So, drawback of vaccination.

1. no vaccination for all the infections and vaacinations is not necessary to all the infections. This is what we studied from chapter to till now we are human we have enough immunity to kill the virus so no need to worry about the infections (communicable disease is curable by body natural immune power itself). Giving vaccination is not contra indication and I am not against the vaccines but we have natural power to tackle the infections.
2. Absolutely no vaccination for the non communicable disease.

Now we can approach towards Homeopathy system.

Then what is the idea ? we connot prepare vaccination against the non infection disease but we can use the science behind the vaccine preparation to eradicate the diseases.

If we send some enemy to the body then the body is preparing some cells to kill the enemy so we are going to use this idea.

How ? we have prepared one substance (medicine) which will act like enemy but harmless but we have to prepare the cherecter of enemy is similar to existing disease. Anyway, the body will prepare the substance to kill the enemy or to clear the enemy ,so the body immune system now will clear the enemy as well as disease since our artificial substance and disease are very similar. So, body will clear the enemy along with disease also cleared. In this way the cure is achived in homeopathy. This princible is worked in curing non communicable disease as well as confused inflammation base communicable disease.

Homeopaths using the same princible to cure non communicable disease many years before vaccine preparation. What it was that ? use the medicine which is having the power to produce same disease. If a person is having head ache in the occiput, then medicine also will produce head ache in the occiput. So, if you give the medicine the person will relive from the complaints. How ? if you have running nose and nose block you have to choose the medicine which is having power to produce the runining nose and nose block so that medicine will cure the running nose and nose block . how ?

When the person suffering with running nose and sneezing long time it means they are having allergy. This runining nose and nose block is induced by our body but usually once the virus is killed then runining nose will be stopped but here something wrong so that body is struggling in stopping that. So we give the medicine which is having the same symptom producing capacity so that the medicine irritates so there by to clear that nose is starts flowing and sneezing to initiate this symtoms body has to come to the already diseased part and induce the same function , since the body is did runining nose and sneezing it will now give the order to stop once the enemy is withdrawn. We are not going to give second dose since we achived what we need.

bronchial constriction is the main symptom of asthma. Now we have to select any chemical or medicine or anything which is having the power to create bronchial constriction. if we identify that then, we can cure the asthma. How ? When you give the bronchial constricting agent to a already bronchial constricted patient it causes further constriction the constriction will be forcibly. So, the bronchus will counter act by our human protecting system by dialatation of bronchus. So, there by the cure is achived. In this way we have to identify many substances which is cabable of producing diseases. This disease symptoms matched with patient symptoms then the substance given to the person to recover from the ailment.

Cure Both Chronic Confused Inflammatory Disease & Failed Feedback Mechanisam.

When the confused inflammatory cells produce lots of disease in different organs and tissues. we have to collect all the symptoms of the present confused inflammations [A]

Together we are using this character of the chronic inflammation to cure and we will make one medicine this medicine is having power to produce exact similar to confused inflammation symptoms [B]

So now if we prescribe that medicine into the sufferer our medicine [artificial enemy] will produce artificial disease this disease almost occupies where ever the chronic inflammatory cells are there and produce similar disease so that person creating an artificial disease (primary action) but last for few hours.

Now the body is identifying this new artificial enemy, so our nerve sensors considered this medicine as a germ and the inflammatory cells will rush to the site where ever the medicine is there and starts their protective functions as well as recovery (secondary rections – cure).

Evanthough the body considered as homeo medicine is the enemy , we are succeeded in bringing the inflammation or recovery process near diseased site.we have preapared the medicine, like it has to act less and short durations, so there by it will disappear from the circulation immediately when curing cells reaching to the disease site. Now the artificial enemy [medicine] is gone but the disease present. So, the brain does the necessary step to complete the remaining process of the inflammation. withdraws the chronic confused inflammation or destroys that and start repair the inflammation site and complete the cure.

All this process is used by homeopathy. THIS IS NOT JUST HOMEPATHY THIS IS THE BEST WAY TO RE-COVER THE HUMAN FROM CONFUSED INFLAMMATION DISEASE.

Here a homeopathic medicine helping the body to recognize, chronic confused inflammation, her is an inflammation which is happening without the brain control. HOMEOPATHIC MEDICINE GUIDE THE INFLAMMATION AND IMMUNITY SYSTEM TO FIND THEIR REMENENTS WHICH IS SCATTERED ALL OVER THE BODY,WHICH IS CAUSING THE DISEASE,SO NOW THE BODY WITHDRAW THIS DISEASE PRODUCING CELLS SO THAT DISEASE IS CURED.

Now we call allopathy doctor he prescribes allopathy medicine which will stop the running nose and stop the sneezing. Result is excess accumulation of histamine so running nose sneezing and allergic symtoms life long then we will go to the same doctor again he will say you are suffering with allergic ruhinitis that is because we have heavy dust and unhealthy admosphere so you have to take life long anti allergic medicine.

When you allow the infection then the runining nose is initiated by the body it will stop that within one or two days. But we forcibly stopped that by strong medicine so the runining nose is not stopped and sneezing is not stopped. The pharmacology is not upto the mark and the sef curing disease made life long suffering now with allopathy medicine.

the working prinicible of the allopathy is opposite cure opposite. means if body does one thing then your medicine will do opposite of the what body doing or what patient symptoms. It means if the patient is having runining nose then medicine will do dry nose, if you have nose block then medicine will relive the nose block. super right it is good, but we are not dealing with in animate object and we are not dealing with no protective object what ever you do is having some impact in living animal which will react to your medicine and how you are achiving your treatment is another importand aspect. You are giving satisfaction by blocking the histamin and inflammation when we do that patient feel no running nose and no nose block but this was done by a body since we interrupted in the mid the body contineuse recovery cycle is broken and since excess histamine is occumilated in the nose cause hyepersensitive to dust and fumes and claimate changes is happen.

It means opposite to disease symptoms it means your opposing the body protective functions that is a mistake so the excess occumilated histamine more powerfull opposite symtoms to the medicine what you used. Now dryness allopathy medicine induced so excess flowing body induces. You are relvied nose block by medicine yes then I will block more powerfully then before.

For Every Action There Is An Equal And Opposite Reaction – Newtons 3Rd Law.

we have allergy but we will go to a allergy specialist he give the same medicine anti histamine. The medicine will do same function and the disease will give more suffering but the medicine will relive that for 6 hours so the patient will have drug addiction.

Some other example of allopathic medicines.

•   when the body produce the disease by constriction medicine will dilate that and gives the relief.

•   If the disease will produce spasm in muscle, Medicine will relax the muscle and give the relief.

•   When the disease will produce excess heart rate medicine will reduce the heart rate.

•   If the disease will produce diarrhea then medicine will produce the constipation.

•   If the disease will produce the heat medicine will produce the cold.

When theoretically speaking antipathy [allopathy] medicines relive the complaints not remove the disease.

So, what we have to do prescribe medicine which has same symptoms patient is having runining nose and your medicine also will irritate the nose and you have to make runining nose so the body will come to the site and do runining nose and clear the inflammation cells from here. So, homeopathy cures and allopathy will make sickness. Not

that MBBS is trained to make sickness and BHMS or homeopaths are made for cure. It all solely depends upon what
prinicible we administer medicine and what science we follow to cure the disease.

100 % a medicine which is following the princible
contraria contraris curanter will make disease this princible
is followed by allopathic medicine – the medicine and disease symptoms opposite.

We are allowed allopathy doctors to govern the entire medical
system now, so he observes and do research then finally giving opinion
about cure . what they going to say they are genuinely report to the world
that non of the disease is curable. We have to take this is the opinion of the
allopathy but we consider this is the opinion of the entire medical field.
So, we are all accepting this, yes the disease are incurable and suffering
with huge collection of the incurable disease in the world.

100 % we can achive the cure if administer similia
similibus curanter – this prinicible is used in homeopathy –
disease symptoms and patient symptoms are similar.

When a person fall infection then allopathy treats
it, then non infection disease starts it means allopathy doctors created mega sick community which is full non infection disease. Now if we use homeopathy medicine like a
vaccine to handle non infection disease also curable in the
same princible of vaccine.

In the vaccine the virus is used as a trick to invite
the curative immune system. In the same way we use the
homeopathy medicine as a trick to invite the body to cure
themselves.

Vaccines invite the immunity to kill the virus;
homeopathy medicine inform the curative center to take
necessory action. Here there is no immune booster in contrast the destructing immune system and destructing inflammation system is recalled by the body so we are cured
from the disease.

The inflammation system (histamine is excess

causing destruction here in nose we inform that to our curative center so body will clear the excess histamine). Our kidney is damaged by immune cells due to allopathic medicine so by giving the signal to higher center we are removing the immune cells from the circulation, because here the immune cells along with inflammation cells will destructing the kidney, we have to remove that. We need a vaccine similar to that but instead of making more immunity here that medicine has to help to clear the unnessory immune cells.

Immunity is good, inflammation is good until when you not using allopathy. once if you used allopathy medicines you have to understand inflammation will kill immunity also will kill if you use that in wrong way. A kniff will kill, a gun will will kill but who is going to be killed who is using that will decide the facts. A gun in the hand of your protector will save, a gun in your enemy will kill you. A immunity and inflammation is cauing all the non infectious disease and because of that only you are suffering allow the inflammation and immunity ro run their function normally don't interfere that (almost I am using this word heare more then 50-100 times).

You need immunity or inflammation or high blood sugar or low sugar , you need high bp or low bp all are sensed and understood by the higher centers (brain and that accordingly), stop inflammation ,clear the immunity everything is decides brain and nervous system homeopaths request that centers to take necessary needed action by acting as a enemy- so the cure is achived similar way like vaccine.

- ❖ Vaccination : same cures, invite immunity – kill the germs
- ❖ Homeopathy : similar cures, invite the nerve center to cure
- ❖ Allopathy : opposite gives the relive. opposite-suppress the nerve center by force, so body

react violently, need to keep suppress the nerve center by regular intake of medicine.

Same (vaacination) needed in some place, same is not working in some place. So, the prinicble of similar used (homeopathy).

Medicine quality for treating non communicable disease

❖ When coming to non communicable disease (excluding infection) we need to choose the medicine which has the power to withdraw confused inflammation and confused immunity and other confused and inflammation chemicals and cells ofinlfmmation.

❖   The medicine needs to rebuild the tissues which is destructed in many places. The medicine has the capacity to remove the dead tissues from body and remove the unnessory growth and proliferation and remove the tumor and destruct the tumors.

❖ The medicine needs to recover the functions of the particular organ or tissues and and reduce the excess function in some place.

All the above cheracters are very easily handled by homeopathy but stopping and removing tumor is less possible.

Role of homeopathy
medicine in infections

At present naturally humans are having capacity

to cure themselves from any infections including HIV and hepatitis unnaturally we don't want to cure ourself from HIV or Hepatitis So when body try to cure by producing fever, we consume a dose of paracetomol and switch of the inflammation.

So, we have sent option that is called vaccinations. Vaccinations will prevent the disease.

what if I have any infection if there is no vaccine or vaccine is there but I have not taken that ?

Homeopathy medicine will support to recover by inviting curing centers and it will work along with inflammation and immunity to kill the germ. If the patient is having confused inflammation the signs and symtoms mostly take you to severe mortality and morbitidy this can be prevented by using homeopathy medicine the necessity of homeopathy here is strongly need.

A death by any infection not because of the germ but because of non functioning or over functioning or mal functioning inflammation and immunity so there is a need of homeopathy and good food and nutrition to handle this situation.

How we can say technique rather then medicinal management ?

The first true single word about this is we come to the stage its enough medicines gives highest main effect and worst side effects so that we in need of searching something harmless and accurate making end to confused inflammation disorders and making collapsed system into normal.

because we find the cause for the disease and we just help the body to take care of their functions by mimicking like a disease , here the medicine not require to work day and night we need to give simple stimulus to disorganized or collapsed system to work in right way so we plan in such way and uses some technique to wake up the system in right way we fool the body as if the enemy is there in so the body is trying to eliminate that we keep this artificial enemy near real enemy so that body is trying to remove the artificial enemy [medicine] as well as real enemy [Disease] and cure achieved by taking responsibility to renovate and recover the collapsed system.

VACCINATION IS A TECNIQUE BUT ANTI ALLER-GIC MEDICATIONS IS MEDICINAL MANAGEMENT, VACCIN-ATION IS TECNIQUE BUT ANTI DIABETICS IS MEDICINAL MANAGEMENT.VACCINATION IS A TECNIQUE SIMILARLY HOMEOPATHY IS USES ALMOST SIMILAR TECNIQUE TO CURE THE PATIENT .SO DON'T TRY TO USE LIKE A MEDI-CINAL MANAGEMENT.SIMILAR TO VACCINATION HOMEO-PATHIC MEDICINE ALSO ENOUGH TO PRESCRIBE SINGLE DOSE AND SINGLE REMEDY TO BRING THE CURE.I HOPE NOW YOU UNDERSTAND HOW SINGLE DOSE WILL WORK CURATIVELY LONG TIME.

We have to understand we are not curing and it is not necessary we are calling automatic curing power within the body and hindering the process just single dose of medi-cine will do that. We no need to prescribe medicine day and night our medicine not necessarily need to work for many hours. Invite the curative human inflammatory system and it will cure the condition.

Need to prescribe another dose when the improve-ment was happened but stopped now so second prescrip-tion if needed otherwise single dose will cure the com-plaints.

single dose stimulate the weak inflammation in right path so that it will recover the system slowly, when the inflammation is cleared from the body still symptoms persists indicates need some more medicine to attract the TRUE INFLAMMATION TO THE DISEASE SITE FOR COM-PLETE THE CURE,THIS IS NOT SOMETHING STRANGE WILL

TAKE FRESH CASE REVIW AND PRESCRIBE NEW MEDI-CINES.WHY IS THIS BECAUSE SOMETIME THE CONFUSED INFLAMMTION WILL BE CLEARED BUT THE HEALING MAY NOT HAPPEN IN THE ULCER IT MAY REQUIRE NEW MEDI-CINES TO COMPLETE THE CURE [COMPLEMENTRY].

so, giving medicine for effect of confused inflammation will act as *palliative* [sleeping pills, bronhodialater, painkillers, anti allergics, hormone supplements, etc] but using technique for removing the confused inflammation completely within the body will bring the cure.

Organ specific medicine:

Majority of the homeopaths also will fail to understand this so they prescribe organ specific medicines or disease diagnosis medicine for treating the disease, its again similar to allopathic medicine action. [it will palliate never cure].

2. DYNAMISATION (THE STORY BEHIND CRUDE DRUGS)

DYNAMISATION OF THE MEDICINES AND MICRO DOSE [MINIMUM DOSE]

I am patient I need recovery without any complications, I am a doctor I have to cure my patient without creating any new disease ? I DON'T WANT TO GIVE THE BURDEN TO MY PATIENT.

Curing power of crude chemical medicine power

Protective functions of the body , sensing the enemy entry, need of repair, completing task and ending the healing all will be communicated through tiny chemical liberations from the wounded site and sensed by electro neuronal transmission in the nerves. So, initiating and running the inflammation and immunity is happen extremely tiny stimulation or order from the nerve and brain in healthy state conducted by minimal electron and ionic changes.

When inflammation is distracted the confused inflammation is formed (Disease developed) disease is started then this confused inflammation is responding further micro stimulation then the elctoro-neuronal transmission in healthy condition. It means confused inflammation attracted so easily even exposure to ac cold weather, sun heat and pressure in the walking all will attract the confused inflammation. Because the disease is hypersensitive then the normal inflammation and immunity. so, it is IMPORTAND THAT THE MEDICINE MUST BE EXTREMELY MINUTE DOSE AND POTANDIZED FORM [DYNAMIC FORM MINUTE AS EQUAL TO MICRO ELECTRICAL NUERO TRANSMISSION]. To meet the C inflammation and to eliminate this.

But almost all pharma industry including allopathy and many including few ayush medicinal system uses massive crud drug administration to optain relief or cure. crude drug which means chemicals and minerals or the herbs given directly to the patient.

If you realise to understand what is crud drug power and true electro neuronal power signalling just few examples given below.

Why heavy and continuease crude medicine used in allopathy ?

1 paracetomol stopping the fever when we compare with fever inducing or fever stopping signal of the hypothalamus. Hypothalamus using 1000-time lesser power then paracetomol molecule to stop fever. It just gives a signal to stop the temperature.

Many doctors thinking they want to stop the inflammation by their medicine and cure the disease directly with their medicine. But it is not possible there is a curing system inside. That curing system is not functioning. So, we are going to recover then the curing systems has to cure and recover the disease. We have only this option. When we try to cure or treat ourself directly then it is may not possible to cure, since body has curing center that's why we need to study physiology and biology. CHRONIC DISEASE IS NOTHING BUT FAILURE OF CURING CENTER IN THE HUMAN BODY. WE ARE GOING TO RECOVER THE FAILED CURING CENTER.

Anyway, we don't have much burden,since allopathy doctors never have and intension to cure, they will only manage the disease by crude drug many thousand time powerfull otherwise the medicine will not work. Why this much heavy powerfull medicine. Since we are not aiming to just give the orders to stimulate or to work or withdraw to work, rather then they give medicine which has to act against the active disease function to compete that medicine has to work more powerfull then disease and when one dose power is exhausted then another dose of medicine. This will continue many years.

Allopathy and other crude medicines are working on the basis of *bulldozar theory* . We have 2 options to stop the buldosar or vehicle or mechine or great powerfull tool. Option one is switch off, so the buldoser will not work the car or bus will not move now the work is completed. But allopathy or crude drug prescriber trying to stop the buldoser when it is running and trying to stop the lorry or the bus or train when they are in running condition (option 2) so we need heavy power to stop the any mechine or vehicle.since you are working against the working bodily functions.

When a patient suffering with severe wheezing then here the bronchus is constricted (boldoser is moving and running). When we prescribe medicine to work opposite direction it means the bronchus has to dialate to relive the symptoms. It means we have to pull the buldoser now it shoud not work and move to reverse direction. Imagain how much energy you need to do this work. Suppose if you stop opposing the buldoser again it moves so we have to keep oppse the buldoser. If the broncho dialater is not working then the constriction is more powerfull so the patient needs to take medicine again to dilate the bronchus and heavy massive crude drug.Bulldozer theory is applicable for management of the disease not applicable to cure.

Suppression it means active disease or natural working fucntions are forcibly tried to controle with heavy drugs by temprorily are called suppression. In many situations this suppression will heve great effect to totally damage and distracting the disease from that place we may consider we have destroyed the target. So that we may assume that the medicine is cured.

(the highest interesting factor I thought only skin disease is suppressed by allopathy medicines but now I realise every medicine in allopathy achive the success only by suppressing natural protecting power)

First question why we have to manage ? why don't you decide to cure that ? curing is not possible without knowing the cause of the disease.

The cause of the disease is prescribing medicine to manage the disease rather then curing the disease. The fuel for disease is optained from the medicine you administer to manage the disease. So , don't manage the disease try to cure which is easy and that will prevent the disease, when there is no fuel the disease will stop automatically.

Managing the disease with crude chemicals not only give the drug addictions and medicine complication this is the cause for the development of the disease of what you manage now. (asthma is managed well by anti histamine and the cause of the asthma is anti histamine, allergy is managed well by anti histamine and this allergy is caused by anti histmine)

Why we have to use micro power of medicine for cure ?

A crude and chemical medicine may not cure the disease. For cure we have to use dynamised medicine not the crude drug. Since the crude drugs will not meet the dynamic disease force. CRUDE MEDICINES it never meets the disease since crud drug will initiate another inflammation and eliminated quickly from the circulation but never eliminate the old confused inflammation. The body react against this crud drugs and it will be removed from the body.

According to your crude drugs may not meet the disease force. yes. Then how the patient getting relif ?. you are managing effect and final product of the disease and managing that you are not meeting the true cause directly and in right way. You will not eliminate the direct cause of the disease even if you know who is making the sickness.

Dynamization theory is not discovered for reducing the complication of the medicine. If the medicine is not dynamized then that may not meet the confused inflammation. This is the only reason for dynamization.

The main aim and intension of cure is removing the bad inflammation unfortunately allopathy doctors prescribing chemical medicines. So, reaction from the body to that chemical medicine is eliminating the medicine through urine is happening but the exhisting disease is remain inside.

When you administer even a crude homeopathy medicine invite another inflammation. Utilise these reactions to cure the disease ? how instead of creating complete new inflammation invite the inflammation recovery part alone ? is that possible ? yes, it is possible. For that we have to use dynamic homeopathic medicines and then we have to decide that body reaction is not opposite like it must be same. Why if you prescribe medicine for asthma patient the medicine must have power to produce constriction already patient is have constriction if we use constriction then patient will die (?) we are using dynamic medicine it is not having power to initiate the violent constriction to the bronchus but inform the higher center that there is a enemy he is going to constrict the bronchus . what will happen of course body has to protect from the homeopathy medicine so the reaction is dilate the bronchus . here we use the curative power with scientific approach. (vaccine theory). So buldoser theory is allopathy fighting opposite to the body reaction switch off theory is running parlel theory homeopathy.

What will happen if we use the crude drug to induce similar symproms patient will die. So that the medicine is diluted. Even if you dilute the atoms in the homeopathy medicine sensed by the sensor of the human body so the reaction will happen but it never makes the suffering to the already suffering individual.

Virus entry – infection

So killed virus or in active virus – (vaccine)—prevention.

So what will happen if you give the active good virus it will make infections, so we are killing the virus and giving that to the humans and incuding the body reaction using that for preventing the disease.

So confused inflammation – disease

So same disease producing power medicine with dilution and dynamysation (homeopathy medicine) --- cure the disease.

But minimizing and diluting the medicine will give the result we have given enough explanation about micro power sensors of the human nervous system in the same chapter.

That's all the reason for dynamysation theory. Those who not yet convinced read the below more explanations.

More explanations

If we want to stop the fever, we can approach in 2 ways one is informing to the nerve that enemy is killed, if the brain understood this then it will stop the fever automatically (option 1-switch off) . This is ideally simple and so eazy and important think is fever is completely stopped by healthy way we no need to prescribe anything again and again.

There is another way, in that we have to block the signal coming from injured site (option 2) , so there is the formation of inflammation and fever will be suppressed temprorily as for as enemy is in the tissue, it will keep send the signal to the brain so we have to keep administering the tablet to block the signals. For longer time and need massive dose. So, this mega dose is not necessary when you using the medicine for precise signs and symptoms. We are just informing to the nerve endings about the situation of the ailment [with extremely tiny dose] nerve ending receive that and order to work the inflammation, so that will continue their work (**Homeopathy**). This is like option 1.

THE OTHERWAY IS BLOCKING THE SIGNALS FROM TISSUES with massive heavy dose of medicine SO THAT TRY TO SUPPRESS THE INFLAMMATION AND IMMUNITY FUNCTIONS [this is like option 2 Allopathy]

Only the dynamized low power homeo medicine help in act as a confused inflammation and fit exact similar to confused inflammation so that body will identify that and remove that. But the crude drug or chemical will invite another true inflammation [like in vaccination] it is never help in clear the highly sensitive confused inflammation. Now are you understand why dynamization.

(we are prescribing medicine to the living object it has power to recieve and react and object the chemicals and crude drugs which we prescribe)

Aim of the treatment is to clear the confused inflammation and recover the functions of the repaired body parts.

Example with crude homeopathy medicine : direct onian extract .

we decide to cure the allergic rhinitis (patient with running nose and sneezing) we will prescribe oniyan extract this will irritate the nasal mucosa so this irritation will causes liberation of histamine this histamine sensed by sensory nerves the signals received by brain will start produce the inflammation inside the nose so running nose, sneezing and minimal head ache will continue along with existing running nose, sneezing. So, a crude extract do single function, means invite the inflammation. so for crude onian extract the reaction of the body is producing an inflammation.

But actually, in confused inflammation need multipolarity action of the true inflammation as well as immunity. why ? because the confused inflammation will do congetion disorder in some part and effusion diseases in some part and functional derangement in some part so need another further more specific and at the same time to cover this multi polarity disorders so that the recovery also will happen in the same multi dimension like removing the congetion in one site and effusion in another site withdrawing the inflammation cells and chemicals in some areas and recovering the functions of the inflammation in some part its like that. So, we are not just inviting another inflammation or recovery inflammation. NEED MORE POWERFULL SPECIFIC RECOVERY OPTION WHICH IS GOING TO CONTINUE FROM THE PLACE HOW IT WAS STOPPED.

So, it is not like one-word answere you need inflammation or not here we no need inflammation but we need to understand the inflammation initiating and controlling system have to come and start to recover their remenents and start to continue their work , from where they stopped.

Again more specificially has to begin where it was now.one patient will have ulcer in the stomach (7th stage of inflammation) and at the same neuralgia (first stage of inflammation) in the face and tumor in the hands (8 th stage inflammation).The medicine we are prescribing have to invite the recovery option for all this stage not just closing the inflammation or just initiating the inflammation.

Example by using Dynamissed onion medicine:

Here we don't want to make another inflammation so we just inform I am enemy entering to your nose, so the oniyan extract is dynamised (potandised-minimised and made equal to the disease power this onion has power to produce running nose, sneezing and itching in the nose similar to disease).

This dynamized extract will be sensed by the nerve ending so the nerve now will not produce another inflammation instead it will clear the confused inflammation completely which is produce the running nose, itching, sneezing. (Because we acted exactly similar to confused inflammation, we induce the nerve to take their function but we are not in the place exactly because dynamized medicine does not have any chemical or mineral to remove) here the nerve has to remove the confused inflammation only.

To catch the confused inflammation the dynamized onion extract acted similar to confused inflammation. so, nerve sending order to remove the both patients is relived. So, that it will work curatively, accordingly never produce one fresh inflammation rather then it will clear the existing inflammation.

Cure it means failed inflammation and immunity system recovered to normal.

THERE IS ANOTHER BENEFIT WHEN WE PRESCRIBE THE DYNAMISED MEDICINE WITH SIMILAR SYMPTOMS SO THE BODY REACTED AND RECOVERD ALLERGIC NOSE. From now patient free from running nose and allergic symptoms. Here we are calling (stimulating) the brain and inflammation system to work and recover their failed function We use the technique, by this technique we demand the body to work .

So, after completion of the work the immune system is recovered from non functioning to good functioning the sneezing and running nose. So, the failed inflammation and immune system recovered from the body. It is not simply cure it is not simly recovery. The failed system is now normal this is very important and understanding. we are inviting inflammation to recover the failed inflammation system to make it normal. We did. It is that *easy comprehend this use this technique free the person falling illness before the disease too advancing it is impossible to recover.*

nose flowing continuously for many days without any enemy is not a real function of the protective function of the nose. The inflammation system is in diseased condition, so we prescribed medicine to recover the malfunctioning of the inflammation now turned into good healthy function [homeopathy].

Suppression means the inflammation and immune functions forcibly stopped and make them failure :

There is another way : When the dust enters the nose, patient start sneezing is a normal response, when he is exposing to the viral then he will have sneezing, is again normal response. In this situation if we prescribe anti allergic that will block the signals from the nose to the nerve so that nose will start sending the signals as there is a enemy in the nose. We prescribed medicine to block this signal [allopathy] so nerve may not feel that so there is no running nose and nasal congestion temporariliy. patient feel relief temporarily.

Here the medicine does not allow the nerve to do their functions, inflammation and immunity is also blocked does not allowed to carry out their functions [suppression].

So, once the medicine is withdrawn the axis of the neuro inflammation is in confusion due to nose pathed with huge collection of inflammation signal chemicals [this chemical blocked by medicines] so that augmented response will happen even to the minute stimulus the affected individual sneeze like anything for simple dust exposure , indicates that neuro-inflammatory axis is collapsed. Here the inflammatory system is collapsed so it will give trouble and disease instead of recovering us from trouble. All happen due to illogical unscientific way to give relief.So the option 2 stop the natural functions and produce the diseases,you have to clearly understood here is the crude drug will suppress the natural functions temprorily so gives the way to disease production it means not only the germs like bacteria or virus is causing disease the crud drugs which is causing the disease,aware this.

WE HAVE TO MAKE A PSUDO DISEASE NOT A TRUE DISEASE, THE CHEMICAL AND CRUDE DRUGS ACT IN PLACE OF BODY REAL INFLAMMATION BUT THE HOMEO-PATHIC MEDICINE ACT LIKE A DISEASE,

vaccinations are making true disease so there by brain react induce true inflammation, we don't want any disease but disease like situation and again it is just enough to stimulate the nerve endings it must not use any real inflammation steps because it may further complicate the situation all we need is to clear the waste no need to make further confused inflammation.

Creating artificial disease by chemical put the patient in great trouble and further sickness, it's enough to mimic like a disease. The presence of the pseudo disease is ideally enough just to stimulate the nerve endings for actions.

Chemical drugs act in place of inflammation so that it needs to be prepared in such way to act longer.

3. CASE TAKING

(patient learn how to narrate and explain your compalints to the doctors and health care workers and Doctors learn how to collect the data of regarding the confused inflammation)

J ust collect all the singns and symptoms of the disease and choose the ritgh remedy which is having similar symptoms is more then sufficient in acute cases. But for chronic cases we need to collect more data.

The routine case history taking need slight changes according to the new invention. Giving importance to trace the histry of medications since birth. Instead of directing the history taking towards diagnosis.

We are going to divert the history collection towards total ailments and discomforts and disorders in general from head to foot, then simply limiting towards only the primary ailments narrated by patient and direction towards diagnosis based on this.

General practitioner other then homeopaths has to learn to get the history of modality modifiying factors of the disease which is very importand. because patient will blink sometimes does not know what is the cause for the disease but the modality gives the clue.at present doctors gives least important but it is need to be added more in future case taking.

We should not forget these worthy points while taking the case   and treating the disease.

1.   Prescribing medicine to recover the disordered natural functions like appetite, thirst, defecation, perspiration, sleeping, emotional, psychological well being all is important and all this function we are recovering during the process of treatment.so we need to collect the data of these same.

2.   giving special importance to vital organ for inflammation and immunity like lymph node, tonsils, adenoid, appendix, spleen, bone marrow and their disorders has been considered and recovered to function normally.in the same mechanism of homeopathic cure [SO WE HAVE TO INCLUDE ALL IN THE CASE RECORD BEFORE PRESCRIBING].

3.   from special sense altered sensation or reasonable altered sensation to strange sensations something not fall under any diagnosis or cannot be correlated with common medical knowledge. We never going to miss the altered sensation all over the body [like in the palm and soles burn-

ing as vitamin deficiency or it will be like that or no medicine for that, crawling sensations', because all this altered sensation is happen due to poring of the inflammation chemicals and it damages nerves minimally or moderately or severely so we are going to consider this extreme tiny alteration in the body before it is going to produce real diagnostic disorder or rare unnamed diagnostic single unpleasant sensations. We have to consider all the special senses are in good health [temperature, pain, tactile, smell, vision].

4. Tiny discolorations simple cracks, rashes here and there and gray hair, baldness caries tooth all fall under confused inflammation effect. Nothing is happening separately as we think this many day like aging cause baldness or aging gives cataract, dental poor hygiene will bring oriental disease all are not true. [observed and verified], most of the disease is caused only by confused inflammation alone.

5.Failed feedback machinimas, failed adaptive mechanisms are given highest importance and helped to recover that.

6.Single or group of symptoms not fall under any diagnosis is possible to recover in fact now the reader must understand we see many diagnostic disease in single person but all this different diagnosis is due to confused inflammation alone this diseases may come periodically or decade by decades of patient life so we need to understand there is no need of diagnosis, we need to consider whole derangements all over the body without considering few important point in the diagnosis.

7.A complete trace of past medical treatment,

by himself or with the help of medical professions which include hospital admission and medicine used for treatment, all medicated soap usage, medicated ointment,shampoos,usage of herbs, health drinks which has medicinal power in it all injections and tablets syrubs, surgery and minor or major invasive procedures and treatment ,,,,etc.

There are lots of **incurable disease** in the world now , because we could not find a right remedy for that we try to find a remedy for effect of confused inflammation it makes again many number of disease [diagnosed disease and single symptoms] discovering medicine to that is long process and again palliative process, but when we understood the real cause for the disease then if we prescribe medicine aimed to just withdraw our confused inflammation chemicals and cells.so you no need to worry about or panicky about incurable disease anymore believe that all the rare uncommon disease are just created by confused inflammatory chemicals.It waste your time for searching something not exist

No need to worry about vitiligo just prescribe the medicine to withdraw a confused inflammatory chemical which is sprayed from sinus to all over the body.so that the further damage to the skin will be prevented immediately afterwards brain will order the skin to repigment.

No need to worry about how the tumor is going to cure just prescribe the medicine for withdraw a confused wound healing cells [which is sprayed over the body from improper wound healing].

The treatment is that simple don't complicate yourself there is no incurable disease except the changes which is not reversible now.

Whether you are going to use homeopathy or allopathy to cure BETTER DON'T CREATE THE DISEASE READ AND UNDERSTAND WHO IS MOST DANGERUS HIV OR ALOP-

ATHY DOCTORS, HEPATITIS OR ALOPATHY DOCTORS.

We feel proud our self yes, we will create cancer ? when you coming to take treatment for common cold we will offer you cancer or tumor as a gift if you say this who will come to take treatment to alopathy.do you think that common cold will damage the person then what we do ?.

Totality of the symptoms

To do this we have to consider all the abnormal symptoms and signs together when we treat it **TOTALITY OF THE SYMPTOMS**. The totality of the symptoms includes.

1.Rheumatism [disease diagnosis] along with sexual weakness [Irrelevant to the diagnosis yet caused by same reason].

2. PSORIYASIS VULGARIS [Disease diagnosis] Along with loss of hunger [irrelevant to the Diagnosis yet caused by confused inflammation], memory weakness [irrelevant to disease diagnosis yet caused by same confused inflammation]. It is not necessarily having same time onset of all signs and symptoms.

The confused inflammation will affect all over the body so need to consider all symptoms.

loss of hunger for long time is a part of disease, similar single symptoms and non diagnostic symptoms we may try to give some medicine to over come individually is not a good idea. like prescribing external application for skin and giving some appetite inducer for lose of hunger.

So, learn characters of the confused inflammation homeopaths reading this is in the name of MIASM.

What is miasma? Instead of just reading about disease diagnosis tracing the confused inflammation and its impacts all over the body and properly classified by major characters this collective data of the chronic inflammation is called miasma. Disease diagnosis is an incomplete confused inflammation data [partial data] or major troublesome signs and symptoms of the c inf. **Miasmatic diagnosis almost a completely traced true picture of the confused inflammation.**

Treating disease diagnosis is clue less no head and no tail .so we have to trace and read all the minute changes in patient body after the interruption of the body protective functions. as for as our diagnosis is limited to one particular organ or body parts or some group of symptoms we clump together with some pathological facts. But actually, speaking the confused inflammation present within the diagnostic terms as well as it produces many damages from head to foot many minor and major ailment some time it may took 10-15 different diagnosis for single person but we does not have any clue to consider all this as a one disease. (one patient will have dandruff,myopia,caries tooth,gerd,constipation,back pain ,,,,,, all are due to confused inflammation.)

When you try treat dandruff it will shift to other part and create some other disease,it will be like that we have to remove that from the root so that we have to trace every minor trivel signs and symptoms of the patient.

Now if the person fall infection [Acute] the symptomatology purely symptoms of infection alone never mingled with confused inflammation [but mixed confused and true inflammation also is possible so that complete cure is possible without any support by a doctor .*if the patient has great many number of confused inflammatory products within body he will give moderate to severe worst prognosis then good prognosis in this situation sometimes need emergency admission of current allopathic medicine to minimize the complications.*

BUT ONCE THE PATIENT RECOVERED IT IS IMPORTAND TO PRESCRIBE HOMEO MEDICINE TO REMOVE ALL THE CONFUSED INFLAMMATION PRODUCTS SO THAT HE IS HEALTHY.ONCE THE CONFUSED INFLAMMTION IS CLEARED NOW THE PATIENT READY TO FIGHT TO THE GERMS WITHOUT MEDICINAL SUPPORT *and the disease also run mild to moderate in severity will not produce any series disease.*

Screening for miasm [confused inflammation] is a essential step for prevention of disease.

Yes, homeopathy can prescribe the medicine in the recovery phase or even in complete silent phase of the disease [what we say healthy state, but until confused inflammation within the person, then he never considered as healthy person].

This is another way of screening all the people all over India and universe now totally under dependency of the allopathic medicine so it is mandatory to do screening by homeopath of course all people having sickness due to confused inflammation need to identify and to cure them is the IDEAL STEP FOR DISEASE FREE UNIVERSE. The people may have diagnosed chronic disease and may not have diagnosed any chronic disease but still the confused inflammation will be there.so the screening has to undergo and it has to treat with proper homeopathic medicine to remove this confused inflammation.

"EVEN WE ARE ALSO SAYING SAME THING PRESCRIBE ANTI INFLAMMATORY AND REMOVE THE CONFUSED INFLAMMATION FROM THE CIRCULATION" allopathy. anti-inflammatory/steroid again produce the confused inflammation and less effect upon the confused inflammation already present. All the anti inflammatory and steroid present in the world will have a power to arrest further production of inflammation never have the power to eliminate the confused inflammation.

Inflammation and confused inflammation are may be similar when pronounce the word but INFLAMMATION is protector of the body characterize the healthy state of the humans, but CONFUSED INFLAMMTION is poison to the human, presence of this indicate diseases and destruction.

We do screening with total health check up and all laboratory tests and scanning all this check up is aimed to detect the diagnostic stand point during this check up many disease are found but even this whole body master check up looks normal But the body still have the confused inflammation present undetectable in future it will make a series diseases and at the time it is detectable by laboratory test.why we have to wait till then.

[The minor trivial symptoms yet marker of confused inflammation like skin cracks in the heels, progressive baldness , caries tooth ,pain in the knee ,pain in the heels , Indigestion , constipation ,numbness in the limbs , lipoma , pimples , sun tan , oily face , pityriasis , milia , excess perspiration in the palms and soles, restlessness, corn, callosity, skin peeling in the palm, nervousness of mild degree, decayed tooth, gingivitis, mouth ulcers ,nose bleeding, nose block, skin discolorations and colored spots, painful defecation, sleeplessness, memory loss, pre menstrual symptoms, gray hair, dandruff, dry skin, reduced hunger, now and then eructation, nail changes, unpleasant sensations like crawling, itching burning, numbness, all of the vision disorders, styes,,,etc,,,etc. similar symptoms described by patient and observed by doctors is there more then thousands of this symptoms will clearly indicate that confused inflammation.Now it is insignificant symptoms but this symptoms will produce the chronic diseases in the place or move anywhere in the body again produce a trivial symptoms or occupies major organ brain,kidney,heart and produce severe life threatening symptoms]

In short what you reading under sub acute/chronic inflammatory disorders in the whole of medicine text is not at all an inflammation all are confused inflammation and all are made by usage of unscientific allopathic medicine. There are many diseases like tumors cancers many rare, uncommon disorders all are just a byproduct of confused inflammation. So, don't prescribe medicine for just patient satisfaction or simply you have medicine for one condition or disease. Just a painkiller just a ointment just a medicated powder or medicated shampoo or just few dose of antibiotic only making all this confused inflammatory disorder .We only making disease in the name of treatment aware this.DONT PRESCRIBE IN ANY SITUATION AGAINST THE PHYSIOLOGY.INFLAMMATION,IMMUNITY, WOUND HEALTING is a strongest and top most functions [physiology] of the body all your medicines aimed at destroying this then lots of disease will arises but you forgot what you did so you are searching cause from extrinsic or food or genetic, this or that,,,,,,etc. and etc. Finally, you are passed out and practicing and retiring without knowing that you are the cause for that disease?

Concomitant symptom:

A symptom usually associated with another symptom but we cannot explain this symptom on the basis of disease diagnosis. This is symptom is highly valuable in homeopathic prescription.

- Nasal bleeding every time a woman about to menstruate.
- Lachrymation with pain in other

parts of body.
- Eructation when pressing painful parts.
- Emptiness in Stomach menses before.
- Ineffectual urging for urination during perspiration.
- Headache after pressing the stool.
- Vertigo coition after.
- Appetite, ravenous, epilepsy, before.
- Coryza [running nose] with polyurea
- Inflammation without pain

A search of concomitant symptoms indicates search of confused inflammation. On the majority of occasions, the scattered confused inflammations stimulated same triggering factors so that different diseases or symptoms but triggered in same occasion or same triggers or giving impression same origin. But before the confused inflammation arrivals it is difficult to explain.

In the above example the first congestive inflammatory chemicals scattered all over the body is presently located in two different sites so that express their presence during menses.

There is good remedy for that so that we can cure and remove this C inflammation.

When allopathy in search if common symptoms of the disease homeopathy in search of **uncommon symptoms** of the along with disease. How we will get uncommon symptoms.

It denotes those symptoms which are Peculiar in their nature & character, where no explanation is possible, which are peculiar to few patients suffering from similar disease, their basis cannot be explained on the basis of pathology. They have their basis in the constitutional make up that determine the psychic of the individual

1.fever with excess thirst is common fever without thirst is uncommon

2.Redness but absence of warmth.

Uncommon symptoms

again explain search of C inflammation symtoms. since an inflammation and disease symptoms reflect common disease nature. But the uncommon symptoms alone express the presence of confused inflammation within the person. When you trace what is uncommon symptoms, they will give all confused inflammation characters only.

But in homeopathy we will say this is not explainable on the basis of pathological basis but the truth is every symptom express presence of the disease alone but we are late in understanding or we read it in different name. Uncommon symptoms help in identifying c inflammation in the clinic.

General symptoms

are high value in homeopathic prescription but here its express diseases arise due to failed feedback mechanism and nerve control.

- Reduced or excess hunger
- Sleep disorders
- Urine related disorders
- Thirst related symptoms
- Perspiration related symptoms
- Sexual function related symp-

toms

•   Thermal environmental relation. Etc.

Homeopathic medicine:

When you see the main characteristics of the drug it has burning sensation ,it has itching ,it has stagnation of blood superficially[congestion].the drug characterizable fit into many acute inflammation which is distracted by allopathy or any other medicine especially if it is sub acute stage and again many superficially acting acute drugs does not have a power to regularize this disordered need some powerful deep acting medicine.

The number of inflammatory chemicals is less but the confused inflammations make the changes within the body tissues so numerous disorders by attacking different body parts and tissues and reacting with external environment so need many drugs to tackle the situations. since symptoms similarity only will attract the confused inflammation disorders.

Each homeopathy drugs symptoms mimic the action of each inflammatory chemicals; millions of symptoms records are there in homeopathic remedy so that we can tackle easily all the confused inflammation symptoms. Removing the confused inflammation and recovering the health is easy if you use the homeopathic medicine.

Prescribing medicine with pathological name or partial attempts either may not give complete cure or never give any improvement because the present disease is happened due to collapse In the protective info and immune disease so the Considering disease particular and prescribing medicine for that will attract the confused inflammation cells and help in eliminate and inflammation in particular but the weak vital force remain uncured may prone to further disease and medicine has to first regularize the system then the regulated system has to identify the disease and clear it so that the cure is achieved a blind prescription of some medicine without understanding the depth of the internal collapse will never give cure.

Example a patient coming with lipoma prescribing homeopathic medicine for lipoma never give cure. because lipoma is indicating that that particular person inflammation system is collapsed so confused inflammation and unwanted dead tissues and misguided cell regeneration together produce the tumor.

So, the selection of medicine is having the power to bring back the altered system we can say we can completely ignore the tumor for prescription. we have to trace from where the and when the system is collapsed [cause like suppressed eruption or suppressed or maltreated ailments] then the collapsed systems what is doing now in the whole body for that we have to take extra care then what patient actually said need to trace all the body parts and tissues to asses the complete disease presence in the body and over all character of the confused inflammation disease it means the disease gets worse or better by what when it appears and when it is disappears . alternating or intermitting nature of the disease .how the patient react to the disease [altered mind,taste,sensations, natural eliminations and excretions ,sleep all altered thinks from health to disease has to be considered both disease particular and general person particular .all this are slowly or initially affected in many cases except in ACUTE CASSES ALL THIS ARE MISSING TO RECOVER. when the recovery is only upon the inflammation means the protective system and immunity will turn into normal but the affected hunger [appetite] loss of sleep, altered mind and other systems in turn creates the disease due to starvation of their functions. anyway, the loss of hunger originated during inflammation but everything recovered but the hunger is not recovered causes mal nutrition and weakness it will produce the disease. similarly, all other issues like sleep, constipation etc. etc.

4.SCIENTIFIC MEASUREMENT / ASSESMENT OF CURE

One line explanation of this protocal differe from usual protocol of allopathic medicine. This PROTO-COL FOR CURING THE DISEASE BRINGING THE HEALTH NOT JUST HIDING THE DISEASE.

People having highest faith in doctors, they thinking doctors doing ideally right treatment. Their belief is, doctors are educated so they know everything. But that is partial truth. Yes, they study all basic chapters in depth and all pharmacology subject more elaborately but they created lots of disease, how?

That's what we are discussing throughout the book. How? because they stop the treatment and struggle in stopping the disease. [confusion is there in what is disease and what is treatment].

They guess managing is more then enough. Then curing. They forced to do their practice and they pampered of their activities no one raised voice against this foolishness.

any treatment must have a rule. that rules must be acceptable to all the doctors. it must follow basic and medical science.it should not be the guess work.

Whether we are curing or suppressing the disease? the assessment is not weather the disease is disappearing or not. But the disappearance itself having rules, that's what we are going to study now.

Allopathy have some check list like disappearance of the bacteria or germs in the blood or in the urine. return of elevated hormones or sugar level to normal. return of bp level to normal bp. This is not the scientific protocol or rules for curing the disease. but this is also a part of recovery, need further more elaboration.

There are many best standard rules are there to cure the disease in homeopathy. This rules and laws need to be utilized by all field of doctors.

only homeopathy has to follow this, not others? those who not believing cure is not on issue but those who believe in cure has to recheck this we are curing or suppressing.

There are 2 important guidelines for assessing the cure of disease. which is there in the homeopathic practice.

Herring law of cure

Simple disappearance of the disease or a symptom is not a cure. No will say that anymore after reading the Character of Confused inflammation and comparing that with real diseases and you will definitely change the aspect of the cure parameters. Then how we can believe that the confused inflammation is shifted to somewhere or we removed it.

This is the standard rules.no it is not like that Homeopaths are discovered confused inflammation [MIASM] but they do not name it is as confused inflammation. so to remove the miasm or confused inflammation we need this scientific measurement.

If we simply follow the diagnostic aspect then there is no need of this Assessment but when we found the miasm or confused inflammation is the cause for the disease now, we can accept the need this observation.

The confused inflammation may not give their presence all time in the blood or scanning and again if follow the standard laboratory investigation as a choice we may remove some disease in the body but shifting and migratory nature it may go in other parts and produce a new disease.

This herring law is actually a simple law we can apply this in the clinic itself we can add additional lab and other testing procedures also.

HERING LAW OF CURE

Herring law of cure will give us standard check list for curing the patient. this is purely scientific based and observed how the nature cure the disease and how the body eliminate the noxious agents from the body. When the disease occurs and spread in a typical fashion and it occupy major organ so this observation says that the disease path so surely a cure must be in opposite direction of how the disease spreads.

A cure must take place from:

1.center to periphery or from internal parts to limbs and skin.

2.from above downwards.

3.from more important organ to less important organs

4.symptoms has to disappear, in the reverse order of their appearance

1.Diseases has to be cured from center to periphery:

When we try to cure the symptoms has to dis appear in the vital organ and then the periphery. If the symptoms disappear in the periphery but the vital organ damage is remaining same indicates wrong direction or consider that disease is within our body.

When we prescribe medicine to an allergic asthmatic person his wheezing symptoms must disappear first instead of sneezing and running nose. An asthma symptom has to dis appear first then the person sneezing and running nose clear.

Wrong direction of cure from periphery to center often occur when using external application all the external applications simply strongly violate the rules for cure. Every external application takes the complaints from periphery to center.

Wrong directions when using external applications.

From skin to internal organs by using many ointments and creams.

From external ear to inner ear.

From nose to lungs.

From joint to heart.

from conjunctiva to Retina.

from vegina to uterus and ovary. [all the 5 examples show wrong directions]

2. The symptoms disappear from above downwards:

A right direction of cure in the urinary tract

A right direction of cure in the reproductive system

WHAT WILL HAPPEN WHEN YOU APPLY EXTERNAL APPLICATION FOR THE GENITAL OR URINARY TRACT INFECTION. The disease progress from urethra to bladder and then to kidney.

Wrong direction of cure---patient will end up with severe chronic kidney disease over the period of time.

What is the right direction of cure in asthma case?

What will happen when you use nasal spray. The allergy moves from nose to lungs an allergic rhinitis patient will become allergic asthmatic patient.

Here there will be confusion to a reader that above downwards. We have to consider nose is the first organ and then proceeding above to adenoid and tonsil and then proceeding above to throat [but it is impossible to go up to brain but here the upper organ is this and then above to all is lung]

The same confusion will happen in GIT Here again

mouth is lower organ it moves up to esophagus then stomach then intestine this is the order.

3.Another important aspect is the disease must dis appear **from most important body parts to least important body parts.**

The patient has come with dermatitis we give the treatment with strong ointment then the patient getting asthma is not a good direction.

Patient is having allergic rhinitis with asthma when we applying ointments makes the huge aggravation of asthma is not a right direction it is a wrong direction.

4. Symptoms disappear in resverse order of their appearance.

Chest burning for 3 years, Head ache for 4 years, Knee joint pain for 5 years.

If the patient gives the duration of their ailment like this, Then the first symptoms disappear from the person must be chest burning and then head ache and the last one is to disappear is the oldest complaints.

Kent observation

Dr Kent has given some 12 observation. Here I am mentioning few.

After medicine prescribed when he come for follow up, we observed this change.

1.LONG AGGRAVATION FINAL SLOW IMPORVEMENT.

beginning of some very marked tissue damages in some organ.

2.AGGRAVATION QUICK, SHORT AND STRONG WITH RAPID IMRPROVEMENT OF THE PATIENT.

this is considered as Homeopathic aggravation yet patient feel comfortable. The prognosis is good.

3.RECOVERY OF THE PATIENT WITHOUT ANY AGGRAVATION

Indicated remedy and dose all are exactly fit to the patient since there is no aggravation and the disease is not having severe structural changes.Prognosis is good.

4.AMILIORATION FIRST AND AGGRAVATION AFTERWARDS:

Either the remedy is superficial or the it could act as a palliative or the patient was incurable and the remedy was somewhat suitable not exactly similar to the patient symptoms.

5.TOO SHORT RELEIF OF SYMPTOMS:

• Medicine action spoiled in the mid.SO REPEAT THE MEDICINE.
• Or in acute condition the high-grade inflammatory reaction of the Orgon. Which is threatened by the process going on.SO MEDICINE TO BE REPETED MUCH OFTEN OR MORE SIMILAR MEDICINE TO BE PREPARED.
• IN CHRONIC CASE, there is a structural change in the organs. USING LOW POWER LIKE LESS THEN 30 DECIMAL AND REPE-TATION SHOULD NOT ADVISIBLE HERE.

Prognosis is bad in chronic case.

6.NEW SYMPTOMS APEARING AFTER THE AD-MINISTRATION OF THE REMEDY indicates medicine is wrong. Medicine has to be antidoted and new prescription after case study is must.

7.OLD SYMPTOMS ARE ABOUT TO RE APEAR: appearance old symptoms are good sign of improvement. So, prognosis is good. Since symptoms appear in the reverse order of their appearance.

8.SYMPTOMS GOES IN WRONG DIRECTION.

indicates medicine is not suitable. so, the medicine has to be antidoted and re case study and new medicine to be administered.

9.SOME PATIENT PROVE EVERY REMEDY WHAT THEY RECIVE.RATHER THEN RECOVER FROM THE DISEASE.

Dr.Hahnemann gives some guidelines to asses the prognosis

Signs of improvement:

Patient feel greater degree of comfort, increased calmness and freedom of the mind, Higher sprit Is the indication of the return of the natural state and again, no appearance of the new unusual symptoms, non of the old symptoms are worse. Diminution of the original symptoms.

Discussion – a wonderful useful scientific observations, but this law is something not only related to homeopaths, Everyone has to follow this when allopathy is found this law, it is useful and we can read this we will observe in this same manner then there will be miracle will happen in the general medical field.

There will be a wonderful cure will happen to all.

In homeopathy we say when a person having skin disease if you treat that external applications then that disease will go inside and make so many diseases. I have read it but I am also studying the allopathic dermatology but except few disease atopic dermatitis and asthma none of other disease is mentioned in the same way.

Homeopathy says when you treat arthritis then

the disease will go inside then it will make cardiac disease. But what general medicine book says arthritis is arthritis and heart attack are heart attack don't confuse both.

Now you can read the the shifting and migratory nature of the confused inflammation everything will be clear for you. A dermatitis if you treat with external application may shift from skin and move inside and create the disease yes. Arthritis and cardiac disease are possibly produced by confused inflammation.

NOW WE CAN UNDERSTAND HOMEOPATHY THROUGH A COMMON MEDICAL TERMINOLOGY AND COMMON MEDICAL BOOK AND HOMEO BOOK easily understandable.

CONFUSED INFLAMMATION IS HIGHLY IN FAVOR OF HOMEOPATHY AND IT WILL GIVE THE GREAT ENTHUSIASAM AND EAGARNESS TO READ FOR YOUNG STUDENTS as well as all doctors.

Allopathy will be chear up that there are lots of new updating and easy understanding, how they can change their treatment everything and everything will be going to be clear.

so, the important discussion like law for cure is the most valid useful tool for curing the sickness. I expect all the doctors must use this.

Do you remove toxins in the body ?

Do you have medicines for body cleansing ? any medicine for Detoxification ?

The question was asked to me, I said we don't have (actually it is there in homeopathy). Then why I said this ? because there is no toxins in the body all the toxins are removed by veins and it purified in the lungs, liver, kidney and waste blood cells are destroyed in the spleen .so there is no need of any toxin removing medicines . This is my belief.

Its true that body eliminate the unwanted chemicals and minerals and metals, poisons. But truth is the body does not have power to destroy the chemicals or blood cells [or] appointed for inflammation/immunity until it completing the task. After completing the task, the cells/chemicals will undergo degeneration by reorder issued by brain. But when we disturb the inflammatory cells / chemicals by anti-pyretic, anti-allergic, steroids strong ointments, medicated soaps, creams,,,,,,,ext. That chemical or blood cells roam around the body till death (by the time it produces lots of disease to human being directly as chronic disease, indirectly by disturbing further inflammation / infection. So, this chemicals and cells ofcourse toxin to the human body. So we have to remove them from body,But scientifically approved harmless way.

Cupping / leaching / venesection

In olden days treatment they believed body is having impure blood because the toxins produced by body is not cleaned well so they tried to clean it by artificial bleeding, but they never mean the chronic inflammatory cells as a toxin they consider all virus and bacteria all the disease in general caused by toxins and impurity in blood.so they cut the veins and make them to bleed,they belived by doing this the impurity and tonsins will be removed from the body.but it helps very minimal [1-2%] after heavy bleeding, because the cells will stuck somewhere and busy in killing germs [in no germ areas] or busy in creating the disease, so they engaged. It is tough to clean them. So, its useless to do venesection. There is a minimal effect doing blood transfusion but it it highly contra indicated taking blood from person suffering from severe auto immune diseases, the confused inflammation disease has to be treated properly before doing transfusion procedur. So it is easy to remove the confused inflammation by proper homeopathy medicine so unnessory cruel treatment is not necessary for producing purification of blood.

Even a women who is menstruating every month is more vulnerable by this confused inflammatory cells, what we expect all the impure disease producing agents will pass through the menstrual bleeding but it is not happening instead of cleaning the toxins and impure blood she suffer as usual like a male ? the confused inflammation cells will produce disease over in reproductive organs and all over the body due to getting attraction by hormonal changes during menses and again repeated hormonal changes will excites the confused inflammatory cells to produce the disease. (but minimal reduction of confused inflammation thorugh menses blood is possible major releief will be there for endotheliyam of the uterus by menses)

HERE THE GUESS IS CORRECT YES THERE IS IMPURITY IN THE BLOOD BUT THE TECHNIC IS HARMFULL & DOESNOT RELIVE YOU.FROM SICKNESS.THE RUST AND MAGNET THEORY IN HOMEOPATHY IS MOST VALID THEN REMOVING THE BLOOD. Need a scientific technique to clear this. Not some useless cruel technique.

So, transfusion of the blood those who are having confused inflammation cells may not have great harm to new recipient. But it has impact when we collect the blood when severe active phase of disease where actually the scattered inflamed cells are not started their work in the tissues it just roaming in the blood. If the recipient is having good health then he will remove that but we can expect fever and other inflammatory signs immediately after the blood transfusion, so we have to allow that other wise confused inflammation will arise newly by prescribing anti pyretic and donor confused inflammation will also start troubling the patient.

OLDEN DAYS TECHNIC TO REDUCE THE SEVERITY OF confused inflammation (success rate is satisfactory)

- EAR PIERCING,
- NOSE PIERCING,
- WALKING IN THE FIRE (during religious festival)
- WEARING ORNAMENTS,
- WALKING AND LYING THORN BED,
- LONG WALKING for religiose purpose like more then 40 kms in a day.
- SUN BATHING ALL WILL ATRACT THE CONFUSED INFLAMMATION CELLS TOWARDS SKIN FROM INSIDE OF THE BODY. So, major organs will escape from severe disease. THE RESON BEHIND WOMEN WEARING MORE ORNAMENTS IS ACTUALLY MEDICAL SCIENCE NOT FOR COSMETICS.
- LYING AND ROLLING AROUND THE TEMPLE

Then why the people wearing ornaments are having the disease why it is not been control the disease?

We are using the ornaments for cosmetic highly glistening most desinful work of gold only we are using. Gold is not having any interaction with human body so that it is highly poor in healing process or doing less help in distract the confused inflammation. But the nickel and lead many covering chains are having high affinity to interacting with human tissues so creating allergy so that confused inflammations reaching to the skin then remain inside the body and damaging the vital organ.

A confused inflammation and immunity chemicals will respond to varies external and internal stimulus like pressure, frictions, cold, heat, emotions,,,,,etc.But the ornaments attract the confused inflammation only by minimal gentle rubbing.so if the confused inflammation is sensitive to pressure, rubbing will come to the neck surface otherwise it may not come to the skin.

There is one great drawback in using this whole olden day's technique that is this technique will bring the confused inflammation to one particular site of the body so this cells again goes inside the body if the sufficient stimulus comes from inside the body. So, Homeopathy never keep the confused inflammation to one particular part but it will clear the cells from the whole body that is the right step.

THE FUTURE PLAN AND ACTIONS

Need many alteration and renovation in the medical and health sector in general. We have read in this book about the discovery and current status of the medical sector. So instead off accepting and adjusting with faulty system we have to explain the necessary alteration in health sector and we have to do that together to rebuild it, for the benefit of good, happy, healthy and peacefull life for all living peoples in the world.

Doctors Must Assure

1.I HAVE NOT CREATED DISEASE

Need strict regulation of the the prescriptions and there by Doctor must assure there is **no new disease while treating the patient**.

2.I KNOW ALL ABOUT THE DISEASE WHAT I AM TREATING.

3.prevention is my main aim.

3.CURING IS ONLY DUTY, MANAGEMENT ONLY ON REQUEST AND DEMAND AND ONLY ON NECESSITY AND THAT IS only in EMERGENCY.

DEMAND THE DOCTOR TO CURE & GIVE THE TARGET TO CURE THE DISEASE :

A doctor must cure his patient. Here the allopathy doctor can be kept as team leader to monitor the progress of the disease. If he attempts to treat patient with allopathy medicine it will make the disease again so he can manage the team and guide the team and observe the disease prognosis with all other AYUSH system doctors.

Need better positive approach towards curing the patient. Doctors in general need to have an idea about how to cure the disease, If any other systems says the incurable disease is curable then all other systems doctors must aware that since curing the disease is main aim of the doctor simply creating gang to making show as if they are best doctor without curing the disease is ideally fall under negligence. Each system has their own over confidence and thinking and teaching others are nothing making groupisam and gangs in the medical field but this gang mostly doing nothing in curing and reliveing the sickness. I hope after all good teaching, the doctors will turn in the aspects of good and positive thinking about curing the patient.

Patient often quarrel with doctors of Homeopaths and AYUSH in India. why you said, you will cure , but you are not cured me . But in allopathy there is no such fights he says very clearly it is incurable from the first day. then why medicine, that is to spoil your stomach and liver and kidney and make new confused inflammation disease and disorder and to earn.

657

4.ALL THE MEDICINE WHICH IS CREATING THE DISEASE WILL BE REMOVED FROM HEALTH AND MEDICAL SECTOR.

Ban allopathy pharmacology and remove the concept of anti inflammation and against immunity.retain essential life saving drugs.

UNTILL THE ALOPATHY IS BANNED TO PRACTICE THEIR PHARMACOLOGY THEY NEVER ALLOW THE PATIENT TO SEND AND TO GET THE CURE FROM AYUSH Doctor. After reading this book, again saying take allopathy and homeopathy parlaly means you are not understanding the writing.

HE WILL PRACTICE HIS SYSTEM AND YOU MUST PRACTICE YOUR SYSTEM MEANS YOU NEVER ACHIVE ANY SUCCESS IN RECOVERING GLOBAL DISEASE BURDEN.

Ask the allopathy doctors to quit their pharmacology and use homeopathy medicine to commit to cure and recovery. Allopathy or AYUSH its not the caste or religion that you are belonging to the special system.You are a doctor,people believing and keeping you near the god so understand that and act accordingly. Take the system what you like to study and try to give the cure.

Follow all the procedure and technique you learned in allopathy but don't use the allopathic medicine.

Homepaths are recommended to stop external application 200 years before itself. All the cases which is labeled as incurable has to be send to the AYUSH [Ayurved-

ham,naturopathy,unani,siddha and homeopathy doctors]. don't manage the cases it is curable. Either doctors must learn the other system or send the cases to AYUSH.

I HOPE ALOPATHY DOCOTORS hereafter WILL HESITATE TO DO ALOPATHY SYSTEM MEDICINE. I HAVE TO WAIT AND WATCH MY JUDGEMENT IS RIGHT OR WRONG.

5.ALL THE SPECIALIST SYSTEM WILL BE MERGED AS REGIONAL SPECIALIST WITH FEW CONVINIENT GROUP FOR ELABORATE STUDY AS WELL ONLY CURE

a.ENT,DENTAL,UPPER RESPIRATORY AND BRAIN OPTHALMOLAGY CONSIDER AS SEPECIALIST-1. Only homeo rarely allopathy medicine

b.IMMUNOLOGY,KIDNEY,GIT, DIET AND NUTRI-TION,INFLAMMATION,HEMATOLOGY,PATHOLOGY---SPE-CIALIST-2 ETC.(maximum homeo-minimum allopathy)

c.ORTHO,DENTAL, UPPER,LOWER LIMB,SPINAL CORD,ACCIDENT AND EMERGENCY RELATED WITH RTA AND OTHER INJURY.ALL NERVOUS SYTESM EXCLUDING BRAIN---SPECIALIST ---3. (maximum allopathy,MODERATE SIDHA AND AYURVEDHA with minimum homeopathy)

d.PSYCHOLOGY AND BRAIN DISORDERS, FORENSIC MEDICINE,SEXOLOGY,GERIATRIC,METERIA MEDICA,PHARMACOLOGY,Poisoning and Toxicology ---4 (maximum homeo,minimum allopathy medicine)

e.CARDIO VASCULAR SYSTEM, IMMUNOLOGY, LYMPHATIC SYSTEMS,INFLAMMATION , AUTO IM-MUNE AND INFLAMMATION DISEASE,HEMATOLOGY.hep-atology,SPLEEN,ORGANON----specialist---5 (maximum homeopathy medicine, with minimal allopathy medicine in an emergency)

f.ENDOCRINE,GYNECOLOGY,ONCOLOGY, OB-STETRICS,PEDIATRICS,(Maximum homoepathy MODEAR-ATE YOGA AND NATUROPATHY, minimum allopathy).

ETC.

5.awards, promotions,increment all on the basis of cure and prevention rate,

depromotion,suspension,prison all on the basis increasing disease burden to the country and making orgon destruction and allowing orgon destructions.

The doctors have to be punished for creating disease , but at the same time has to be honored when he is curing the Disease and repairing the collapsed system into good functional system. Announcing Awards for curing the cases will encourage the doctors.

Non of the police or militance or other officials will be appreciated for keeping their work pending and making many new crime or offence.But in medical field allopathic Doctors not questioned, why this many disease why this many incurable cases.

A Patient going to orgon transplant then the regular treatment doctor warned and educated about prevention aspect need punishment if he/she repeats the same.

Organ transplant for chronic diseases reveal highest worst treatment and even not fit for management of the disease itself but it has considered as normal he says simple it is incurable, we also believed that but it is not true. Yes, the irreversible pathological changes never return to normal then what you did till the condition progressed into irreversible pathology.When the house or town in the fire if you maintain the fire then what will happen to your belongings it will become irreversible why don't you prevent fire why don't you reduce the fire why don't you stop the fire then what you are doing here.Allopathy maintain the fire for that we are paying.dont forget this.

No one is asking question to the allopathy why you are treating the cases where you don't know any medicine to cure or recover or even maintain in many cases ? This is the cause for India bulging with incurable cases.

He cheats the public saying simple that he is specialist in the enterohepatic or so many other specializations. He never uses the word even forgetfully that he can cure. When you say that we will cure. You will be committed and you will be the responsible so you have to answered he never says that.

MEDICAL STUDENTS & YOUNG PROFESSIONALS

The aim of this book is educating the medical world about the new invention. Solving the problem of the medical world. What is right in medical practice and what we have to do for improving the standard of medical sector and increasing the *success rate in curing the disease and preventing the disease.* So, with few modifications this book **needs to be kept as syllabus for medical professions of all doctors and health sectors .**

Think why the students not given importance to AYUSH & alternate system . Because allopathy is popularity-based medicine. This attitude has to be changed. He is popular in creating disease this is obsolutely opposite to what a young enthusiastic medical student thinking, opposite to the opinion and expectation of general public and shocking news to the health sector,yes allopathy doctors are creating so many diseases that's what we discussed in this book.

ASK THE STUDENTS FIRST TO CHOOSE THE PATH EITHER THEY WANT TO MAKE THE DISEASE AND MAINTAIN THE DISEASE OR THEY WANT TO CURE THE DISEASE AND THEN ALLOW THEM TO STUDY.KEEP THE UPPER LIMIT FOR HOW MANY OF THEM IS ENOUGH TO MANAGE

THE DISEASE AND HOW MANY OF THEM NEED TO CURE THE DISEASE BASED ON THAT FILL THE SEATS IN THE COLLEGE AND BUILD NEW COLLEGE.

When studence says, I will study allopathy but I will cure the disease means it is not a right answere, because allopathy educating the doctors all the disease is incurable.THE AIM OF STUDY AND PRACTICE IS TO CURE PATIENT .WHAT METHOD SCIENTIFICALLY CURE THE PATIENT HAS TO BE ALLOWED TO CURE.HIDE ALLOPATHY.

But here after homeopathic students will desire to do homeopathy and they will also clear in their confusion and they also get their allopathic disease texts and pathology and preventive medicine written by homeopath (ALL IS THERE IN THIS BOOK and covered organon) so that they will not have dilemma ? or confusion what to follow homeopathy or allopathy to understand the core of the problem.

And more ever there is no modern concept (allopathic concept) of the disease any more the confused inflammation theory is applicable to all AYUSH as well as allopathy.so this is another step in integrating all system together. No different opinion from different school.

AYUSH teaching against allopathy unfortunately they demanded to read allopathy text for learning the diagnosis and disease characters and prevention aspect but now this struggle is cleared.

Everybody is having their own thought about the health & disease. Its not true. There are many mode of prescriptions either medicine and disease is opposite [antipathy, allopathy] in working plan or similar in working plan [homeopathy].when you plan to cure the patient you have to choose homeopathy, when you have to save the patient in an emergency and accidents you can choose alopathy. forget about conversion of allopathy into homeopathy OR

Homeopathy into allopathy. But each individual states and country must understand we have more then enough emergency menagers and no curative doctors this in turn will increase the emergency since no one is educated about cure the disease. It means allopathy strongly object that the disease is incurable he is occupying in many countries fully he can manage the disease in an emergency he will not cure the disease .

So, the country leaders must watch and reduce the number of allopathy doctors and increase number of homeopathy and ayush system doctors.

There are many rumers and false teaching about AYUSH system of medicines and mostly AYUSH hidden from the studence those willing to become doctor. There are many AYUSH doctors joined just because they never got MBBS seats so they joined here. This is something foolish decision. There are lots of inferiority complex in AYUSH doctors they compare all the time with allopathy and underestimate themselves.This low confidence will be more in some state the top most state which is insult the AYUSH department is Tamilnadu.

Many country governments is almost removed the alternative system of medicine (like homeopathy and herbal and acupuncture, ayurvedha, etc). These countries will face many troubles in giving healthy and peacefull life to the citizens. So, value and promote those who prevent disease and cure the disease and promte health.

For some people wants to earn crores the entire country people has been brain washed to study allopathy and to take allopathy medicine. These countries will be the topper in allopathy medical shops.Topper in allopathy medicine sales. No doubt the people will have heavy and seriuse life long disease.

These country and state should be given special

importance to monitering whole of health sector and allopathy . ALLOPATHY IS THE CAUSE FOR DISEASE KEEP THAT IN MIND AND CLOSE THE NUMBER ALLOPATHY COLLEGE USE THAT FOR AYUSH SYSTEM OF MEDICINE.OTHERWISE IT IS HIGHLY IMPOSSIBLE TO SAVE THE PEOPLE.

Allopathy pharmacology is making disease and not single disease and it makes whole pathology of the medical field, so it has to be banned, with few exceptions.

a lot many renovation and reforms need for medical field.

We have to accept that we are in confusion and clueless how the disease is coming so I hope I made better understanding about the disease and I expect medical field in general will grow fast in the right direction. Doctors will show interest in doing research and more ever they can judge easily what is going to happen to the patient and he can easily comprehend the situation and he can rightly guess what will be outcome or result so kindly bear my scolding since you did a mistake and I am fearing you should not continue the mistake until some rules and regulations imposed on you from your higher medical officials and association or government. comeforward to experience the rightness and spreading the healthiness to the public. So, I am scolding and warnining,don't get frustration or wounded because of that. I know you did the mistake since you are guided in such way you are did your duty. But I have given enough explanation now, so don't contineue the mistake again and do your duty in the same way like save the suffering community with good scientifically and biologically, physiologically accepted way. I hope you will learn how to cure the patient very quickly; I have highest faith on you.

I hope I have removed a great wall between homeopathy and allopathy helped to merge these 2 systems. it means first step in integrative medicine.

Do service to suffering humans and save them PREVENT PUBLIC FALLING IN SICKNESS, IN THE NAME OF TREATMENT.

Thank you.

DR.K.DEIVAMANI.BHMS.

Chennai,Tamilnadu-INDIA.

Reference : The book has been written by the knowledge of collective datas of all my medical study and gathered knowledge by seeing patient but still used some specific books for the reference.

Guiton physiology.

Principles of internal medicine by HORRISONs. (18th edition)

Organon of medicine – 5th edition - Dr.Hahnemann.

Social preventive medicine by DR.PARK (24th edition).

Pathology DR.Robbin

wikipedia

WHO official website.

global burden of disease (GBD)

BOOKS BY THIS AUTHOR

Maruthuva Kandupidippum, Puratchiyum

Tamil version of the same research and revolution in the field of medicine.

Thotru Noy Thaduppu Maruthuvam (Infectious Disease And Prevention)

available in only in tamil soon i will write in english and publish in kindle. written major infections and homeopathy managment focused mainly preventive aspect.